The
MENOPAUSE
Comprehensive Management

Fourth Edition

Dedication

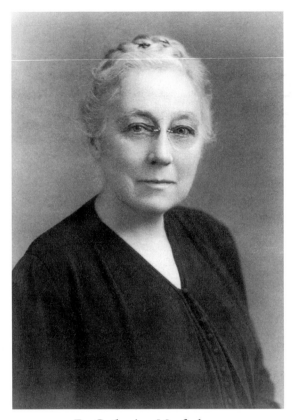

Dr Catharine Macfarlane

This edition is dedicated to the late Dr Catharine Macfarlane who was Professor of Gynecology at the Woman's Medical College of Pennsylvania. She made her outstanding contribution to women's health when she established in 1936 the first general clinic dedicated to regular preventative examinations for women after midlife.

After meeting Marie Curie, Dr Macfarlane introduced and used radium to treat cervical cancer in 1903. Thus, with the advent of effective medical care, she was determined that women's health should not be ignored following the reproductive years. Nationally known and much honored, she championed the rights of women physicians throughout her illustrious career. I am proud to have been a colleague and friend of Dr Macfarlane during her last productive years.

The photograph of Dr Catharine Macfarlane has kindly been supplied by Archives and Special Collections, MCP Hahnemann University, Philadelphia, USA.

The MENOPAUSE
Comprehensive Management
Fourth Edition

BERNARD A. ESKIN, MD, MS

Professor, Obstetrics/Gynecology
and Reproductive Endocrinology/Infertility

Director, Menopause and Geripause Center

Clinical Associate Professor, Psychiatry

Professor, Pharmacology

Medical College of PA-Hahnemann University
School of Medicine, Philadelphia, USA

The Parthenon Publishing Group
International Publishers in Medicine, Science & Technology

NEW YORK   LONDON

Library of Congress Cataloging-in-Publication Data

The menopause : comprehensive management/
by B. A. Eskin. – 4th ed.
  p. cm
  Includes bibliographical references and index.
  ISBN 1-85070-090-7 (alk. paper)
  1. Menopause. I. Eskin, Bernard A.
  [DNLM: 1. Menopause. WP 580 M548 1999]
RG186.M48 1999
618.1′75–dc21   99-045757

British Library Cataloguing in Publication Data
Eskin, Bernard A.
  The menopause : comprehensive management. –
  4th ed.
  1. Menopause
  I. Title
  618.1′75

ISBN 1-85070-090-7

Published in the USA by
The Parthenon Publishing Group Inc.
One Blue Hill Plaza
PO Box 1564, Pearl River
New York 10965, USA

Published in the UK and Europe by
The Parthenon Publishing Group Limited
Casterton Hall, Carnforth
Lancs. LA6 2LA, UK

Typeset by AMA DataSet Ltd., Preston, UK
Printed and bound by Butler & Tanner Ltd.,
Frome and London, UK

Contents

List of contributors

Mason C. Andrews, MD
Eastern Virginia Medical School
Department of Obstetrics and Gynecology
The Jones Institute for Reproductive Medicine
601 Colley Avenue
Norfolk, VA 23507-1627
USA

Hugh R. K. Barber, MD
Cornell University School of Medicine
122 East 76th Street
New York, NY 10021
USA

Brian M. Berger, MD
Harvard Medical School
Beth Israel Medical Center
Boston IVF
1 Brookline Place, Suite 602
Brookline, MA 02445
USA

Bhagu R. Bhavnani, PhD
Department of Obstetrics and Gynecology
St. Michael's Hospital
30 Bond Street, Room 735A-South
Toronto, Ontario M5B 1W8
Canada

William P. Castelli, MD
Boston University of Medicine and Framingham
    Cardiovascular Institute
Metrowest Medical Center, Inc.
115 Lincoln Street
Framingham, MA 01702
USA

Karen L. Dahlman, PhD
Department of Psychiatry
Mount Sinai School of Medicine
The Mount Sinai Medical Center
One Gustave L. Levy Place
New York, NY 10029-6574
USA

Nina S. Davis, MD
Department of Urology
Washington University School of Medicine
The Everett Clinic
3901 Hoyt Avenue
Everett, WA 98201
USA

Alan H. DeCherney, MD
Department of Obstetrics and Gynecology
University of California Los Angeles
10833 LeCont Ave 27-117
Center for Health Sciences
Los Angeles, CA 90095-1740
USA

Linda K. Dunn, MD
Department of Obstetrics and Gynecology
Chestnut Hill Hospital
8835 Germantown Avenue
Philadelphia, PA 19118
USA

Bernard A. Eskin, MD, FACOG
Department of Obstetrics/Gynecology and
    Reproductive Endocrinology
Medical College of PA-Hahnemann University
3300 Henry Avenue
Philadelphia, PA 19129
USA

R. Don Gambrell Jr, MD
Department of Physiology and Endocrinology
Medical College of Georgia
School of Medicine
903 15th Street
Augusta, GA 30912-3000
USA

Jesse J. Hade, MD
Department of Obstetrics and Gynecology
University of California Los Angeles
10833 LeCont Ave 27-117
Center for Health Sciences
Los Angeles, CA 90095-1740
USA

Debra S. Heller, MD
Department of Pathology
UMDNJ – UH-E141
150 Bergen Street
Newark, NJ 07103-2406
USA

Jennifer Hoblyn, MD
Department of Psychiatry
Mount Sinai School of Medicine
The Mount Sinai Medical Center
One Gustave L. Levy Place
New York, NY 10029-6574
USA

Stephen B. Levine, MD
Case Western Reserve School of Medicine
Center for Marital and Sexual Health
232 Chagrin Blvd
3 Commerce Park, Suite 350
Beachwood, OH 44122
USA

Richard C. Mohs, MD
Mount Sinai School of Medicine
Psychiatry Service
VA Medical Center
130 West Kingsbridge Road
Bronx, NY 10468
USA

Frederick Naftolin, MD, PhD
Department of Obstetrics and Gynecology
Yale University School of Medicine
FMG 335
New Haven, CT 06520-8063
USA

Puthgraman K. Natrajan, MD
Department of Physiology and Endocrinology
Medical College of Georgia
School of Medicine
903 15th Street
Augusta, GA 30912-3000
USA

Kelly Parsey, MD
UMDNJ-Piscataway
340 Changebridge Road
PO Box 1000
Montville, NJ 07045
USA

Laura E. Post, MD
Department of Internal Medicine
Eastern Virginia Medical School
Health Services
2159 Lynnhaven Parkway
Virginia Beach, VA 23456
USA

Mona R. Sutnick, EdD, RD
2135 St. James Place
Philadelphia, PA 19103
USA

Ian H. Thorneycroft, PhD, MD
Department of Obstetrics and Gynecology
University of Southern Alabama
251 Cox Street, Suite 100
Mobile, AL 36604
USA

Bruce R. Troen, MD, PhD
Jefferson University School of Medicine
Medical Research Center
Lankenau Hospital
100 Lancaster Avenue
Wynnewood, PA 19096
USA

Foreword

The Fourth Edition of *The Menopause: Comprehensive Management* promises to retain the high standard of professional and intellectual rigor that has been the hallmark of the previous three editions. However, as time passes, so have the 'cast of characters' and we see new names and new subjects appearing that are appropriate for the changing place of aging women in our society. But, at a time when others are cashing in on women readers' avid interest in the subject, this remains a textbook rather than a book for patients. As such, it serves as an important source of well-documented information for those who occupy themselves with the health and care of the increasing numbers of menopausal women. The book has appropriately broadened; the contents reflect rather a holistic bent. Lifestyle and social and sexual issues *per se* are featured and this is an apt general text for all sectors of medicine and menopause care-givers.

The time between publication of the Third Edition and the approaching third millennium has been filled with scientific progress which has resulted in changes to the profile of aging individuals and the problems they undergo and are willing to consider as preventable or remediable. Chapters on geripause, sexual capacities at midlife, infertility in the older woman, exercise, urological problems, cognitive changes and nutritional aspects and alternative therapies for the menopause, all are relevant to these changes in our aging sisters and the accommodation they will make with the world in which they will live.

With sound editing, up-to-date references and seasoning engendered by the previous editions, this pioneering textbook continues to show the longevity and long horizon envisioned by its Editor. Thus, the Fourth Edition is not 'old wine in new bottles'. It is, in fact, a healthy cocktail that acknowledges the change that our society and our health needs have developed with aging.

Yale University School of Medicine

Frederick Naftolin

Acknowledgements

I am grateful to Parthenon Publisher David Bloomer, Editor Nat Russo and his associate Frieda Volpone for their friendship and assistance. Many thanks to my Managing Editor Jean Wright for expediting the publication of the book.

I personally thank my wife, Lynn, for her patience and understanding of the time spent on this edition. I am particularly appreciative of her work in collating and typing much of the matter of all the editions of this textbook.

Preface

Bernard A. Eskin

This concept and textbook were conceived over 20 years ago. The original chapters of the First Edition (1980) were directed towards redefining the 'menopausal syndrome' and describing the symptoms that were considered significant. Ours was the initial attempt to clarify the differences between aging and menopause as they influenced woman's health.

In that First Edition, there was a comprehensive compilation of symptoms and signs related to reproductive cessation due to the sex hormonal loss that occurs in middle-aged women. Evidences of increasing longevity were characterized, with particular emphasis on the extending span of life after menopause. The characteristics of aging and how to separate them from menopausal alterations were debated. This early textbook and its successors have been praised, quoted, reprinted and updated over these 20 years, abetted by considerable research by many.

As a memorial, each of the editions have been dedicated to scientists who, during their lifetimes, were instrumental in advancing woman's prerogatives in health care. Dr James H. Leathem (First Edition) was an endocrinologist who focused on sex hormone research, particularly the aging ovary, and introduced antihormones. Dr Charles W. Lloyd (Second Edition) initiated new insights into sexual dysfunction and aging in women. Dr Robert B. Greenblatt (Third Edition) introduced sex hormone replacement after menopause with attention towards androgens as well as estrogen therapy. Dr Catharine Macfarlane (Fourth Edition) directly influenced women's health care by providing early oncologic interventions and the first preventative medicine clinic for women's problems. I am proud to have studied or worked with all of these innovators.

The original premise of this book has been to serve as an accurate reference and a current resource. The transitional period prior to the onset of the menopause was introduced in an earlier edition. During this phase, subtle decreases in sex hormones parallel clinical changes and may be recognized by some women in their mid-thirties. In this edition, I introduce the geripause, which represents the phase after menopause at ages 68–85 (early) and 85–100 years (late). These complete the lifetime of woman's sex hormonal levels (see Figure in Epilogue).

The textbook is divided into four major sections: Aging and the Menopause, Endocrinology of the Menopause, Clinical Problems in the Menopause, and Therapy of the Menopause. Each section is subdivided into a number of chapters that describe a major entity.

Section I

Aging and reproductive loss continue to be closely bound. Using well-proven hypotheses and new experimental data, these separate factors are explored. Genetic discoveries, including DNA fingerprinting, gene localization, gene therapy with cloning and *in vitro* fertilization, provide new methods of intervention. The geripause is introduced and important public health and statistical clinical findings follow. New mechanisms for assessing the health of the older gestational woman are presented with monitoring and treatment that have reduced fears and dangers. However, the physiological needs of pregnancy remain impressive and special care is required. Pathology describes both the aging characteristics and the tissue changes that are seen in hormonal deficiency. Estrogenic loss and aging deficits do not reduce potential sexual gratification. A unique holistic and mental health approach to sexuality for the mature woman is provided.

Section II

The thyroid gland is a most subtle, but highly affected gland for the maturing woman; it requires careful evaluation and particular notice, since it imitates so many medical conditions. Next, the perimenopause shows a considerable amount of hormonal change as an antecedent to full deprivation of the sex steroids. With the menopause there is the overwhelming demise of reproduction, yet complete collapse of the hypothalamic–pituitary–ovarian axis does not occur. New techniques, particularly assisted reproductive technology (ART), surrogate pregnancies, and primordial cell cloning, can provide substantial mechanisms for enabling older women to maintain gestational options.

Section III

There are many clinical problems that may be associated with the menopause that may be serious or affect the quality of life. While not always caused by estrogen deprivation, they are closely associated with decreased ovarian activity. Most evident have been the bone changes characteristic of osteoporosis. Cardiovascular disease becomes particularly manifest when reduced estrogen occurs but is further in evidence with menopause and geripause. Exercise has become an agreeable method of providing mental and physical well-being, but is particularly important in cardiovascular and bone issues. Gynecological and urological complaints are particularly evident, caused by the atrophic changes. Malignant breast disease increases markedly after menopause; thus, a careful appraisal is necessary. Cognitive changes have been a new challenge for neurologists and improved interventions are underway. Dietary advice has mostly concerned weight loss; however, besides this cosmetic loss, we should be involved in the development of healthier and more desirable foods. The many alternative dietary therapies available for women in the menopause have been presented here.

Section IV

The final section describes the pharmaceuticals available, emphasizing hormonal replacement therapy. Hormonal agents vary chemically and have different pharmacodynamics, side-effects and complications. Replacement therapy with estrogen has become more acceptable in the interim since the Third Edition. Since the number of delivery systems for these medications has increased, a section is devoted to these techniques. Sex steroids prompt a fear of cancer and many trial evaluations have been made. These results and conclusions are given.

Much has been done since the last edition and, hopefully, the trend towards improving the quality of life for women during the post-reproductive phases will continue into the next century.

'While Medicine has done much in the century that is nearly ended, the future will show more marked influence year by year...'

Journal of the American Medical Association
1899;32:1261–3

Section I
Aging and the menopause

1

The menopause and aging

Bernard A. Eskin

Introduction

Reproductive aging is an aggregate of many factors. The effectiveness of the entire endocrine system, including the gonads, deteriorates as a result of systemic aging. In the chapters that follow, the anatomical and endocrine decline that occur during the years of transition, pre- and post-menopause, and geripause are presented. These modifications are the results of the progressive aging within tissues, the reduced ability of cells to respond to stimulus and modifications of the intrinsic factors which activate cells.

The philosophical debate continues concerning the etiology of reproductive aging. Is aging the result of target organ degeneration with tissue loss or regression of neurotransmission from the central nervous system? From the most recent data it becomes apparent that these conditions coexist. In women, the obvious losses of first, reproduction and later, menses are results of many biological and chemical changes brought about by aging.

Why aging occurs remains unknown and its course still unalterable. Most research has been directed towards describing the anatomical and physiological changes; however, manipulation into the genetic code provides a vestige of penetration. The recent gene insertion for the protein component of telomerases in senescent human cells re-extends their telomerases to lengths typical of young cells[1]. Intracellular and molecular biological techniques have brought new insight by describing the biochemical alterations of growth and metabolism seen in the elderly. From these observations, many new hypotheses have evolved, mostly generated by animal research. The accelerated interest shown during the 1990s is the result of an increased visibility of the aged segment of our population and their spiralling social and economic impact.

The need for improving the quality of life for postmenopausal women has become a serious matter in medical care for the turn of the century. Longevity has naturally improved, and with it, quality has become considerably more important. Of note has been the entrance of many human 'old age' illnesses requiring intense clinical research and care. The 'baby boomer' generation is now over 50 years old, with new demands. The scientific promise of a 100 plus age carries with it the demands for parallel quality years.

Regardless of the fact that much has been written concerning the aging processes related to biological reproduction, the relevant questions in correlating aging and menopause remain the same. These are:

(1) Does menopause affect life expectancy?

(2) Does aging cause reproductive failure and menopause?

(3) Is the rate of cellular senescence increased with reproductive senescence?

Practically, clinical problems that must be considered are:

(4) Is cellular deterioration due to lack of estrogen?

(5) Do the available replacement therapies prevent any sequelae of aging?

These questions are considered and discussed throughout this book. In this chapter, the direct questions relating to the aging phenomenon are addressed in light of both knowledge and hypotheses that have accrued. After a general review of the basic theories of aging, specific information concerning aging and reproduction is presented. The readers are then asked to judge our conclusions and form their own.

General theories of aging

Molecular chemical research and genetic expression experience of intracellular changes caused by aging have led to several theories[2-4] (Table 1). These theories recognize a series of events within the cell which prevent the orderly processes of growth and metabolism and remain formidable despite all the most recent knowledge. No single theory for human aging satisfies totally all the biological phenomena that occur. This categorization of theories has remained.

Genetic

The 'genetically determined' theories consider biological life to have a predetermined longevity and perhaps quality of living owing to persistence of the individual genetic code. Genetic expression, therefore, is a result of preformed biological conditioning provided by a preconceived template[5]. This hypothesis has remained extant over many decades because of results obtained from epidemiological statistics by life insurance actuaries, intraspecies records and longevity data for identical versus non-identical twins. Computer-tabulated research indicates that the primary basis for longevity of an individual strain, or a species, appears to be the sum of the genetic material incorporated in the fertilized egg at the climactic moment when the spermatozoon meets the unfertilized egg.

Programming

Within the cell there are biochemical factors that occur genetically which have been chemically pre-programmed. Evidence of the DNA code biochemically visualizes this theory. This concept provides a mechanism by which the genetic theory can function. Stepwise changes occur within these cells leading to degeneration within the cytosol or nuclear materials on a pretimed basis. Although not universally true, this thesis is more widely applicable than most others. Concurrently, this theory provides opportunities for treatment with optimism for the reversal of some aging conditions. Early results show that mechanisms may evolve which inhibit or modify the genetic signals that cause health hazards.

Somatic mutations

The mutation theory refers to environmental insults, i.e. extrinsic effects on the cells in the body. Practicably, examples might be the results of radiation, medication or normal biological reactions. This theory seems compatible with other approaches to aging, as most species are vulnerable to fairly random molecular events. The nature of the mutation is influenced by the factors that affect cell function. This theory is applicable particularly to reproductive tissues, such as in the ovary, where serious alterations could result in the transmission of mutations to succeeding generations. Cloning provides evidence, to date in animals, that all cells are transmissable and, thus, liable to extreme manipulation. A concept that appears viable is that cloned anlage that have aged maintain the level of cellular disintegration from these older tissues. Since the female gamete is present from birth, arrested in the first meiotic division, irreparable modifications may occur by environmental damage.

Autoimmune

Autoimmune protection is reduced or lost with aging. The immune factors circulating throughout

Table 1 Theories of cellular aging

(1) Genetic

(2) Programmed aging

(3) Mutation theory

(4) Autoimmune

(5) Cross-linkages

(6) Extracellular factors

(7) Combination

the body can then overwhelm the individual cells, causing cellular destruction. In addition to the autoimmune loss, there is a marked decline with aging in both availability and activity of the total immune systems. Thus, there is a decrease in defense against infections, immune complex diseases and carcinogenesis, all of which contributes further to an acceleration of the intracellular aging processes. The potential effect of the loss of cellular resistance to the immune system has become an important condition. In the geripause age, a new series of heretofore casual diseases may become more threatening. Upon losing immunological safeguards, the affected cells are destroyed or modified by infiltration of the lymphatics and circulating lymphatic cells.

Cross-links

The cross-linkage theory deals with a complex series of biochemical events which can inhibit the function of the cells through the aging process. There is evidence that some molecules present in the cytoplasm of old tissue cells comprise atypical or transformed components of DNA, RNA and peptides, covalently bound together. This reflects age-dependent deterioration of molecules with possible loss of continuity or bonding weakened by age. Tissues could lose differentiation by that mechanism with possible reduction in function.

One concept postulates that aging is a specific biological function which promotes the progressive evolution of sexually reproducing species. Like any other important function, aging is mediated by several molecular mechanisms working simultaneously. Three such mechanisms have been postulated to date:

(1) Telomere shortening due to suppression of telomerase at early stages of embryogenesis;

(2) Age-related activation of a mechanism that induces the synthesis of heat shock proteins in response to denaturing stimuli;

(3) Incomplete suppression of generation and scavenging of reactive oxygen species (ROS).

None of these phenomena can kill the organism, but only weaken it, which becomes crucial under extreme conditions[6].

Extracellular factors

The impact of extracellular factors upon cellular performance is impressive. Extrinsic as well as intrinsic factors contribute to organizational decline during aging. Most apparent is a condition which disturbs the cells by changing the proper sequence of biochemical events, such as incorrect neurogenic or trophic stimulation. Transport mechanisms as well as membrane energy and chemistry reactions could be restricted. When aging affects enzyme systems, for example, an inappropriate reaction occurs which disturbs the entire cell.

Combination theories

These hypotheses can be combined to satisfy the individual conditions. Within the cell molecular physiology, aging could effect a series of disruptions which radically prevent outside stimuli from reacting in an expected manner. The cell response may not only be diminished, but if it is effectual, it may result in developmental 'errors'. Therefore, this leads to intracellular disease states, such as seen in histological dysplasias and neoplasias, and tissue and organ degradation.

Medawar[7], as quoted by Strehler[2], described aging as the result of genetic and stochastic processes. The latter represents the accumulated sum of the effects of recent stress, injury or infection. These are environmental in origin and thus, in a paradoxically technical sense, the effects of 'nature'. While we have added many scientific data to these general theories in the subsequent half century, the basis of aging remains 'genetic versus environmental'!

Alterations in aging in all endocrine tissues

The theories of aging described pertain to intracellular changes seen in all elements of the body, although many investigators consider them to be appropriate only to those tissues we associate with clinical aging, i.e. skin, neurological and vascular tissues, muscle and bone. Anatomical and physiological modifications caused by the aging process have been established in these specific areas.

The endocrine system is unique in that, besides obvious losses of tissue growth and metabolism, secretory activity may be inhibited, modified or even completely reversed by the aging process. Secretions generally required for normal physiological function of other parts of the body may be lost[8]. Particularly applicable is a reduction in muscle strength which leads to frailty[9].

A series of histological modifications occurs in the endocrine glands owing to aging which are not unique[8]. Connective tissue increases in the gland capsule and connective tissue elements replace secretory cells. In the endocrine cell, mitotic rate decreases and fragmentation of mitochondria and nuclear damage often appear.

Thus, alterations in the endocrine tissues with aging relate to both secretory and target organ functions[10]. The changes are:

(1) Primary loss of functional tissue by hypoplastic or atrophic changes in secreting cells;

(2) Decrease in secretory rate as a result of these cellular changes;

(3) Decrease of metabolic clearance of hormones produced;

(4) Decrease in end-organ response to the hormones.

Menopause and longevity

There have been several research programs which compare longevity after menopause in the woman with that in other mammalian females[11-14].

Women live the longest after menopause relative to their total life span, when compared with all other mammals. During the 20th century, longevity for women has increased two-fold. Maximum reproductive age has been unaffected by this increased life expectancy[15]. Thirty-three per cent (33%) of a woman's life remains after the cessation of menses; conversely, in the monkey, the mouse, the rat and other mammals unless genetically altered this period is short, usually 10–15% (Figure 1)[14]. The reproductive span in one strain of mice

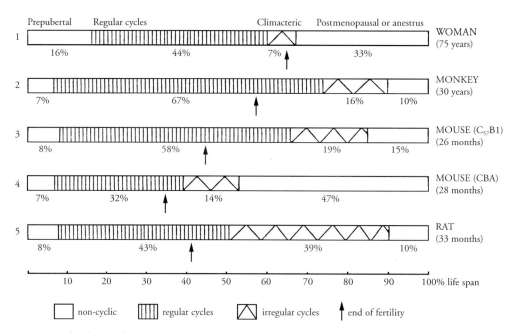

Figure 1 Reproductive cyclic activity expressed as percentage of total life span. From reference 14, with permission

(CBA) has been genetically reduced, compared with other mouse strains[16]. In these mice the total life span was unchanged; only the percentage of time in the postcyclic period was increased (47%). These data provide evidence that the life span is unassociated with postreproductive percentiles (Figure 1). Interestingly, a review from medieval times until early this century showed that the effects of senescence rarely became a consideration because of the short life span seen in women in those eras[13,17]. Considerably more astounding is the promulgation of research seen in *Drosophila melanogaster* which promoted the 'disposable SOMA' theory: that longevity requires investments in somatic maintenance which reduce the resources available for reproduction. A recent series of statistical historical studies has indicated that a trade-off existed[18].

The four representative periods of the life span in all females were defined as prepuberty, regular reproductive cyclic activity, irregular cyclic activity and postmenopausal or senile anestrous phase[14]. Clinically, these have been defined more elaborately as prepuberty, puberty, active reproductive, decelerating reproductive, perimenopause (premenopause) and postmenopause[19]. A statistical analysis of these phases has been compiled to ascertain the relative proportions of the life span

of each using actuarial longevity projections (Figure 2).

Conclusions reached by Jones[14] show several characteristic features:

(1) The proportion of the life span spent in sexually immature condition is by far the greatest in women;

(2) Under the sheltered conditions afforded by industrial civilization or laboratory existence all females become infertile well before the end of the total life span;

(3) The end of the reproductive life span in women occurs shortly after reproductive cycles stop;

(4) The proportion of the life span in primates characterized by total absence of reproductive cycles is the longest in humans (Figure 1).

For practical reasons, much of the basic biological research in gerontology has been limited to small mammals. Specifically, in recent years the relationship of aging to the reproductive cycle has been studied in mice[16] and rats[20]. Human ovaries differ from those of most other mammals because they continue to secrete hormones which are capable of maintaining subclinical cycles for a comparatively

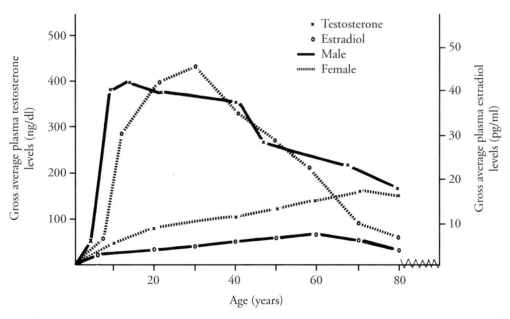

Figure 2 Plasma levels of estradiol and testosterone in human females and males according to age

long time after overt reproduction ceases. The reproductive cycles may be re-established in old rats by the use of 1-dopa; however, no evidence of a statistically valid extension of the life span has resulted from this treatment.

The distinguishing histological and endocrine characteristics of the human ovary are discussed in the chapter on pathology. The number of oocytes remaining in the ovary may account for cyclicity as well as fertility at an unexpectedly older age. Since the number of viable oocytes in women at a given range of years (such as 40–44) may vary as much as 100-fold, the age of menopause is an individual response[21,22].

Surgical menopause by bilateral ovariectomy with or without hysterectomy does not appear to change the longevity of the woman, when the surgery is performed for benign disease. Using the evidence available, there appears to be no reduction in duration of life with premature ovarian failure. Since both of these conditions are treated with estrogen replacement because of potential medical problems, we must rely on prior interpretation of these results. Although there has been no extension of reproductive life, the longevity of the female is currently 75–78 years and may increase to 85 years during the coming two decades[23]. Initial responsibility has been placed on the improved conditions for childbirth and perinatal health.

Longevity seems to be a combination of conditions. It would appear from present statistics available that, in the woman, it is not related to the time of menopause. From these data, the length of the postmenopausal period relates to the mean life span in the human female and can be documented in lower mammals[24]. Conversely, extension of cyclic reproduction by ovulatory techniques would not seem to be a potential mechanism for lengthening the life span. Both basic and clinical research into cyclic extension, fertility notwithstanding, shows no lengthening of life span. The commentary of Weismann[11] continues to be as valid as it was almost 100 years ago[23]:

'Death itself, and the longer or short duration of life, both depend entirely on adaptation. Death is not an essential attribute of living matter; it is neither associated with reproduction, nor a necessary consequence of it . . .'

Aging as a cause of reproductive failure

In the human, reproduction may serve as a biological model for aging. This is particularly true in the female, where decreasing sex hormone production eventually results in the demise of a dynamic physiological system (Figure 3)[25]. The gradual reduction in estrogen secretion due to fading follicular growth and development in the ovary has been shown. An age-related decline in the process of folliculogenesis results in reduced oocyte quality. The well-characterized age-related increase in meiotic non-dysfunction is one symptom of compromised oocyte growth[26].

Appropriate levels of estrogen cause both negative and positive feedback stimuli to the hypothalamic–pituitary axis, which maintains cyclicity in the reproductive process. Secondary to this major goal, estrogen maintains sexual endorgan tissue structures. In the aging woman, when ovarian estrogen secretions are reduced, available extra-ovarian levels continue to prevent many degenerative changes for a limited time. When body estrogen is completely depleted, senescence of the secondary sexual organs occurs.

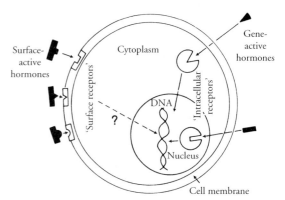

Figure 3 Subcellular location of receptors for different hormone classes. Cells consist of an outer surface membrane, enclosing the soluble cytoplasm and the DNA-containing nucleus. Hormones whose receptors are located on the membrane include pituitary hormones, insulin, epinephrine and glucagon. Receptors for steroids and thyroid hormones are found inside the cell, in the cytoplasm and the nucleus. Hormones of this latter category act more or less directly on the genome. Surface-active hormones may in some cases act indirectly on the genome, although their initial actions are on the cell membrane. From reference 25, with permission

In a man, testosterone appears to maintain a threshold level well into the seventh decade, while his estradiol levels are slightly increased. The woman has a mild increase in androgen blood titers with the elevation of serum testosterone. These are usually the result of persistent activity of the extragonadal steroid pathways (Figure 3) and a limited aromatization.

Alterations in reproductive tissues with aging

Ovaries differ from other endocrine organs in women because they function for only a limited period during the life span. Other endocrine glands continue to secrete throughout life and require therapeutic replacement when they become deficient. The aging cellular events and apoptosis (programmed cell death) described for all the endocrine glands pertain similarly to the reproductive system. The reproductive aging process seems to occur over a short period of time as a result of a predetermined series of events. Most likely, this is precipitated by both ovarian and pertinent neuroendocrine failure, then further enhanced by the obsolescence of the tissues throughout the reproductive axis. The ability to maintain the regulation of the various reproductive functions is complicated and results in the onset of premenopause.

This biological aging occurs in the female reproductive organs. Hormonal secretion diminishes almost linearly, and hormonal effectiveness is depressed further by reduced end-organ responses. The ovarian effluent decreases invariably from a peak in the reproductive years, through the perimenopausal era, and into the geripause, the postmenopausal reproductive senescence (Figure 2). This new descriptive term is introduced here to represent the late postmenopause (after age 65). This period is becoming longer and more significant as we enter the 21st century (see Chapter 2). The once well-honed reproductive system shows well-documented evidence of decreasing efficiency and activity at each level.

Most of the research done by biologists and endocrinologists has been with regard to singular biological levels of the reproductive axis. Thus, it is difficult to determine where the reduction in activity begins or whether it has a multiple-level origin. Receptor systems exist at target cells for both pituitary hormones (follicle stimulating hormone, FSH; luteinizing hormone, LH) in the ovary, and steroid hormones (estrogen, progesterone, androgens) in the target cells. These differ as pituitary hormones are proteinaceous and act on surface receptors and steroid hormones respond with intracellular (cytosol or nuclear) receptors (Figure 4)[27]. The functional efficiency of the systems is an elemental factor in cellular aging[28].

Hypothalamic and pituitary senescence

The central nervous system initiates the cyclic reproductive response when a 'mature' hypothalamic–pituitary axis reacts to estrogen feedback. At puberty, this lessening of the resistance by the hypothalamus provides the first cyclicity. In monitoring the roles of the various levels as they may be implicated, the hypothalamic–pituitary axis appears to be most vulnerable.

Aging of the hypothalamic–pituitary–ovarian axis parallels that of other organ systems. Longitudinal analyses have not been done, and are necessary to ascertain whether these measures will predict reproductive reserve before irreversible dysfunction occurs[9]. The hypothalamus and pituitary glands must remain efficient to provide reproductive cyclicity, as programming for ovulation is provided by this axis. Cytological studies in postreproductive animals and postmortem studies on postmenopausal humans have yet to reveal any modifications that could be associated with aging. Additionally, the initial rise in gonadotropins in the menopause would seem to make the consideration of pituitary senescence difficult to accept. The later postmenopausal decreases in gonadotropins are more consistent with the atrophism of the secreting cells[29].

A theoretical possibility, which has research support, shows that aging of the neuroendocrine reproductive system causes a reversal of its pubertal onset[30,31]. In order to provide ovulation, the pituitary must have the qualitative capability to cause a negative feedback on gonadotropin release at a moderate estrogen increase and a severe positive effect (surge) at a higher level. The feedback

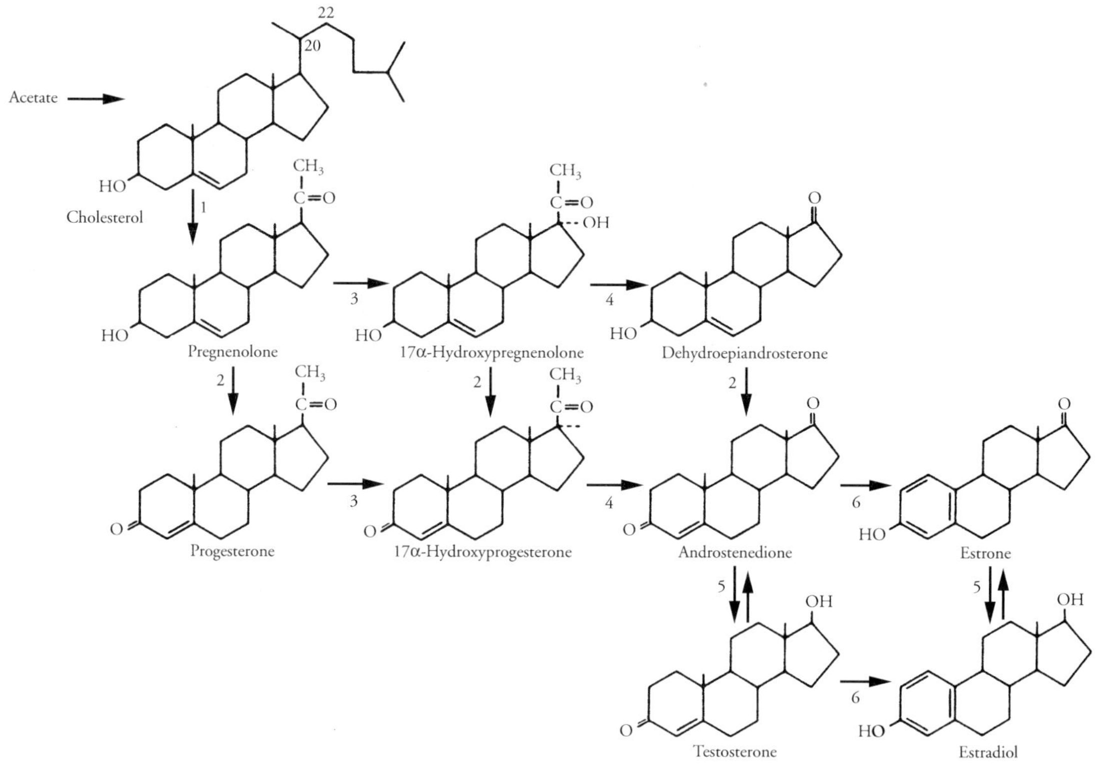

Figure 4 Steroid biosynthetic pathways. The following enzymes are required where indicated: (1) 20-hydroxylase, 22-hydroxylase and 20,22-desmolase; (2) 3β-ol-dehydrogenase and o⁴-o⁵ isomerase; (3) 17α-hydroxylase; (4) 17,20-desmolase; (5) 17β-ol-dehydrogenase; (6) aromatizing enzyme system. From reference 27, with permission

mechanism in women appears to become less efficient in the later reproductive phases.

This may be responsible for the increased infertility seen in women who have waited until their late thirties to begin child-bearing[32,33]. Thus, it becomes apparent that aging reverses an important feedback function rather than causes a direct pituitary disruption. This subtle differentiation in pituitary activity seems less intrusive on the general endocrine health of menopausal women.

The neuroendocrinology of aging has been well reviewed[34-37]. Clinical experiments with epinephrine or progesterone, or by stimulation of the preoptic area of the hypothalamus, showed that ovulation could be restimulated in the senescent rat[38,39]. There have been several recent studies on the effect of agonal therapy with l-dopa and bromergocryptine in recycling rodents in the postestrus (senescent) period. These therapies, considered to have a releasing hormone action similar to a dopamine surge, cause secretion of a pulse of gonadotropin from the pituitary which stimulates ovarian tissue more readily than the existing intrinsic hormones. The significance of this effect remains difficult to define[34,39]. At present, these results have not been confirmed by controlled studies with humans, although elderly women treated with l-dopa or bromergocryptine for Parkinsonism have been noted on occasions to cycle after the menopause.

Absence of primordial or sensitive follicles
Convincing histological evidence has shown that the aging cells lose the ability to regrow and develop into active follicles even with adequate stimulation[40,41]. The remaining follicles tend to have a reduced sensitivity to the intrinsic gonadotropin, which may be due to the biological character of the older follicles or a reduction in gonadotropin receptor in the cells[42].

The hormonal pathway involved in steroid synthesis has been hypothetically shown to be dependent upon a two-cell response. The two cells involved are the granulosa and theca cells, which surround the follicles that are developing during each cycle. Several studies have shown that the steroid pathway requires both of these cells for the formation of estrogen. Androgens result from the cholesterol to pregnenolone responses (Figure 5)[43], and intermediate androgens such as dehydroepiandrosterone and androstenedione are formed within the theca cells. Androgens are transported from the theca cells to the granulosa cells where aromatizing enzymes produce estrogens. The estradiol and estrone are then secreted into the vascular system.

Estrogens and gonadotropins are required for the formation of receptors for gonadotropins. Estrogen has the capacity to form both FSH and LH receptors on either of the cells; LH has the ability to form FSH receptors, particularly on the granulosa cells; and FSH has the capability of forming both FSH and LH receptors on either cell (Figure 6). In addition, it appears that estrogen forms its own estrogen receptors on any of these cells involved. During the aging phenomena, many of these responses are not adequate or effective with a resulting reduction in follicular growth and development[41,44].

In addition, many of the enzymes are reduced in numbers and effectiveness during the aging process. This causes the hormone pathway to malfunction and, in fact, may bring about an increase in intermediate hormonal release. When aromatization does not occur, intermediate androgens continue to be formed and secreted directly into the blood. The increase in the amount of androgens present may cause serious clinical symptoms in women.

Functional loss of stroma occurs in biological aging intracellularly with increased fibrosis[38,45]. Because of this, there is diminished active cellular milieu needed to produce the steroid fractions required for appropriate hormonal secretions[46,47]. This may also be a reason for the enzyme letdown that has been described (Figure 3).

Alterations in sensitivity to gonadotropins

As stated above, these changes may be due to reduced gonadotropin receptors by modification or loss[48]. These proteinaceous receptors act on the surface of the cells and may respond by providing the specific enzyme systems required for intracellular biochemical pathways. The expected steroidogenesis in the ovary leading to the secretion of estrogens may be interrupted by receptor alterations[49]. The changes that occur could be precipitated by factors such as toxicity, mutations or immunological damage. The results of the loss of gonadotropin activity would be a sex steroid shift in the secretion of intermediary metabolites (Figure 4). Some of these androgenic steroids are clinically active and may be responsible for postmenopausal symptomatology.

Sensitivity of the follicle to gonadotropins has been considered a requirement for the function of the secretory cells. In the ovary, the loss of receptor at the molecular level reduces the activity of the gonad and its vitality for further responsiveness.

It has become evident that gonadotropins may be qualitatively altered and, thus, less effective at the specific target cell[50,51]. Some studies have indicated environmental effects that cause central

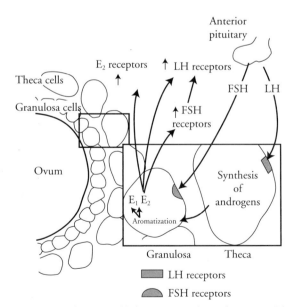

Figure 5 The two-cell theory: granulosa–theca steroid pathway; follicle stimulating hormone (FSH) luteinizing hormone (LH) activity on cell receptors. From reference 43, with permission

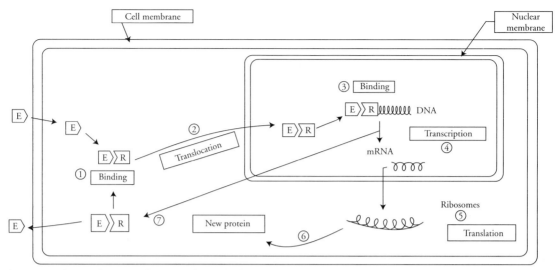

Figure 6 The mechanism of action of estradiol. Estradiol enters through the membrane by diffusion and is (1) bound to the receptor. The complex is (2) translocated to the nucleus where it is (3) bound to the chromatin material. The DNA (4) transcription to mRNA results in (5) ribosomal translation in the cytoplasm. New protein (6) is formed and utilized in cell metabolic processes. The estradiol–receptor complex leaves the nucleus (7) where it is dissociated to estradiol (which presumably leaves the cell) and receptor protein, which is reused in the binding process

nervous system changes capable of influencing the hypothalamic discharge and, by that means, of modifying gonadotropin release[52].

Steroid receptor loss
One important theory depends on reduced receptor response with biochemical modifications in the cytosol protein necessary for estrogen action. Research from many laboratories, including our own[13,53,54], shows modifications in the aging cell that may limit capability for the specific steroid action expected. While the appropriate estrogen is present, a decrease in target cell sensitivity depresses the reproductive organs and requires an increased estrogen level for restoration of activity[50]. Since estrogens act also on the ovary, the reduction in end-organ response causes the ovary to decrease steroid output resulting in an impasse.

This short summation of the arguments for reproductive failure and aging serves to introduce the many controversies. Cessation of reproductive activity is secondary to the loss of many physiological and biochemical events and occurs either genetically or environmentally. Any level of the reproductive system may be causative, although ovarian senescence appears to be the most

common. The effect of estrogen and estrogen receptors on the aging organs is discussed in the following section.

Cellular senescence as a result of menopause

Gonadal secretion of estrogen and progesterone wanes and the ovulatory ability of the ovary decreases. The loss of these hormones, which are responsible for secondary sexual characteristics in women, causes changes that are initially subtle, but which cannot be easily separated from those resulting from aging. The clinical symptomatology seen is remarkably variegated (Table 2). The signs and symptoms of the disorders that appear to be the result of estrogen deficiency are not limited to the reproductive system. Estrogen affects tissues throughout the body, and receptors for this steroid have been isolated in non-sexual tissues.

These clinical conditions show a different hormone threshold level for each individual. The variation appears to be due to end-organ response rather than steroid level. Radioimmunoassay studies in aging women show that metabolic clearance rates are modified, and almost always decrease when estrogen production wanes. This might be responsible for a progressively higher level of circulating steroid, which could lead to tissue pathology, especially if exogenous hormone is also being given. However, most gerontologists feel that intracellular control occurs, which modifies the response to the estrogen stimulus[50].

Estrogen has been described as decreasing initially between the ages of 26 and 29; however, most evident effects are seen in the decelerating reproductive (36–42), perimenopausal (42–51) and postmenopausal (51–65) years[19]. As estrogen decreases, menstrual problems evolve such as amenorrhea (cessation of menses), oligomenorrhea (prolongation of cycles), hypomenorrhea (reduction in amount of bleeding) and menorrhagia (heavy menstrual bleeding).

Ovarian hormones are quantitatively and qualitatively transformed in aging (Figure 2). Intermediate steroids increase and may act peripherally to bring about the clinical changes with advancing age[19]. The effect of progesterone, which is still measurable in the postmenopausal serum, has been under considerable investigation for therapeutic use, an area that is discussed in the final section of this book.

Tissue effects of sex hormones

Data on intracellular receptors for estrogen and progesterone in hormone-specific target tissues (i.e. breast, uterus, pituitary, etc.) have accumulated since the initial hypotheses were presented in 1967[55,56]. These reproductive hormone–target cell responses depend on unidentified intracellular binding proteins having attributes which include high specificity and affinity for each steroid (Figure 7)[25]. When estrogen or progestin passes through the membrane into the cell cytosol, a complex consisting of steroid and receptor protein is formed, which can then be translocated as a unit from the cytoplasm through the nuclear membrane into the nuclear compartment[57]. Receptor transformations occur within the nucleus and, under specific conditions, nuclear mRNA synthesis results. Following this, mRNA translation in the ribosomes can lead to protein synthesis. Thus, the initial steroid has caused a series of intracellular events to occur which stimulate the affected tissues to growth and development, according to the set pattern generated by the chromosomal genes (genome) of the nucleus[57]. Receptor research has shown that the steroid receptor system may be more simplistic and may be present on the cell nuclear membrane, thus reducing the complexity involved with a cytosol protein receptor[58,59] (Figure 3).

Some steroids related to estradiol cause incomplete responses because the duration of residence in the nucleus is altered[46]. It has been hypothesized that the endogenous estrogens – estrone, estradiol

Table 2 Disorders related to estrogen deficiency

Directly
Atrophic vulvovaginitis
Urethral syndrome
Skin, hair and breast changes

Indirectly
Hot flushes
Osteoporosis
Psychosexual problems
Functional cardiac diseases

Probably
Psychological conditions and trauma
Atherosclerotic heart disease
Lipid metabolism

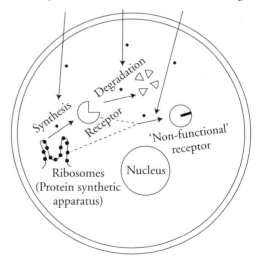

Control by hormones and/or other biochemical agents

Figure 7 Theoretical positions where hormones or other biochemical agents could control receptor changes during aging. From reference 25, with permission

and estriol – have a different response according to the target organ, and the metabolic action may depend on the time that the steroid–receptor complexes of these estrogens remain in the nucleus. When the complex remains within the nucleus for a longer time, a greater effect on the cell results. Metabolism and growth may follow even when the cell has evident resistance to the stimulating complex, if prolonged binding to the nuclear substance can occur[60].

The quantity of receptor available in the cytosol of the target cells is an important condition which can regulate the response by a cell to a specific steroid hormone. The levels of the receptors are specific to target tissue and appear to be unalterable. However, estrogen therapy increases the number of receptors available for estrogen action[61]. Another possible source of receptor supply is from those reclaimable after the receptor complex has effected the nuclear response. After such exposure to estrogens, the estrogen receptor moves to the cell nucleus and gradually dissociates, returning to the cytoplasm in a free condition, and, thus, can be recycled (Figure 6). The number of free estrogen receptors available is an important control for further activity of the cell by this steroid[55].

On the other hand, certain non-steroidal antiestrogens act as antagonists to the cell metabolism by competing for the available receptors[62]. Some of these antiestrogens act initially in a manner similar to estrogens by stimulating the same metabolic and regulatory pathways that cause uterine and endometrial growth. The responses may be lessened because of the reduced efficiency of the estrogen employed.

Another means of endogenous control over steroid receptor levels is the influence that one steroid exerts on the receptor levels of others. For example, estrogens can induce progesterone receptors in human breast cells, while progesterone can impair the replenishment of the estrogen receptor in the rat uterus. This type of effect reduces the sensitivity of the uterus to subsequent estrogen exposure after a single estrogen bolus. This cross-reaction may be due to an inhibition of receptor synthesis or to increased inactivation. Progesterone has been seen to be secreted in the postmenopausal woman. If progesterone is an antago-

nist to estrogen reception, obviously it can cause the estrogen to be even less effective.

Mechanisms available at present to change receptor responses are essentially limited to five alternatives (Table 3). One of the important factors in the study of aging concerns the innate loss of receptors in the cells of the aging reproductive tract[49].

There has been rapid progress in the field of receptors for reproductive hormones. Estrogen receptor analysis to determine estrogen-responsive tumors has been utilized in breast cancer therapeutics for several years[63]. Antiestrogen therapy for estrogen-dependent cancer has been effectively used. Research into receptors and neoplasia in aging has shown some interaction, but still requires further data[54]. Several studies have recently characterized a second estrogen receptor by immunohistochemical techniques. Laboratory studies in capillary endothelial cells in human prostate, cerebellum and capillary endothelial tissues of the heart have identified estrogen receptor-β. This antipolyclonal estrogen β receptor still requires a simpler technique before the general elaboration of its qualities can be done. Meanwhile, the defined estrogen receptor has been redesignated as estrogen receptor-α[64].

Current investigations show that receptor loss with aging results in decreased intracellular metabolism. Thus, when estrogen receptors decrease, there may be a loss of function at specific reproductive target cells and other less obvious tissues in the body. With cellular aging, peripheral endocrine changes occur, which in themselves can be responsible for the deterioration of many bodily systems besides reproduction.

Table 3 Determinants of estrogen response

(1) Levels of receptors in target tissue

(2) Hormone quality and quantity

(3) Interference by other steroids

(4) Temporal effect of the complex in the nucleus

(5) Measurement of how readily the receptor complex separates from the hormone and whether it can provide reusable receptors

Changes in receptor systems in aging

The conditions for secretion from the follicular cells in the ovary have been described. In the two-cell theory (Figure 5), the theca and granulosa cells receive signals presumably through gonadotropin membrane receptors for LH and FSH. The two cells respond in tandem by secreting steroids into the circulating system. Thus, the active ovary has appropriate secretory cells which are stimulated by gonadotropins secreted from the pituitary. These hormones signal the ovarian cells through receptor systems on the membranes. This results in the secretion of estrogens, primarily as estradiol, and other intermediate steroids including progesterone (Figure 4). Estrogens and progesterone, thus secreted, act at the appropriate target organs and require their own intracellular or nuclear receptors for response. Additionally, estrogens provide specific ovulatory functions in the scheme of follicular growth through the presence of estrogen receptors in the ovary[36].

Specific research into estrogen receptor systems is ongoing, and has shown that they are not limited to the ovary and secondary sexual tissues, but are also found to a lesser degree in other tissues. Advances in the measurement of estrogen α receptors provide several new medical applications[65]. Successful production of non-specific antisera to purified estrogen receptor has led to the development of sensitive radioimmunoassays for this receptor. Rapid and accurate estrogen α receptor determinations have become available for the diagnosis of reproductive disease states and for evaluating cancer treatment.

New information on eukaryotic gene structure has shown that mutations involving the intermediate sequences of steroid-hormone regulation may be phenotypically silent. These may not influence the expression of the signal under usual circumstances. However, in aging and cancer or other genetically effected illnesses, gene structure could be altered and the mutations effected by these previously silent responses would become evident[65].

The mechanisms for intracellular systems for the estradiol α receptor have been described (Figure 7). These receptor systems appear to control steroid hormone action. However, a recent question has arisen whether these receptors are present directly on the nuclear membrane[58] rather than only effected through a specific cytoplasmic receptor. Another receptor system, the eosinophil binding system, which may be responsible for some of the early estrogen responses – for example water inhibition, increased vascular permeability and histamine release – has also been described[66].

Until the advent of receptor biochemistry, no therapy could be conceived to consider how target cell action might be affected by the vicissitudes of histological aging. Molecular biological research, which is now being actively done in many laboratories and has begun to show the changes that occur within the cells as a result of the aging of receptor systems, has been summarized[49]. As indicated above, steroids appear to have intracellular or nuclear receptors, while other hormones such as gonadotropins have surface receptors (Figure 4). Hormones require a receptor system in order to transmit the specific biochemical purpose. While the specific mechanisms of translation in the nucleus are not fully understood, several steps appear to be necessary for activation of the chromatin material. These biochemical events may be changed by aging and may be responsible for reduced or modified hormonal behavior[25,67]. The ability of many of the hormones to stimulate DNA synthesis and cell division has been observed to decrease with aging[36].

Changes in cell responsiveness during aging have been ascribed to a wide variety of hormones and neurotransmitters, and a great number of target cells and tissues. This has been described in various animal species as well as in man, and for a wide variety of physiological and biochemical processes[60]. In this research, the time and rate of change with age varies, depending upon the variables noted. In this book, the basic mechanisms by which hormones and neurotransmitters act at the cellular and molecular levels under normal conditions, independent of the aging process, are presented[49,50]. Any of the changes that occur within the cell can mediate hormone and neurotransmitter action and modify it according to the age of the individual[68]. This could result in altered hormonal and neurotransmitter responsiveness with a completely different end result. The major emphasis at present is on the differentiation between changes in receptor and postreceptor events causing altered functional responses during the aging process[50]. In addition, the ability of a number of hormones to stimulate DNA synthesis and cell division has been observed to decrease with aging.

In an earlier review, 200 different receptor systems were studied as a function of age during the adult portion of the life span[69]. The various types of receptor alterations were cataloged and reported as they occurred during the aging process. In general, 50% of the studies reported showed reduced receptor concentration with increased age, 35% reported no changes whatsoever, 10% found increased receptor concentrations with increased age and 5% reported changes in affinity which were generally decreased with increased age. Discrepancies were noted in independent work from many other laboratories over many years. The need for resolution of these controversies by standardization of experimental models and methodology was recognized. Reasonably close, if not causal, relationships between receptor and response loss exists in about 35 cases. Since it is apparent that correlations alone do not establish causality, receptor loss may not necessarily be totally responsible for reduced responsiveness in some of these systems[49]; however, the importance of receptor dysfunction remains unquestionable.

The mechanisms of hormone receptor loss from target cells during aging have been investigated[25,49,50]. Molecular processes that are altered during aging result in decreased cellular concentrations of functional hormone receptors. These include abnormal synthesis (assembly), degradation (disassembly), possible presence of receptors in a non-functional state, and the negative state, and the negative effect of other hormones and biochemical agents on the processes (Figure 7). These destructive events could account for the reduction in activity shown in cells effected by toxic substances as well as aging.

Using radioactive labelling, the concentrations and affinity of receptors were determined in aging tissues in rats. Steroid hormone concentrations appear to be reduced during aging in a number of tissues, including brain, fat, liver, muscle and prostate gland. The binding affinity is not changed, but seems to depend on the ability of the tissues to maintain normal receptor concentrations and not

on the ability of the receptors to respond. This finding is not universal to all of the hormones studied, but may be a response undetectable by present research techniques[69]. Glucocorticoids have shown a reduction of 60% in the ability to control nutrient transport and metabolism between maturity and senescence in rodents[70]. This is paralleled by a 60% reduction in glucocorticoid receptor concentrates. Estrogens have been shown to have a reduced ability to provide certain enzymes required for the proper transmission of nerve impulses in the brain. Estrogen receptor concentrations in the brain were also noted to have decreased with aging, an important preliminary finding.

Starting with the perimenopausal period, estrogen concentrations decrease in both production and serum levels. Estrogen appears to have ubiquitous activity in the cells throughout the body, and the primary method of expression is through intracellular estrogen receptors. If receptors decrease with aging, a further reduction in cellular activity would result. Not all the cells of the body appear to age equally, and a differential in the receptor systems may be responsible for the uneven results which have been seen.

In our laboratory, we have isolated iodinated proteins in breast tissues, which act within the cytosol and appear to be required for normal estrogen receptor action[71]. Estradiol receptor protein changes occur qualitatively and quantitatively in the cytosol in breast tissue from rats made iodine deficient[72]. Progesterone receptor is also affected by a lack of iodine, and varies indirectly with the estradiol receptor levels[73]; thus, iodine appears to be a determinant of receptor availability and action in rat breast tissues[74]. When older rat models were used, dietary deficiency or blockade of iodine caused histological atypism in the mammary tissues, which was sharply increased compared with that seen in younger animals[54]. These abnormal mammary glands were also seen to show differences in receptor levels according to advancing age.

Studies of the effects of aging on estrogen metabolism in the rat uterus have revealed several variables in receptor responses. The probability of non-functional receptors in aged uteri has been described, although it is particularly difficult to separate these receptors from the functional molecules. The likely explanation for apparent steroid receptor loss during aging in the rat uterus is an altered control of the biosynthetic pathway rather than a change in the molecular structure of the receptor itself. Further research being carried out in several laboratories is studying postreceptor responses[50]. Measuring RNA polymerase II activity following estrogen administration, the absolute magnitude of response was not shown to diminish with age. Impaired responsiveness of senescent nuclei was seen in the presence of mature receptor preparations. This would show that aging may affect cellular components and/or processes in the scheme of estrogen action distal to cytoplasmic receptor activation, and the number of molecular sites in which this could occur has been described, but not discriminated. Age-associated defects for estrogen stimulation occur at various levels in the transduction apparatus of the cells found in the rat uterus. These may range from quantitative and possibly qualitative deficits in the receptors themselves to nuclear changes involved in the activation of the RNA polymerase II[60].

While the receptor aging studies were mostly in rodents, the data seem remarkably similar to the information known in the human. Difficulties in quantitation and evaluation of the research have led to the conflicting evidence. There has been indirect evidence of reduced estrogen receptor protein in the breasts of menopausal women; whether this is due to aging or estrogen loss is controversial[63]. Uterine endometrial cell loss has been previously reported[75,76]. The evidence that the loss of estrogen and progesterone may reduce cell metabolism in various tissues of the body seems likely. Research is active in this field, as both neurotransmitters and receptors are fundamental to end-organ expression of hormones.

Summary

Aging has been considered by gerontologists for many years to be a response to both neurogenic and endocrine system decline[3]. It appears that the question of whether reproductive loss due to aging stems from depletion of stimulation in the central nervous system or from failure of target tissue action, or perhaps anywhere along the intermediate axis. This remains unanswered and, thus, a matter for current research. These problems in aging and reproduction require competent solution if treatment and/or quality and longevity in the postmenopausal period of life is expected to improve.

Cellular deterioration and estrogen

Non-reproductive somatic cells go through a series of events that promote growth and development. Such cells range from cell populations that are consistently proliferating (skin, gastrointestinal lining, blood-forming elements) to those which are non-growing (nervous tissue, muscle)[4]. As discussed above, the endocrine system lies between these extremes as it requires constant input for preparation and secretion of the specific hormones involved.

When estrogen diminishes, intracellular activity decreases in estrogen-dependent tissues. These tissues appear to be limited to primary and secondary sexual organs as well as specific areas of the central nervous system. Atrophism is most apparent in the vulvar, vaginal and urethral regions, also as a result of cellular aging. Cellular changes are detailed in Chapter 4 and the clinical problems in later chapters.

When estrogen replacement is given, the affected tissues are still not fully restored, indicating that end-organ failure continues regardless of available hormone. Secretions from the higher endocrine centers (pituitary and hypothalamus) increase initially, responding to the changes and feedback from the cellular milieu at the target organ. These modifications in molecular structure in the estrogen-dependent cells cannot be defined by present research techniques. However, new enzyme models with rat uteri have shown anion differences[60]. The need to prove that these models also represent similar responses in women remains an important step for further clinical research.

It is apparent that non-reproductive tissues are affected on an individual basis, according to receptors that are present. Whether specific estrogen receptors are required cell stimulators in these organs is unknown. Several clinical problems which focus on symptoms in the skeletal and central nervous systems have been studied.

Osteoporosis, neurovascular phenomena (such as hot flushes) and cardiovascular diseases are the serious postmenopausal conditions encountered. Cardiac protection by estrogen seems clinically evident, and some basic research has enlightened this area[77,78]. The combination of both a neuro-endocrine and a neurocardiac basis for protection by estrogen in the presynaptic ganglia of the heart has been added to the many theories[79,80].

However, no estrogen receptors have been measured in bone, and the effects of estrogen on nervous tissue have remained difficult to define. Recent studies[58] show the possibility that there may be nuclear receptors that are not measurable at present in specific estrogen receptor-β form. These systems may be the reasons for a lack of correlation in these tissues when effects are compared with laboratory receptor measurements.

Estrogen replacement and aging

If estrogen is responsible for cellular senescence of reproductive tissues, replacement therapy should be fully effective as a restorative measure. However, the legendary 'fountain of youth' remains elusive. Treatments of many kinds have been used in an attempt to turn back the clock. At present, gerontologists strive to improve the quality of life as longevity increases. The use of hormones, from the mystical transplants of Brown-Sequard in the 19th century to the `estrogen forever' phase of the early 1970s, remains obscure.

Estrogen increases estrogen receptors and, therefore, enhances bodily cellular responses under their control[61]. Nevertheless, aging itself reduces endocrine activity by the deterioration of the secretory mechanisms, and decreases the metabolism within the responding cells by modifying receptors and other unknown factors. Estrogen appears to have specific effects on the central nervous system, hypothalamus and pituitary gland perhaps through catechol estrogens. Further modifications of these higher centers by aging may be restrictive or even non-responsive to the needs of the reproductive system.

Estrogen has been described as providing clinical improvement, and the following chapters discuss the advantages and disadvantages of its use. Experimental work with estrogen, estrogen analogs and intermediate sex steroids in an effort to change intracellular pathways and receptor action is under way. Estrogen replacement therapy remains the most potent method for improving the quality of life for the menopausal woman[81]. Pharmaceutical research is dedicated to producing therapeutic hormones that are safer and more effective.

Progesterone as a therapy for the menopause may serve as a substitute for estrogen in certain target organs. The clinical use of progesterone to protect some estrogen-dependent tissues from neoplastic changes during estrogen therapy in the postmenopause continues to be suggested. Changes in central nervous system stimuli, as seen by secondary hypothalamic pulses, appear to be the basis for hot flushes. The resulting elevations of gonadotropin (LH) are considered by some to be responsible for a limited response. This hypothalamic thermal action is being treated by anti-gonadotropic-releasing hormone substances as an alternative to estrogen[82].

Throughout the research and clinical history of estrogen replacement, there has been no evidence that estrogen or other hormonal therapies are effective in deterring aging. On the other hand, aging can block the effect of estrogen in reproductive tissues and other hormone-affected tissues. Estrogen, while initially useful in the perimenopause, can change only modestly the atrophism of aging in the postmenopausal period. Thus, aging is intrusive on reproduction and our present knowledge does not provide complete replacement therapies that can revitalize the system.

Conclusions

(1) Menopause does not appear to affect longevity nor is it affected by increased life expectancy.

(2) Cellular aging is a direct cause of reproductive failure which leads to the menopause.

(3) Estrogen-dependent tissues have an increased rate of senescence in the perimenopause and menopause.

(4) Intracellular deterioration is more dependent on aging than menopause, or the lack of the sex steroids.

(5) Aging of the reproductive stimulatory centers is responsible for reduction in target cellular activity and eventual intracellular demise.

(6) Hormonal replacement has limitations in reparation of the aging cells.

The success of sex hormone therapy in aging is dependent on responsive cell metabolism in the individual, focally distributed around the body. The use of estrogen replacement therapy must be considered on the basis of individual effectiveness versus risk.

References

1. Miller PB, Soules MR. Correlation of reproductive aging with function in selected organ systems. *Fertil Steril* 1997;68:443–8
2. Strehler BL. *Time, Cells, and Aging*, 2nd edn. New York: Academic Press, 1974
3. Rockstein M. *Theoretical Aspects of Aging*. New York: Academic Press, 1974
4. Shock NW. Physiologic theories of aging. In Rockstein M, ed. *Theoretical Aspects of Aging*. New York: Academic Press, 1984:119–28
5. Fossel M. Telomerase and the aging cell. *J Am Med Assoc* 1998;279:1732–5
6. Skulachev VP. Aging is a specific biological function rather than the result of a disorder in complex living systems: biochemical evidence in support of Weismann's hypothesis. *Biochemistry* 1997;62:1191–5
7. Medawar PB. *An Unsolved Problem of Biology*. London: Lewis, 1951
8. Leathem JH. Endocrine changes with age. In Ostfeld AM, ed. *Epidemiology of Aging*, DHEW Publication 75-711. Washington, DC: DHEW, 1972:224–32
9. Fiatarone MA, O'Neill EF, Ryan ND, *et al*. Exercise training and nutritional supplementation for physical frailty in very elderly people. *New Engl J Med* 1994;330:1769–75
10. Gusseck DJ. Endocrine mechanisms and aging. *Adv Gerontol Res* 1972;4:105
11. Weismann A. *Essays Upon Hereditary and Kindred Biologic Problems*. London: Oxford University Press, 1981
12. Tietze C. Reproductive span and rate reproduction among Hutterite women. *Fertil Steril* 1957;8:89
13. Young JZ. *An Introduction Into the Study of Man*. Oxford: Clarendon Press, 1971
14. Jones EC. The post-reproductive phase in mammals. *Front Horm Res* 1975;3:1
15. Brody JA, Grand MD, Frateschi LJ, *et al*. Epidemiology and aging: maximum reproductive age unaffected by increased life expectancy in the twentieth century. *Aging* 1998;10:170–1
16. Thung PJ, Boot LM, Muhlbock D. Senile changes in the oestrous cycle and in ovarian structure in some inbred strains of mice. *Acta Endocrinol* 1956;23:8
17. Amundsen DW, Diers CJ. Age of menopause in medieval Europe. *Hum Biol* 1973;45:605
18. Westendorp RG, Kirkwood TB. Human longevity at the cost of reproductive success. *Nature (London)* 1998;396:743–6
19. Eskin BA. Menopause: hormones and drug therapy during reproductive senescence. In Cooper RK, Walker RF, eds. *Experimental and Clinical Interventions in Aging*. New York: Marcel Dekker, 1983:85–117
20. Bloch S. Studies on climacterium and menopause in albino rats. III. Histological observations on the aging genital tract. *Gynecologica* 1961;152:414
21. Block E. Quantitative morphologic investigations of the follicular system in women. Variations at different ages. *Acta Anat* 1952;14:108
22. Maszmann L. Epidemiology of climacteric and post-climacteric complaints. *Front Horm Res* 1973;2:22
23. Fries JF. Aging, natural death, and the compression of morbidity. *N Engl J Med* 1980;303:130–5
24. Keefe DL. Reproductive aging is an evolutionarily programmed strategy that no longer provides adaptive value. *Fertil Steril* 1998;70:204–6
25. Roth GS. Altered biochemical responsiveness and hormone receptor changes during aging. In Behnke J, Finch G, Momeut G, eds. *The Biology of Aging*. New York: Plenum Press, 1978:291
26. Volarcik K, Sheean L, Goldfarb J, *et al*. The meiotic competence of *in vitro* matured human oocytes is influenced by donor age: evidence that folliculogenesis is compromised in the reproductively aged ovary. *Hum Reprod* 1998;13:154–60
27. Goebelsmann U. Steroidogenesis. In Mishell DR Jr, Davajan V, eds. *Reproductive Endocrinology, Infertility and Contraception*. Philadelphia: FA Davis, 1979:42–54

28. Lamberts SWJ, van den Beld AW, van der Lely A-J. The endocrinology of aging. *Science* 1997;278: 419–23

29. Metcalf MG, Donald RA, Livesey JH. Pituitary-ovarian function in normal women during the menopausal transition. *J Endocrinol* 1980;87:191

30. Eskin BA. Clinical consideration of age-related changes in serotonin and norepinephrine metabolism of reproductive function. *Neurobiol Aging* 1984;5:151

31. Atit R, Eskin BA, Walker RF. Comparison of gonadotropin secretion in women and female rats during aging. *Age, J Am Aging Assoc* 1986;9:10

32. Simon JA, Bustillo M, Thorneycroft IH. Variability of midcycle estradiol positive feedback: evidence for unique pituitary response in individual women. *J Clin Endocrinol Metab* 1987;64:789

33. Eskin BA, Trivedi RA, Weideman CA, Walker RF. Positive feedback disturbances and infertility in women over thirty. *Am J Gynecol Health* 1988;2:110

34. Finch CE. Neuroendocrinology of aging: a view of an emerging area. *Biol Sci* 1975;25:645

35. Finch CG, Tanzi RE. Genetics of aging. *Science* 1997;278:407–11

36. Wilkes MM, Lu KH, Hopper BR, Yen SSC. Altered neuroendocrine status of middle-aged rats prior to the onset of senescent anovulation. *Neuroendocrinology* 1979;29:255

37. Morrison JH, Hof PR. Life and death of neurons in the aging brain. *Science* 1972;278:412–19

38. Clemens JA, Ameromoni Y, Jenkins T, Meites J. Effects of hypothalamic stimulation, hormones, and drugs on ovarian function in old female rats. *Proc Soc Exp Biol Med* 1969;132:561

39. Miller AE, Riegle GD. Serum LH levels following multiple LHRH injections in aging rats. *Proc Soc Exp Biol Med* 1978;157:494–9

40. Greenblatt RB, Colle ML, Mahesh VB. Ovarian and adrenal steroid production in postmenopausal woman. *Obstet Gynecol* 1976;47:383

41. Meredith S, Butcher RL. Role of decreased numbers of follicles in reproductive performance in young and aged rats. *Biol Reprod* 1985;32:788–94

42. Butcher RL. Effect of reduced ovarian tissue on cyclicity, basal hormone levels and follicular development in old rats. *Biol Reprod* 1985;32:315–21

43. Eskin BA. Physiology of gonadotropins LH/FSH. In *Issues in Reproductive Endocrinology*. New York: Medical Arts Press 1984:99

44. Page RD, Butler RL. Follicular and plasma patterns of steroids in young and old rats during normal and prolonged estrous cycles. *Biol Reprod* 1982;27: 383

45. Thung PJ. Ageing changes in the ovary. In Bourne J, ed. *Structural Aspects of Ageing*. New York: Hafner, 1961:109

46. Mattingly RF, Huang WY. Steroidogenesis of the menopausal and postmenopausal ovary. *Am J Obstet Gynecol* 1969;103:679

47. Vermeulen A. The hormonal activity of the postmenopausal ovary. *J Clin Endocrinol Metab* 1976;42: 247

48. Channing CP, Tsafriri A. Mechanism of action of luteinizing hormone and follicle stimulating hormone on the ovary *in vitro*. *Metabolism* 1977;26: 413

49. Hess GD, Roth GS. Receptors and aging. In Johnson JE, ed. *Aging and Cell Functions*. New York: Plenum Press, 1985:149–85

50. Roth GS, Hess GD. Changes in the mechanisms of hormone and neurotransmitter action during aging: current status of the role of receptor and postreceptor alternatives. *Mech Aging Dev* 1982;20: 175

51. Cooper RL, Roberts B, Rogers DC, Seay SG, Conn PM. Endocrine status versus chronological age as predictors of altered LH secretion in the aging rat. *Endocrinology* 1984;114:391–6

52. Cooper RL. Pharmacological and dietary manipulations of reproductive aging in the rat: significance to central nervous system aging. In Cooper RL, Walker RF, eds. *Experimental and Clinical Interventions in Aging*. New York: Marcel Dekker, 1983: 27–44

53. Moudgil VK, Kanugro MS. Effect of age of rat on the induction of acetylcholinesterase of the brain by 17-beta estradiol. *Biochim Biophys Acta* 1973;329: 211

54. Krouse TB, Eskin BA, Mobini J. Age-related changes resembling fibrocystic disease in iodine-blocked rat breasts. *Arch Pathol Lab Med* 1979; 103:631

55. Jensen EV, Suzuki T, Kawashina T. A two-step mechanism for the interaction of estradiol with rat uterus. *Proc Natl Acad Sci USA* 1968;59:632

56. Shyamala G, Gorski J. Interrelationships of estrogen receptors in the nucleus and cytosol. *J Cell Biol* 1967;35:125A

57. Jensen EV, Mohle S, Brecher PI, DeSombre ER. Estrogen receptor transformation and nuclear RNA synthesis. In O'Malley BW, Means AR, eds. *Receptors for Reproductive Hormones*. New York: Plenum Press, 1973:122–36

58. Gorski J. Evolution of a model of estrogen action. *Rec Prog Horm Res* 1986;42:297–9

59. Anderson JN, Peck EJ, Clark JH. Estrogen-induced uterine responses and growth. *Endocrinology* 1975; 96:160

60. Roth GS. Effects of aging in the mechanisms of estrogen action in rat uterus. *Adv Exp Med Biol* 1986;196:347–60

61. Little M, Szendro P, Teran C, Hughes A, Jungblut PW. Biosynthesis and transformation of microsomal and cytosol estradiol receptors. *J Steroid Biochem* 1975;6:493

62. Clark JH, Peck EJ, Anderson JN. Nafoxidine, mode of action on estrogen receptor systems. *Nature (London)* 1974:251:446

63. McGuire WL, Carbone PP, Vollmer EP. *Estrogen Receptors in Human Breast Cancer*. New York: Raven Press, 1975

64. Lindner V, Kim SK, Karas RH. Increased expression of estrogen receptor beta in RNA in male blood vessels after vascular injury. *Circ Res* 1998;83: 224–9

65. Chan L, O'Malley BW. Mechanism of action of the sex steroid hormones. *N Engl J Med* 1976;294: 1322

66. Tchermitchin A, Tchermitchin X, Galand P. Correlation of estrogen-induced uterine eosinophilia with other parameters of estrogen stimulation produced with estradiol and estriol. *Experimentia* 1975; 31:993

67. Roth GS, Adelman RV. Age related changes in hormone binding by target cells and tissues: possible role in altered adaptive responsiveness. *Exp Gerontol* 1975;10:1

68. Snyder DL, Johnson DM, Eskin BA, *et al*. Effect of age on cardiac norepinephrine release in female rats. *Aging Clin Exp Res* 1995;7:210–17

69. Roth GS. Hormone receptor changes during adulthood and senescence: significance for aging research. *Fed Proc* 1979;38:910

70. Roth GS, Livingston JN. Reductions in glucocorticoid inhibition of glucose oxidation and presumptive glucocorticoid receptor content in rat adiposities during aging. *Endocrinology* 1976;99:831

71. Eskin BA, Sparks CE, LaMont BI. The intracellular metabolism of iodine in carcinogenesis. *Biol Trace Element Res* 1979;1:101

72. Eskin BA, Jacobson HI, Bolmarich V, Murray JA. Breast atypia in altered thyroid states: intracellular changes. *Senologia* 1977;4:114

73. Eskin BA, Mitchell MA, Modhera PR. Mammary gland hormone receptors in iodine deficiency. *Proc Endocrinol Soc* 1985;67:24

74. Eskin BA. Iodine and breast cancer: an update 1982. *Biol Trace Element Res* 1983;5:399

75. Gosden RG. Uptakes and metabolism *in vivo* of tritiated estradiol-17 beta in tissue of aging female mice. *J Endocrinol* 1976;68:153

76. Nelson JF, Holinka CF, Finch CE. Loss of cytoplasmic estradiol binding capacity during aging in uteri of 57/6 mice. *Proc Endocrinol Soc* 1976;58:349

77. Grodstein F, Stampfer M. The epidemiology of coronary heart disease and estrogen replacement in post-menopausal women. *Prog Cardiovasc Dis* 1995; 38:199—210

78. Hulley S, Grady D, Bush T, *et al*. Randomized trial of estrogen plus progesterone for secondary prevention of coronary heart disease in postmenopausal women. *J Am Med Assoc* 1992;280:605–13

79. Eskin BA, Snyder DL, Gayheart P, Roberts J. The protective effect of estrogen on the cardiac adrenergic nervous system. In *Cardiovascular Disease in Women*. Dallas: American Heart Association, 1997:23–30

80. Martino MA, Eskin BA. Estrogen and the post-menopausal heart: advances in protection. *Female Patient* 1999;24:19–28

81. Eskin BA. Sex hormones and aging. In Roberts J, Adelman RC, Cristofalo VJ, eds. *Pharmacologic Interventions in the Aging Process*. New York: Plenum Press, 1978:207–24

82. Yen SSC, Tsai CC, Naftolin F, Vandenburg G, Ajabor L. Pulsatile patterns in gonadotropin release in subjects with or without ovarian function. *J Clin Endocrinol Metab* 1972;34:671

2

Geripause

Bruce R. Troen

Introduction

A demographic revolution is occurring that will change the landscape of medical care. The growth in numbers of people aged 65 years and older is greater than that of the general population, and the most rapid increase is occurring in the group aged 85 years and above. This pattern will be maintained and even accelerate in the next 35 years. Therefore, not only are there more elderly, but there are more of the oldest old. The ramifications of such a population shift are profound and will force us to reassess our notions of 'old age' and the approach to delivering medical care to these patients. This will be especially important for women, who are a significant majority of those 65 and older. Until recently, the phases of maturity for a woman comprised child-bearing age (premenopausal), followed by the menopause (or a perimenopausal period) and ending in a postmenopausal state. It is now clear that the term postmenopausal insufficiently describes the years after the menopause. Instead, the postmenopausal period is more the penultimate stage of life and is increasingly often the prelude to a prolonged epoch for many women – the geripause. In order to provide the best possible care, we must approach the geripausal/geriatric patient in a manner which recognizes that the patient's physiology and response to stress and illness are markedly different than at earlier times in life.

Demography

The average/median life span (also known as life expectancy) is the age at which 50% of a given population survives, and maximum life span potential (MLSP) represents the longest lived member(s) of the population or species. The average life span of humans has increased dramatically over time, yet the MLSP has remained approximately constant and is usually stated to be 90–100 years (Figure 1)[1]. In 1900 the average life expectancy at birth for humans was 47 years[2]; as of 1996 it was 76 years[3]. Of note, the longest lived human for whom documentation exists was Jeanne Calment, who died at the age of 122 in August 1997. As causes of early mortality have been eliminated through public health measures and improved medical care, more individuals have approached the maximum life span. As depicted in Figure 1, this has resulted in a rectangularization of the survivorship curve. Evidence for the continuation of this trend is the increase in life expectancy at the age of 65 by 3.3 years since 1960[2]. In 1997, people reaching the age of 65 had an average life expectancy of 17.6 more years (19.0 for females and 15.8 for males). As of 1991, 85-year-olds had an average life expectancy of more than 5 years[2]. Life

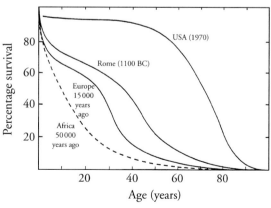

Figure 1 Human survivorship curve at different periods in history. From Cutler RG. In *Principles of Geriatric Medicine and Gerontology*, 1985, with permission from The McGraw-Hill Companies[1]

expectancy at birth has also continued to increase (Table 1)[3]. Of note, life expectancy at birth varies depending upon gender and race: in 1996 it was almost 80 years for white females, 74 years for black females, 73 years for white males and 66 years for black males (Table 1). Continued increases in life expectancy in the next century, the greater life expectancy for women and the tendency for women to marry men older than themselves lead to the projection that 70% of 'baby boom' women will outlive their husbands and can expect to be widows for 15 or more years.

At present, approximately 12% of Americans are age 65 or older. Although the entire US population grew by 45% between 1960 and 1994, the elderly population in general rose 100% and the population of those aged 85 and over grew 274%[2]. The number of people 100 years and over has doubled since 1980. As of 1997, those 65 and older numbered 34.1 million and accounted for 12.7% of the US population[4]. During the next 35 years, the number of people aged 65 and older will more than double, and the number aged 85 and older will triple[4]. Women account for a significant majority of the elderly population. In 1997, there were 20.1 million women and 14.0 million men aged 65 and over. This imbalance increases with age: almost 60% of those aged 65–69 are females, over 70% of those 85 and over are female and approximately 80% of centenarians are women[2]. The older population will continue to grow significantly in the upcoming decades (Figure 2).[2].

Table 1 Life expectancy at birth by race and sex: USA, 1940–96. Data from reference 3

| | All races | | | White | | | All other | | | | | |
| | | | | | | | Total | | | Black | | |
Year	Both sexes	Male	Female	Both sexes	Male	Female	Both sexes	Male	Female	Both sexes	Male	Female
1996	76.1	73.1	79.1	76.8	73.9	79.7	72.6	68.9	76.1	70.2	66.1	74.2
1990	75.4	71.8	78.8	76.1	72.7	79.4	71.2	67.0	75.2	69.1	64.5	73.6
1980	73.7	70.0	77.4	74.4	70.7	78.1	69.5	65.3	73.6	68.1	63.8	72.5
1970	70.8	67.1	74.7	71.7	68.0	75.6	65.3	61.3	69.4	64.1	60.0	68.3
1960	69.7	66.6	73.1	70.6	67.4	74.1	63.6	61.1	66.3	NA	NA	NA
1950	68.2	65.6	71.1	69.1	66.5	72.2	60.8	59.1	62.9	NA	NA	NA
1940	62.9	60.8	65.2	64.2	62.1	66.6	53.1	51.5	54.9	NA	NA	NA

NA, data not available

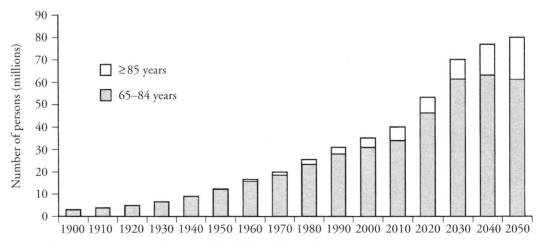

Figure 2 Number of persons ≥ 65 years: 1900–2050 (millions). Data from reference 2

Growth slowed during the 1990s because of the relatively small number born during the Great Depression of the 1930s. By 2010, the first group of 'baby boomers' will reach the age of 65. Consequently, between the years 2010 and 2030, the older population will mushroom, when the 'baby boom' generation reaches age 65 and beyond[5]. Between now and 2030, the number of people aged 65 and older will double and account for 20% of the population. By 2050 and 25% of the elderly will by 85 and older. One can appreciate further the increasing longevity of those who reach the age of 65 by considering the following: 14% of 65-year-olds in 1960 were expected to reach the age of 90, 26% of 65-year-olds in 2000 will be expected to reach the age of 90 and 42% of 65-year-olds in 2050 will probably live to the age of 90[2].

Normal aging

There is evidence supporting at least five common characteristics of aging:

(1) Increased mortality with age after maturation: in the early 19th century, Gompertz first described the exponential increase in mortality with aging owing to various causes, a phenomenon that still pertains today[6]. In 1995, the death rate for all causes between the ages of 25 and 44 was 189.5/100 000 and for the ages of 65 and over was 5069.0/100 000: a more than 25-fold increase[7].

(2) Changes in biochemical composition in tissues with age: there are notable age-related decreases in lean body mass and total bone mass in humans[8,9]. Although subcutaneous fat is either unchanged or declining, total fat remains the same[9]. Consequently, the percentage of adipose tissue increases with age. At the cellular level, many markers of aging have been described in various tissues from different organisms[10]. Two of the first to be described were increases in lipofuscin (age pigment)[11] and increased cross-linking in extracellular matrix molecules such as collagen[12,13]. Additional examples include age-related changes in both the rates of transcription of specific genes and the rate of protein

synthesis, and numerous age-related alterations in post-translational protein modifications, such as glycation and oxidation[14,15].

(3) Progressive decrease in physiological capacity with age: many physiological changes have been documented in both cross-sectional and longitudinal studies[16-18]. Declines in various organ systems include: cardiac output and heart rate in response to stress, peripheral blood vessel compliance, bone mineral density, cartilaginous resiliency, creatinine clearance, renal blood flow, maximum urine osmolality, forced vital capacity and expiratory volume, maximal oxygen uptake, intestinal motility, visual accommodation and acuity, color sensitivity, depth perception, high-frequency perception, speech discrimination, T-cell immune response, total sleep time and time in rapid eye movement (REM) sleep, and psychomotor performance. These decreases occur linearly from about the age of 30; however, the rate of physiological decline is quite heterogeneous from organ to organ and individual to individual[19,20]. As described in detail elsewhere in this book, women experience a dramatic decline in estrogen at the time of the menopause. Growing evidence suggests that testosterone, dehydroepiandrosterone and growth hormone levels also decline with age[21].

(4) Reduced ability to respond adaptively to environmental stimuli with age: a fundamental feature of senescence is the diminished ability to maintain homeostasis[22]. This is manifest not primarily by changes in resting or basal parameters, but in the altered response to an external stimulus such as exercise or fasting. The loss of 'reserve' can result in blunted maximum responses as well as in delays in reaching peak levels and in returning to basal levels. For example, the response of heart rate and cardiac output to exercise and sympathetic nervous system stimulation are significantly reduced in the elderly[23].

(5) Increased susceptibility and vulnerability to disease: the incidence and mortality rates for many diseases increase with age and parallel

the exponential increase in mortality with age[24]. For the five leading causes of death for people over 65, the relative increases in death rates compared to people aged 25–44 are: heart disease 92-fold; cancer 43-fold; stroke > 100-fold; chronic lung disease > 100-fold; and pneumonia and influenza 89-fold[7]. The basis for these dramatic rises in mortality is incompletely understood, but presumably involves changes in the function of many types of cells that lead to tissue/organ dysfunction and systemic illness.

Health status

Increasing age is accompanied by poorer health, as manifest by higher disease rates and increasing levels of frailty and disability. More than a quarter of those over 65 categorize their own health as fair or poor[25]. The leading causes of death in the elderly are listed in Table 2[3]. Cardiovascular disease caused

the most deaths in this age group in 1996. Cancer was responsible for the second highest number of deaths. Given the growth of the elderly population, the number of incident cancers is projected to more than double in the first part of the 21st century[26]. Most people over 65 report at least one chronic ailment, including (in descending prevalence) arthritis, hypertension, heart disease, diminished hearing, cataracts, orthopedic impairment, sinusitis and diabetes (see Table 3)[25]. Cerebrovascular disease rates quadruple, heart disease rates triple and arthritis and hypertension rates double between the perimenopausal era (24–64) and the geripause (> 65). Women suffer from higher rates of arthritis and hypertension, whereas men have higher rates of heart disease and hearing impairment. Several conditions that do not explicitly appear in Table 3 merit mention. There are more than 1.3 million osteoporotic fractures a year in the USA, including 500 000 in the spine, 250 000 in the hip and 240 000 in

Table 2 Leading causes of death in people 65 years and over in the USA in 1996. Adapted from reference 3

Cause	All people		Men		Women	
	%	Rate*	%	Rate*	%	Rate*
Cardiovascular	35.7	1808	35.2	1983	36.2	1686
Cancer	22.3	1131	25.6	1442	19.6	915
Cerebrovascular	8.2	415	6.6	374	9.5	443
COPD and allied conditions	5.3	270	6.0	338	4.8	223
Pneumonia and influenza	4.4	221	4.2	236	4.5	212
Diabetes	2.7	137	2.5	139	2.9	136
Accidents and adverse effects	1.8	91	1.9	110	1.7	78
Alzheimer's disease	1.3	62	0.9	49	1.5	71
Renal	1.2	62	1.2	70	1.2	56
Septicemia	1.0	51	0.9	50	1.1	52

*Rate per 100 000 population; COPD, chronic obstructive pulmonary disease

Table 3 Chronic conditions by age (years) in the USA in 1996: rate per 1000 persons. Data from reference 25

Condition	All 45–64	All ≥ 65	Male ≥ 65	Female ≥ 65
Arthritis	233	490	405	550
Hypertension	223	403	349	442
Heart disease	121	308	367	224
Hearing impairment	145	284	362	268
Deformity/orthopedic impairment	176	178	166	187
Chronic sinusitis	179	153	135	167
Diabetes mellitus	64	126	124	128
Cerebrovascular disease	15	71	80	65

the wrist[27]. This results in significant morbidity (manifest often in decreased mobility) and economic cost. Up to 50% of women above the age of 50 are osteopenic and of those 18% are osteoporotic[28]. One-third of all women and one-sixth of all men who reach the age of 90 suffer a hip fracture; 26% of hospital discharges for hip fracture in 1994 were for men[28]. Urinary incontinence affects 15–30% of community-dwelling elderly and up to 50% of those in long-term care facilities[29]. Perimenopausal-aged women experience more stress incontinence, whereas urge and mixed incontinence predominate in the elderly[30]. Incontinence is associated with isolation, depression and the risk of institutionalization. Dementia is one of the most common causes of disability in the elderly. More than 25% of those 85 and over and more than 50% of those 95 and over suffer dementia[31]. Alzheimer's disease accounts for two-thirds or more of dementia, with a prevalence in community dwellers of 10% of those over 65 years and 47% of those older than 85[32]. Because women have a longer life expectancy, they experience a higher rate of dementia. It is interesting to note that out-patient screening for breast and cervical cancer is decreased in women with a higher number of chronic conditions[33].

Many of the elderly suffer from multiple conditions, and these restrict the activities of older people. Over 50% of those 65 and over report at least one disability, with a third experiencing severe disabilities. Women spend approximately twice as many years disabled prior to death as do their male counterparts[34]. With increasing age, disabilities and difficulties in performing activities of daily living (ADLs) and instrumental activities of daily living (IADLs) become more prevalent (Table 4)[35]. ADLs include bathing, dressing, eating and ambulation[36]. IADLs include meal preparation, shopping, managing money, using the telephone, doing housework and laundry, ability to travel and taking medication[37]. It is important to note, however, that more than 70% of people 65 and over report their health status as good, very good or excellent, despite the prevalence of chronic conditions in this group[25]. Furthermore, despite the prevalence of chronic conditions and increasing disability, more than 90% of the elderly live in the community and 75% of those 85 and older still live at home.

Approach to the elderly patient

There is a tremendous amount of variation in the manner in which individuals age and respond to illness. Consequently, knowledge of a patient's baseline function and health is critical for accurate diagnosis and therapy. Problems that merit special attention in the elderly are listed in Table 5.

There is often altered presentation of disease in the elderly; severe or life-threatening illnesses may be manifest by vague, non-specific or even trivial symptoms. Such symptoms may represent an abrupt change in the patient's health. For example, the patient could cease to go shopping, refuse to arise from bed or fall more often than usual. Non-specific symptoms that may represent specific illnesses include confusion, self-neglect, falling, incontinence, apathy, anorexia, dyspnea and fatigue. Furthermore, symptoms that appear to represent illness within one organ system can actually indicate change in another. Delirium in the elderly infrequently results from acute central nervous system pathology. Rather it is most commonly a sign of systemic illness that is secondarily affecting the brain. Delirium is also a much more common harbinger of physical illness in older people than is fever, pain or tachycardia. Many

Table 4 Disability prevalence with age. Data from reference 35

Age (years)	Any disability	Severe disability	Difficulty with ≥ 1 ADL	Difficulty with ≥ 1IADL	Needs personal assistance with ≥ 1 ADL or IADL
45–54	24.5	11.5	3.1	4.5	3.3
55–64	36.3	21.9	6.0	8.1	6.1
65–79	47.3	27.8	10.5	15.3	11.5
≥ 80	71.5	53.5	27.5	40.4	34.1

ADL, activity of daily living; IADL, instrumental activity of daily living

presentations of pathology represent change in the older patient's homeostatic reserve and could also reflect changes in sensitivity to pain and other stimuli (for example, a patient with acute and/or chronic cognitive impairment). Examples of altered presentations of specific illnesses in the elderly include:

(1) Depression without sadness;

(2) Infectious disease without leukocytosis, fever or tachycardia;

(3) Silent surgical abdomen;

(4) Silent malignancy ('mass without symptoms');

(5) Myocardial infarction without chest pain;

(6) Non-dyspneic pulmonary edema;

(7) Apathetic thyrotoxicosis.

Often the elderly will not volunteer information about symptoms because of misconceptions about normal age-related changes versus disease-related phenomena. These 'hidden illnesses' in the elderly include sexual dysfunction, depression, incontinence, musculoskeletal stiffness, hearing loss and dementia. To ferret out these problems, in addition to alcoholism in the elderly, physicians and other health-care workers must proactively question patients. Because specific disease diagnoses may not allow for accurate diagnoses in the elderly, it is often more useful to consider the presenting problem, such as those grouped under the 'Is of geriatrics' (Table 6)[16]. Of particular note is iatrogenesis because of the advantages and disadvantages that must be weighed in proceeding with diagnosis and treatment, particularly in frail older individuals.

History

Obtaining a history from an older patient may take more time and may require eliciting information from family members and friends. Nevertheless, the patient should remain the primary source, except in the case of advanced cognitive impairment. If a patient's responses are inappropriate and/or inconsistent, then evaluation of cognitive status should be undertaken (see below). The initial interview should be conducted with the patient

Table 5 Common issues in the elderly

Function
Polypharmacy
Ambulation
Cognition
Depression
Urinary incontinence
Constipation
Alcohol
Elder mistreatment

Table 6 The Is of geriatrics. Adapted from reference 16

Iatrogenesis
Immobility
Immune deficiency
Impairment of vision/hearing
Impotence
Impoverishment
Inanition (malnutrition)
Incoherence
Incontinence
Infection
Insomnia
Instability
Institutionalization
Intellectual impairment
Irritable colon
Isolation (depression)

dressed, seated and facing the interviewer at eye level. Given changes in vision, hearing and speech discrimination, it is important to talk directly without the use of jargon to the patient and to insure that the patient understands. This includes allowing enough time for the older patient to respond. It is critical to obtain a thorough medication history, including over-the-counter medications and home remedies. Adverse drug reactions and interactions are particularly common among the elderly and are directly proportional to the number of medications being taken owing to the high incidence of disease. Age alone is not an independent predictor of adverse drug reactions[38]. It is very helpful to have the patient bring all of his or her medicine to the physician's office ('brown bag' technique). It is essential to determine the patient's compliance and perceived effects of the medications. Special emphasis also needs to be placed on the social history, health-care maintenance,

Table 7 Activities and instrumental activities of daily living

Activities of daily living (basic self-care)	Instrumental activities of daily living (community interactions)
Mnemonic DEATH	Mnemonic SHAFT
Dressing	Shopping
Eating	Housework
Ambulating	Accounting
Toileting	Food preparation
Hygiene	Transportation

functional capabilities, nutritional history, alcohol consumption and the review of systems. Explicit inquiries about urinary signs and symptoms (especially incontinence for women and hesitancy for men) should be included in the review of systems. Functional assessment includes determination of ADLs and IADLs (Table 7)[36,37]. For those patients who depend upon a care-giver, screening for elder mistreatment should be considered[39]. Elder abuse includes physical neglect, psychological abuse and/or neglect, financial or material abuse/ neglect, or violation of personal rights.

Physical examination

For very frail patients, multiple sessions for a complete physical examination may be required. If back pain, deformity or significant arthritis exists, time in the supine position may need to be limited. This is particularly pertinent for osteoporotic and/or arthritic patients undergoing pelvic examination. During general observation of the patient and assessment of vital signs, special attention should be given to the presence of ADL deficits, poor hygiene, dishevelled appearance, systolic hypertension, orthostatic hypotension and the patient's weight. The timed 'Up & Go' test helps to determine functional mobility[40]. The patient is asked to rise from a seating position, walk 3 m, turn around, and return to sit in the chair. A time of less than 20 s suggests good mobility, whereas times over 30 s suggest potential problems. During this test, the patient's gait should be assessed. Lower extremity function in the elderly (balance, gait, strength and endurance) can predict short-

term mortality and nursing-home admission[41]. Visual and aural acuity should be assessed. Decreased hearing can occur as a result of wax accumulation in the ear. The skin should be assessed for ulcers and neoplasms in sun-exposed areas. Cardiovascular palpation is less reliable when kyphoscoliosis exists. Systolic murmurs associated with benign aortic sclerosis are common. However, diastolic murmurs and the presence of an S_3 gallop are always important and merit further consideration and work-up. Arterial insufficiency results in hair loss, bruits and decreased pulses, whereas venous disease more commonly leads to stasis, skin changes and edema. A baseline pulmonary examination is particularly important, as rales may not indicate infectious disease or congestive heart failure. Breast masses may be easier to palpate owing to lack of estrogenic stimulation. If the patient is unable to lie flat, the abdomen may appear falsely distended. There can be a palpable liver edge without hepatomegaly, and peritoneal signs may be blunt or even absent in the frail elderly. Often one can palpate a distended bladder, an aortic aneurysm and even a sigmoid colon fecal impaction. A rectal examination can assess fecal impaction, and sacral reflexes, and obtain stool for hemoccult testing. A speculum examination of the vagina may be painful and difficult, owing to the absence of estrogen. Extremities should be examined for arthritis and deformities. It is also important to assess toes and toenails. A mini-mental status examination should be performed in all older patients to establish a baseline. A documented mental status will help to determine the acuity of any change and, therefore, the necessary work-up. The Folstein mini-mental status examination[42] remains the bulwark in screening for dementia and delirium, although other tools such as the clock-drawing and timed-change tests have shown promise in recent studies[43,44]. Behavioral changes and/or sadness should prompt screening for depression, using the Geriatric Depression Scale[45], or explicitly asking the patient about sadness/depression[46].

Conclusion

As described above, the number of people 65 years and older will continue to increase dramatically well into the 21st century. The physiology of the elderly and their response to pathology markedly differ from those of younger individuals, including women who are premenopausal and perimenopausal. Furthermore, the most explosive growth will occur in the group of people 85 years and older. We are beginning to learn that these 'old' old may represent a distinct subgroup in the elderly population. Indeed, in the not too distant future, we may use the term 'elderly' to refer to those 85 and over. Despite the prevalence of chronic illness and the rapid age-related increase in mortality in those 65 and over, there is some evidence to suggest that future cohorts may be healthier. Manton and colleagues report that age-related disability declined between 1982 and 1994[47]. In addition, since 1953, Americans have engaged in healthier behaviors: per capita tobacco consumption has declined by 40%, butter consumption is down by one-third, use of whole milk and cream is down one-quarter, and the use of saturated animal fats in cooking is down by 40%[48]. It is possible that such behaviors, often associated with the 'baby boomers' as they have matured, may reduce future rates of chronic diseases. These changes, along with advances in health-care, may continue to fuel the increase of life expectancies that has been driving the rectangularization of the survivorship curve. It is unknown what impact there will be on health-

Table 8 Geriatric principles. From reference 49

Assess each patient individually
Assess cognitive and functional status
Disease often presents atypically
Disease often presents as a change in functional status
Rule out organic causes of behavioral changes first
Pathogenesis of symptoms is often multifactorial
An ounce of prevention is worth a pound of cure
Beware iatrogenesis
Take a holistic approach
Be the patient's advocate
Do NOT be ageist

care utilization. Health-care providers face the challenge of assimilating a geriatric database into their care of the elderly and not falling prey to the myth of hopelessness in treating older patients. Indeed, there is likely to be greater success for some preventive strategies due to the increased incidence and prevalence of diseases in the elderly. Furthermore, since the elderly can manifest dramatic symptoms and signs in response to relatively minor perturbations in their physiology, targeted therapies that result in small 'objective' improvements in an organ system can lead to dramatic benefits for the patient. A proactive approach that incorporates the 'Geriatric principles' in Table 8[49] will begin to lay the foundation for enhanced care of patients in the geripause.

References

1. Cutler RG. Evolutionary perspective of human longevity. In Hazzard WR, Andres R, Bierman EL, *et al.* eds. *Principles of Geriatric Medicine and Gerontology*. New York: McGraw-Hill, 1985:16
2. Hobbs FB, Damon BL. *65+ in the United States*, Current Population Reports. Washington, DC: US Bureau of the Census, 1996:23–190
3. Peters KD, Kochanek KD, Murphy SL. *Deaths: Final Data for 1996*, National Vital Statistics Reports 47. Hyattsville, Maryland: National Center for Health Statistics, 1998
4. Administration on Aging. *Profile of Older Americans: 1998.* http://www.aoa.dhhs.gov/aoa/stats/profile/default.htm
5. Day JC. *Population Projections of the United States by Age, Sex, Race, and Hispanic Origin: 1995 to 2050*, Current Population Reports. Washington, DC: US Bureau of the Census, 1996:25–1130
6. Gompertz B. On the nature of the function expressive of the law of human mortality and on a new mode of determining life contingencies. *Philos Trans R Soc London* 1825;115:513
7. Rosenberg HM, Ventura SJ, Maurer JD, *et al. Births and Deaths: United States, 1995*, Monthly Vital Statistics Report 45. Hyattsville, Maryland: National Center for Health Statistics, 1996:31–3
8. Riggs BL, Melton LD. Involutional osteoporosis. *N Engl J Med* 1986;314:1676–86

9. Shock NW, Greulich RC, Andres R, *et al. Normal Human Aging: the Baltimore Longitudinal Study of Aging.* Washington, DC: US Department of Health and Human Services, 1984

10. Florini JR. Composition and function of cells and tissues. In *Handbook of Biolochemistry in Aging.* Boca Raton: CRC Press, 1981:

11. Strehler BL. In *Time, Cells, and Aging.* New York: Academic Press, 1977

12. Bjorksten J. Cross linkage and the aging process. In *Rothstein M*, ed. *Theoretical Aspects of Aging.* New York: Academic Press, 1974:43

13. Kohn RR. Aging of animals: possible mechanisms. In *Principles of Mammalian Aging.* Englewood Cliffs, NJ: Prentice-Hall, 1978

14. Finch CE. Introduction: definitions and concepts. In *Longevity, Senescence, and the Genome.* Chicago: University of Chicago Press, 1990

15. Levine RL, Stadtman ER. Protein modifications with aging. In Schneider EL, Rowe JW, eds. *Handbook of the Biology of Aging.* San Diego: Academic Press, 1996:184–97

16. Kane RL, Ouslander JG, Abrass IB. Clinical implications of the aging process. In *Essentials of Clinical Geriatrics.* New York: McGraw-Hill Health Professions Division, 1999:3–18

17. Shock NW. Longitudinal studies of aging in humans. In Finch CE, Schneider EL, eds. *Handbook of the Biology of Aging.* New York: Van Nostrand Reinhold, 1985:721

18. Taffet GE. Age-related physiologic changes. In Cobbs EL, Duthie EH, Murphy JB, eds. *Geriatric Review Syllabus.* Dubuque, IA: Kendall/Hunt Publishing Company, 1999:10–23

19. Lakatta EG. Changes in cardiovascular function with aging. *Eur Heart J* 1990;11(Suppl C):22–9

20. Lindeman RD, Tobin J, Shock NW. Longitudinal studies on the rate of decline in renal function with age. *J Am Geriatr Soc* 1985;33:278–85

21. Roshan S, Nader S, Orlander P. Review: aging and hormones. *Eur J Clin Invest* 1999;29:210–13

22. Adelman RC, Britton GW, Rotenberg S, *et al.* Endocrine regulation of gene activity in aging animals of different genotypes. In Bergsma D, Harrison DE, eds. *Genetic Effects on Aging.* New York: Alan R Liss, 1978:355

23. Lakatta EG. Cardiovascular aging research: the next horizons. *J Am Geriatr Soc* 1999;47:613–25

24. Brody JA, Brock DB. Epidemiological and statistical characteristics of the United States elderly population. In Finch CD, Schneider EL, eds. *Handbook of the Biology of Aging.* New York: Van Nostrand Reinhold, 1985:3

25. Benson V, Marano MA. *Current Estimates from the National Health Interview Survey, 1995,* Vital Health and Statistics 10. Hyattsville, Maryland: National Center for Health Statistics, 1998

26. Polednak AP. Projected numbers of cancers diagnosed in the US elderly population, 1990 through 2030. *Am J Public Health* 1994;84:1313–16

27. Christiansen C. Consensus development conference: diagnosis, prophylaxis, and treatment of osteoporosis. *Am J Med* 1993;94:646–50

28. Looker AC, Orwoll ES, Johnston CC Jr, *et al.* Prevalence of low femoral bone density in older US adults from NHANES III [see Comments]. *J Bone Miner Res* 1997;12:1761–8

29. Resnick NM. Urinary incontinence. *Lancet* 1995; 346:94–9

30. Thom D. Variation in estimates of urinary incontinence prevalence in the community: effects of differences in definition, population characteristics, and study type. *J Am Geriatr Soc* 1998;46: 473–80

31. Ebly EM, Parhad IM, Hogan DB, Fung TS. Prevalence and types of dementia in the very old: results from the Canadian Study of Health and Aging [see Comments]. *Neurology* 1994;44:1593–600

32. Evans DA, Funkenstein HH, Albert MS, *et al.* Prevalence of Alzheimer's disease in a community population of older persons. Higher than previously reported [see Comments]. *J Am Med Assoc* 1989; 262:2551–6

33. Kiefe CI, Funkhouser E, Fouad MN, May DS. Chronic disease as a barrier to breast and cervical cancer screening [see Comments]. *J Gen Intern Med* 1998;13:357–65

34. La Croix AZ, Newton KM, Leveille SG, Wallace J. Healthy aging. A women's issue. *West J Med* 1997; 167:220–32

35. McNeil J. *Americans with Disabilities: 1994-1995,* Current Population Reports. Washington, DC: US Bureau of the Census, 1997:P70-61

36. Katz S, Downs TD, Cash HR, Grotz RC. Progress in development of the index of ADL. *Gerontologist* 1970;10:20–30

37. Lawton MP, Brody EM. Assessment of older people: self-maintaining and instrumental activities of daily living. *Gerontologist* 1969;9:179–86

38. Denham MJ. Adverse drug reactions. *Br Med Bull* 1990;46:53–62

39. Swagerty DL Jr, Takahashi PY, Evans JM. Elder mistreatment. *Am Fam Physician* 1999;59:2804–8

40. Podsiadlo D, Richardson S. The timed 'Up & Go': a test of basic functional mobility for frail elderly persons. *J Am Geriatr Soc* 1991;39:142–8

41. Guralnik JM, Simonsick, EM, Ferrucci, L, *et al.* A short physical performance battery assessing lower extremity function: association with self-reported disability and prediction of mortality and nursing home admission. *J Gerontol* 1994;49: M85–94

42. Folstein MF, Folstein SE, McHugh PR. 'Mini-mental state'. A practical method for grading

the cognitive state of patients for the clinician. *J Psychiatr Res* 1975;12:189-98

43. Esteban-Santillan C, Praditsuwan R, Ueda H, Geldmacher DS. Clock drawing test in very mild Alzheimer's disease. *J Am Geriatr Soc* 1998;46: 1266-9

44. Froehlich TE, Robinson JT, Inouye SK. Screening for dementia in the outpatient setting: the time and change test [see Comments]. *J Am Geriatr Soc* 1998; 46:1506-11

45. Yesavage JA, Brink TL, Rose TL, *et al.* Development and validation of a geriatric depression screening scale: a preliminary report. *J Psychiatr Res* 1982; 17:37-49

46. Mahoney J, Drinka TJ, Abler R, *et al.* Screening for depression: single question versus GDS [see Comments]. *J Am Geriatr Soc* 1994;42:1006-8

47. Manton KG, Stallard E, Corder LS. The dynamics of dimensions of age-related disability 1982 to 1994 in the US elderly population. *J Gerontol A Biol Sci Med Sci* 1998;53:B59-70

48. Longino CF. Myths of An Aging America. *American Demographics* 1994, August

49. Rosenblatt D. *Geriatric Gems*. Ann Arbor, MI: University of Michigan Geriatrics Center, 1995

3

Pregnancy in perimenopausal and menopausal women

Linda K. Dunn

Introduction

The pregnancy rate in the developed world is declining as a result of improved contraceptive methods, the availability of abortion and improving employment opportunities for women. At the same time, the proportion of pregnancies in women aged 35 and older is increasing, partly because of voluntary delays in conception and partly because of an increase in infertility.

There have always been women aged 35 and older who have conceived and delivered. In the past, the majority of these women were multiparous and often of high parity, with a unique set of maternal and fetal risks related to the number of prior pregnancies and the mothers' underlying health. These earlier reports could not have anticipated the revolution in child-bearing as a result of assisted reproductive technology. Now women in their late forties and beyond can become first-time mothers. This chapter, as part of a book on the menopause, focuses on the pregnancy experience of women aged 40 and older reported in the literature of the 1990s, augmented by summaries of the earlier literature regarding the obstetric outcomes of women spontaneously pregnant in the perimenopausal years.

Fertility

Women voluntarily deferring pregnancy should be advised about the age-related decline in the ability to conceive. A French study of women receiving donor insemination because of male factor infertility demonstrated a small decrease in fecundity after the age of 30 with a greater decline after the age of 35[1]. Studies by Virro and Shewchuk in 1984[2] and Stovall and colleagues in 1991[3] produced similar results. These studies have been criticized because these women may have entered the insemination program because of a combination of documented male subfertility and some unrecognized aspect of female infertility. In defense of these studies, possible confounding factors such as coital frequency and known causes of female infertility were controlled.

Most of these women were nulliparous. Studies of Hutterite women who use no contraception and are often highly parous have indicated that pregnancy interval increases with age, suggesting decreasing fertility[4]. Decreased coital frequency or declining male fertility may also have contributed to the longer intervals between pregnancies.

Whatever the combination of causes, the studies suggest a 20–30% decline in the ability to conceive for women over 35, compared to women younger than 35.

Spontaneous abortion

The incidence of spontaneous abortion in clinically recognized pregnancies increases progressively as maternal age rises[5,6]. The incidence for women aged 40 and older is 25–30%, compared to 10–15% in younger women. A portion of the increase is certainly due to the increase in aneuploid conceptions as maternal age advances. From recent work with donated ova, it has been learned that older women can achieve and deliver pregnancies almost as successfully as the younger women who donated the eggs[7]. Therefore, aging of the oocyte must also be a significant cause of early pregnancy loss in older gravidas. There may also be a contribution to spontaneous abortion caused by flagging progesterone production as the menopause nears.

Aneuploidy and anomalies

There is a marked increase in aneuploid conceptions as maternal age increases. However, there is no increase in malformations not resulting from chromosome abnormalities. Baird and colleagues[8] studied the British Columbia Health Surveillance Registry, reviewing 577 000 live births. They identified 27 000 children with birth defects, having excluded all those children born with chromosome abnormalities. The incidence of birth defects did not vary with maternal age.

The most common trisomies observed in liveborn children include: trisomy 21 (Down syndrome); trisomy 18; trisomy 13; 47,XXX; and 47,XXY (Klinefelter syndrome). Down syndrome is the most common trisomy in man with a population incidence of 1 in 700. The incidence varies with maternal age such that a 20-year-old woman has a risk of 1 in 2000 of delivering a Down-syndrome baby, a 35-year-old woman has a risk of 1 in 350, and a 40-year-old woman a risk of 1 in 100. These are the figures often given to pregnant women by their care-givers during discussions of prenatal diagnosis. Providing only this information is insufficient, because the incidence of all trisomies is increased. In complete counselling, women should be told that the risk of delivering a live-born child with any trisomy is *double* the risk for Down syndrome alone. This additional information still does not provide complete counselling for women considering chorionic villus sampling or amniocentesis. These women need to be additionally informed of the risk that the test results will be abnormal. Because 30% of Down-syndrome fetuses and 70% of trisomy-18 fetuses deliver as late spontaneous abortions or result in still-birth, the risk of an abnormal test result is higher than the risk of delivering an aneuploid child. For women who will be 35 years old at the time of delivery, the risk of an abnormal test result is 1 in 100, and for a 40-year-old the risk is 3 in 100 with steep increases in risk for women older than 40. In a study in Utah of pregnancy outcomes in women 45 and older, the overall aneuploidy rate was 9.9%[9]. This population of women was unlikely to accept prenatal diagnosis. The delivery of aneuploid infants is a serious risk for women aged 40 and older, but preventable with acceptance of prenatal diagnosis and therapeutic abortion. In women undergoing oocyte donation, the risk for aneuploidy depends on the age of the donor, not the recipient, so these women have a much lower risk. In addition, women in assisted reproductive programs have the option of preimplantation diagnosis for aneuploidy with transfer of euploid embryos.

Medical complications

Since reports from the 1960s, two medical complications of pregnancy have been consistently shown to occur more frequently in older mothers. Not surprisingly, these two co-morbidities are diabetes and hypertension[10-20]. The incidences of type 1 and type 2 diabetes increase with age, so pregestational diabetes is one aspect of the problem. In addition, obesity increases with age and contributes to the increased incidence of gestational diabetes. Both pregestational and gestational diabetes contribute to increases in macrosomia, dystocia and Cesarean section. The incidence of diabetes varies by screening criteria and method of detection, and has been reported to be approximately 2% in older women in the less recent literature, compared to younger women with an incidence of approximately 1%. In the more recent literature, the rate of diabetes in women aged 40 and older during pregnancy is reported to be approximately 9%, with rates in a younger cohort of approximately 2%.

The incidence of hypertensive disorders, including chronic hypertension, pregnancy-associated hypertension and pre-eclampsia, is considerably higher than the incidence of diabetes. Rates recorded in the same studies cited for diabetes[10-20] range from 7.5 to 33% for hypertensive complications in women 40 years and over. In women 45–63 years of age in an oocyte donor program, women with pre-existing hypertension were excluded. When those women in excellent health became pregnant, six out of 36 (17%) with continuing pregnancies developed pre-eclampsia[21]. In Dildy and colleagues' study of primarily multiparous Utah women pregnant after age 45, the incidence of pre-eclampsia was 10.1%[9]. In Sauer and co-workers' oocyte donation group of 17 women aged 50 and over, eight developed gestational hypertension or pre-eclampsia for an incidence of 47%[22].

These studies of both multiparous and nulliparous women from the USA, Europe and Israel present a remarkably consistent record of hypertensive complications which are somewhat higher in nulligravidas and progressively increase with age. With careful management, the potential complications of eclampsia, stroke and coagulopathy can be avoided, but the problems of low birth weight and abruption are unavoidable despite scrupulous maternal care.

Obstetric complications

It is fascinating to read discussions of the Cesarean section rate in women aged 40 and older. All published studies reviewed for this chapter document higher rates in this age group, usually at least double the rates for the general obstetric population for the reporting institutions. These rates are presented in Table 1. The rising Cesarean rate over time is evident. The two studies from Finland during the same time period reflect regional variations in obstetric populations or in obstetric practice. Striking is the performance of the oldest groups. In Dildy and colleagues' primarily multi-

parous population aged 45 and older, the rate is 31.7%, which is comparable to Narayan and co-workers' experience with multiparous women over 50 who had a rate of 28.6%. In contrast, in the assisted reproductive groups of Sauer and associates and Antinori and colleagues in women 45 and older, the rates were 59% when labor was permitted and obviously 100% when it was not. Consistent in these reports is the marked increase in abdominal delivery in older women. The reasons are both legitimate and complex.

First of all, the incidences of malpresentation are very high (11%)[20] in women aged 40 and over, whether or not they are parous. Contributing factors to malpresentation may include high parity, myomas and prematurity. Second, the incidence of placenta previa is increased ten-fold (from 0.2 to 2%)[19]. This increase is true for nulliparous and multiparous women. Third, the increased incidence of both gestational and pregestational diabetes may lead to macrosomia in some patients. Fourth, there are increases in fetal growth restriction and placental dysfunction secondary to maternal hypertensive disorders. These complications are more commonly associated with non-reassuring fetal heart rate patterns during labor. Most important, there are marked increases in dysfunctional labor and dystocia in older gravidas, despite appropriate labor augmentation and expert anesthesia.

Table 1 Reported Cesarean section rates (%) for women ≥ 40 years old

| Authors | Year | Country | Rate | | | |
			≥ 40 years	≥ 45 years	≥ 50 years	Overall
Higdon[23]	1960	USA	8.2			3.8
Posner et al.[10]	1961	USA	8.0			3.0
Koren et al.[11]	1963	Israel	6.0			3.1
Kajanoja and Widholm[13]	1978	Finland	31.0			12.0
Caspi and Lifshitz[12]	1979	Israel	9.7			4.0
Kujansuu et al.[15]	1981	Finland	16.7			8.3
Narayan et al.[24]	1992	UK			28.6	—
Sauer et al.[22]	1995	USA			59.0	—
Antinori et al.[21]	1995	Italy		100.0		—
Dildy et al.[9]	1996	USA		31.7		17.0
Bianco et al.[19]	1996	USA	38.9 (nullip.)			18.3
			24.7 (multip.)			8.9
Gilbert et al.[20]	1999	USA	47.0 (nullip.)			22.5
			29.6 (multip.)			17.8

nullip., nulliparous; multip., multiparous

Some authors have credited physician factors for some of the increase in the rate of Cesarean section in older gravidas[17]. Other authors have disagreed, citing data indicating that oxytocin is used for longer and in higher doses prior to eventual abdominal delivery in these women[25].

Perinatal outcomes

All of the references cited above which discuss increases in medical and obstetric complications in older mothers also document increased risks for the fetus and neonate. These risks are particularly prevalent for women 40 years of age and older. Significant improvements in neonatal care have lowered these risks over time. Two relatively small studies suggest that improved care for mothers and babies has resulted in similar perinatal mortality rates for women younger than 35 and women 35 and older[16,26]. However, two very large studies (McGill Neonatal Database and the Swedish Medical Birth Register) continue to show increasing perinatal mortality rates as a function of maternal age[27-30]. Maternal hypertension and diabetes were controlled for in each of these population studies. Both studies document an increase in preterm-birth and in low-birth-weight infants, and both indicate a doubling in the perinatal mortality rate for older mothers, compared to women younger than 35. In the Swedish study, the late fetal death rate for women 40–52 years of age was 6.5/1000 and the early neonatal death rate was 4.7/1000. The fetal death rate was significantly raised, compared to the younger women, but the neonatal death rate was not significantly raised.

Maternal mortality

Maternal deaths are defined as 'deaths that occurred during a pregnancy or within 42 days of the end of a pregnancy and for which the cause of death was listed as a complication of pregnancy, childbirth, or the puerperium (International Classification of Diseases, Ninth Revision, codes 630–676)'[31]. There has been a steady decline in maternal mortality rates since 1930, when the US rate was 670 deaths per 100 000 live births. The rate fell to 7.2 per 100 000 in 1987 and then increased

to 10.0 in 1990, the last year for which complete data are currently available[32].

The most important risk factors for maternal death are age and race. There has always been, and continues to be, a large and disturbing increase in maternal death in black women. With regard to age, the curves are parallel with steep increases after the age of 35 (Figure 1)[33]. The leading causes of maternal death are hemorrhage, embolism and hypertensive disorders of pregnancy. Recent increases have been noted due to cardiomyopathy and infection. Age is a significant risk factor for both hypertension and cardiomyopathy.

The Healthy People 2000 goal for maternal mortality is 3.3 deaths per 100 000 live births. This goal will not be reached and has been restated as a goal for 2010. With the increase in pregnancies in older women, reaching the goal will be especially challenging. Reaching the target will require attention to the very high rate of maternal death in black women. Based on World Health Organization (WHO) reports, 20 other countries have maternal mortality rates lower than in the USA[31]. Information from Sweden[34] documents exactly the same major causes of death, suggesting that the

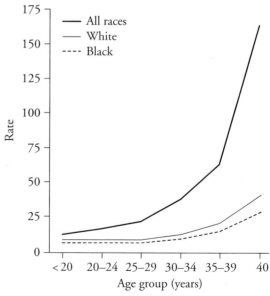

Figure 1 Pregnancy-related mortality rate per 100 000 live births by age and race. From reference 33

pathology is similar but that differences may exist in the organization and accessibility of services.

It is important to note that maternal deaths are considered to be under-reported, with the true incidence 1.3–3.0 times what is reported. Important sources of error are women whose deaths are attributed to diseases such as malignancy, or heart failure or renal failure, which were aggravated by pregnancy. Death certificates may omit mention of a recent pregnancy. These chronic diseases occur more frequently in older women.

Pregnancy by oocyte donation in menopausal women

Several centers have reported the use of donor oocytes for infertile women over age 40 and women who have undergone a natural menopause. When these women are compared with younger women participating in assisted reproductive programs and with women of the same age using their own oocytes, the natural decline in fertility with age seems to disappear[35]. Implantation rates, clinical pregnancy rates and completed pregnancy rates approach those of younger women.

The women accepted into these programs have been subject to intense medical scrutiny prior to attempted conception, to reduce as much as possible the risks reviewed in this chapter. Sauer and colleagues[36] report medical screening of the wife with stress electrocardiogram (ECG), mammography, chest radiography, glucose tolerance testing, extensive blood work and a Pap smear. Both partners were required to be tested for human immunodeficiency virus (HIV), syphilis and hepatitis. In addition, the wife had a pelvic ultrasound scan, a hysterosalpingogram and an endometrial biopsy on hormone replacement. The husband had his semen analyzed and cultured, and the sperm were evaluated with a hamster egg penetration test. Of 18 patients screened, four women were excluded, two because of abnormal ECGs, one because of diabetes and one because of multiple large myomas. Of the 14 couples enrolled, nine achieved pregnancy. Two women miscarried. At the time of the report in 1993, three had delivered and four pregnancies were ongoing. There were two sets of twins.

In 1995, Sauer and colleagues reported further on oocyte donation for older women, confining the report to women 50 and older[22]. Fifty-five women were screened and 19 were excluded: six for myomas, three because of malignancies, three because of abnormal treadmill ECGs, three because of diabetes, three because of psychological problems and one because of multiple sclerosis. Of the 36 couples enrolled, 17 conceived and delivered. Nine of the pregnancies were multiple: two quadruplet gestations reduced to twins, one triplet gestation and six additional sets of twins. As discussed above in the section on 'Medical complications', eight patients developed hypertensive complications. Other than gestational age and birth weight, there is no information about the neonates.

Antinori and co-workers report from Rome on 44 pregnancies achieved with donor oocytes in 113 women aged 45–63[21]. Remarkable is that 300 women were excluded from participation after medical, biochemical and psychological screening similar to Sauer's. The reasons for exclusion in decreasing order of frequency were hypertension, smoking, heart disease, psychological reasons, obesity, myomas, breast disease, coagulation disorders, thyroid dysfunction, encephalopathy, diabetes, and liver and renal disease. This list would be familiar to any primary-care physician who cares for mid-life women. Despite passing this rigorous evaluation, six of the women with ongoing pregnancies developed hypertension, one requiring delivery at 25 weeks. There were ten spontaneous abortions, suggesting that donor oocytes cannot completely reverse the biological effects of aging. Ten of the pregnancies were multiple. All patients were delivered by elective Cesarean section.

The remarkable advance in assisted reproduction as a result of donor oocytes provides the opportunity of successful pregnancy to a group of women who could never have imagined parenthood in the past. The small studies reported to date suggest that, with rigorous medical selection, a group of women most likely to benefit and least likely to have serious complications can be selected. Whether or not encouraging conception is wise in menopausal women, particularly considering that half these pregnancies are multiple, is a question for society to address.

Summary

With delays in child-bearing by fertile women and new treatment strategies for infertile women, many more women aged 40 and over are becoming pregnant, many of them for the first time. These women are at increased risk for spontaneous abortion, aneuploidy, pregnancy-associated hypertension, gestational diabetes, Cesarean section, still-birth, low-birth-weight infants and death. Despite these risks, the outcomes of pregnancies in healthy women over age 40 approach the outcomes of younger women, primarily as a result of careful antepartum surveillance and partly as a result of improvements in neonatal care. Preconception counselling and medical screening are recommended. Women aged 45 and older, those with underlying medical problems and those with multiple gestations should seek tertiary obstetric care.

References

1. Schwartz D, Mayaux MJ. Female fecundity as a function of age: Results of artificial insemination in 2193 nulliparous women with azoospermic husbands. Federation CECOS. *N Engl J Med* 1982;306:404–6
2. Virro MR, Shewchuk AB. Pregnancy outcome in 242 conceptions after artificial insemination with donor sperm and effects of maternal age on the prognosis for successful pregnancy. *Am J Obstet Gynecol* 1984;148:518–24
3. Stovall DW, Toma SK, Hammond MG, *et al*. The effect of age on female fecundity. *Obstet Gynecol* 1991;77:33–6
4. Tietze C. Reproductive span and rate of reproduction among Hutterite women. *Fertil Steril* 1957;8: 89–97
5. Hansen JP. Older maternal age and pregnancy outcome: a review of the literature. *Obstet Gynecol Surv* 1986;41:726
6. Wilson RD, Kendrick V, Wittmann BK, *et al*. Spontaneous abortion and pregnancy outcome after normal first-trimester ultrasound examination. *Obstet Gynecol* 1986;67:352
7. Navot D, Bergh PA, Williams MA. Poor oocyte quality rather than implantation failure as a cause of age-related decline in female fertility. *Lancet* 1991;337:1375–7
8. Baird PA, Sadovnick AD, Yee IM. Maternal age and birth defects: a population study. *Lancet* 1991;337: 527–30
9. Dildy GA, Jackson GM, Fowers GK, *et al*. Very advanced maternal age: pregnancy after age 45. *Am J Obstet Gynecol* 1996;175:668–74
10. Posner LB, Chidiac JE, Posner AC. Pregnancy at age 40 and over. *Obstet Gynecol* 1961;17:194–8
11. Koren Z, Zuckerman H, Brzezinski A. Pregnancy and delivery after 40. *Obstet Gynecol* 1963;21:165–9
12. Caspi E, Lifshitz Y. Pregnancy at 40 years of age and over. *Israel J Med Sci* 1979;15:418–21
13. Kajanoja P, Widholm O. Pregnancy and delivery in women aged 40 and over. *Obstet Gynecol* 1978;51: 47–51
14. Horger EO, Smythe AR. Pregnancy in women over forty. *Obstet Gynecol* 1977;49:257–61
15. Kujansuu E, Kiuinen S, Tuimala R. Pregnancy and delivery at the age of forty and over. *Int J Gynaecol Obstet* 1981;19:341–5
16. Prysak M, Lorenz RP, Kisly A. Pregnancy outcome in nulliparous women 35 years and older. *Obstet Gynecol* 1995;85:65–70
17. Edge VL, Laros RK. Pregnancy outcome in nulliparous women aged 35 or older. *Am J Obstet Gynecol* 1993;168:1881–5
18. Bobrowski RA, Bottoms SF. Under appreciated risks of the elderly multipara. *Am J Obstet Gynecol* 1995;172:1764–70
19. Bianco A, Stone J, Lynch L, *et al*. Pregnancy outcome at age 40 and older. *Obstet Gynecol* 1996;87: 917–22
20. Gilbert WM, Nesbitt TS, Danielsen B. Child-bearing beyond age 40: pregnancy outcome in 24 032 cases. *Obstet Gynecol* 1999;93:9–14
21. Antinori S, Versaci C, Panci C, *et al*. Fetal and maternal morbidity and mortality in menopausal women aged 45–63 years. *Hum Reprod* 1995;10: 464–9
22. Sauer MV, Paulson RJ, Lobo RA. Pregnancy in women 50 or more years of age: outcomes of 22 consecutively established pregnancies from oocyte donation. *Fertil Steril* 1995;64:111–15

23. Higdon AL. Pregnancy in the woman over forty. *Am J Obstet Gynecol* 1960;80:38–42

24. Narayan H, Buckett W, McDougall W, *et al.* Pregnancy after 50: profile and pregnancy outcome in a series of elderly multigravidae. *Eur J Obstet Gynecol Reprod Biol* 1992;47:47–51

25. Adashek JA, Peaceman AM, Lopez-Zeno JA, *et al.* Factors contributing to the increased cesarean birth rate in older parturient women. *Am J Obstet Gynecol* 1993;169:936–40

26. Ezra Y, McParland P, Farine D. High delivery intervention rates in nulliparous women over age 35. *Eur J Obstet Gynecol Reprod Biol* 1995;62:203–7

27. Fretts RC, Schmittdiel J, McLean FH, *et al.* Increased maternal age and the risk of fetal death. *N Engl J Med* 1995;333:953–7

28. Fretts RC, Usher RH. Causes of fetal death in women of advanced maternal age. *Obstet Gynecol* 1997;89:40–5

29. Cnattingius S, Forman MR, Berendes HW, *et al.* Delayed childbearing and risk of adverse perinatal outcome: a population based study. *J Am Med Assoc* 1992;268:886–90

30. Cnattingius S, Berendes HW, Forman MR. Do delayed childbearers face increased risks of adverse pregnancy outcome after the first birth? *Obstet Gynecol* 1993;81:512–16

31. Maternal mortality – United States, 1982–1996. *Morbid Mortal Weekly Rep* 1998;47:705–7

32. Berg CJ, Atrash HK, Koonin LM. Pregnancy-related mortality in the United States, 1987–1990. *Obstet Gynecol* 1996;88:161–7

33. Koonin LM, MacKay AP, Berg CJ, Atrash HK, Smith JC. Pregnancy-related mortality surveillance – United States 1987–1990. *Morbid Mortal Weekly Rep* 1997;46(Suppl 4):22

34. Högberg U, Innala E, Sandström A. Maternal mortality in Sweden, 1980–1988. *Obstet Gynecol* 1994;84:240–4

35. Sauer MV, Paulson RJ, Lobo RA. Reversing the natural decline in human fertility. An extended clinical trial of oocyte donation to women of advanced reproductive age. *J Am Med Assoc* 1992;268:1275–9

36. Sauer MV, Paulson RJ, Lobo RA. Pregnancy after 50: application of oocyte donation to women after natural menopause. *Lancet* 1993;341:321–3

4

Pathology of the menopause

Debra S. Heller

Introduction

Menopause is defined as the permanent cessation of menses due to loss of ovarian follicular activity. A woman is considered menopausal when she has not had a menstrual period for a year. The perimenopausal period, when ovarian function declines, generally extends for 2–8 years prior to and 1 year after the last menstrual period. The median age of menopause in the USA is 51 years[1]. At the turn of the 19th century, female life expectancy coincided with the menopause. At the turn of the 20th century, many women live more than a third of their lives, over 30 years, after the menopause[2]. It is predicted that over 50 million women will be postmenopausal after the year 2000[3]. Apart from natural menopause, many women experience surgical menopause. During this period, many changes occur in a woman's body. This chapter reviews pathology associated with the menopause.

Female reproductive tract

Some of the most profound physical changes at menopause occur in the reproductive tract. Estrogen deficiency, aging, previous birth trauma and genetics play roles in the physiological changes and potential disease states of the menopause. In one 2-year study of gynecological admissions[4], 10.04% of the women were postmenopausal. The most common diagnoses were postmenopausal bleeding (32.72%) due either to atrophy or hyperplasia in almost equal proportion, vaginoperineal lacerations with cystorectocele, with or without incontinence (10.9%), cancer (11.21%; of these 25.45% were endometrial or ovarian), benign ovarian cysts (11.21%), uterine prolapse (9.3%), endometrial polyps (9.09%), leiomyomata (3.93%)

and cervical cancer (3.93%). The most common category was uterine pathology (68.78%), followed by ovarian pathology (15.15%), prolapse-related (10.9%), vulvar (2.72%) and vaginal (1.51%).

Vulva

Changes in the vulva are related to age and estrogen deficiency. There is a decrease in the number and coarsening of the texture of the pubic hair, as the hair follicles age. The labia majora decrease in size, with loss of elastic and fatty subcutaneous tissue. Histologically, there is thinning of the epidermis and dermis[5]. Vulvar conditions seen with increasing frequency in this age group include the non-neoplastic epithelial disorders lichen sclerosus and squamous cell hyperplasia. Paget's disease of the vulva and squamous cell carcinoma are also more common in postmenopausal women. Any suspicious lesion of the vulva must be biopsied.

The non-neoplastic epithelial disorders of the vulva, according to the International Society for the Study of Vulvovaginal Disease (ISSVD), comprise lichen sclerosus, squamous cell hyperplasia and other. These conditions often present with pruritus. Lichen sclerosus leads to gross thinning and whitening of the vulva, with narrowing of the introitus. Histologically, there is loss of rete pegs, thinning of the epithelium and a zone of dermal homogenization with variable chronic inflammation (Figure 1). Squamous hyperplasia may be secondary to an uninterrupted itch–scratch cycle. Histologically, there is hyperkeratosis, acanthosis and chronic inflammation (Figure 2). Both conditions are often treated with topical steroids.

Paget's disease of the vulva is most often an *in situ* lesion. It may be associated with underlying adenocarcinoma in the vulva, as well as extra-genital carcinomas, and these should be searched for. Grossly, the vulva appears red and velvety, with white patches. Histologically, the large Paget cells can be seen at the dermal-epidermal junction, percolating up (Figure 3). Excision is the treatment of choice; however, the lesion tends to recur, possibly because of the microscopic margins often extending beyond the grossly visible ones.

The most common malignancy of the vulva is squamous cell carcinoma (Figure 4). While the incidence is increasing in the premenopausal age group in association with human papillomavirus, the majority of cases are still seen in elderly women. Recent advances in surgical therapy, with separate vulvar and groin incisions, has led to decreased postoperative morbidity in these women.

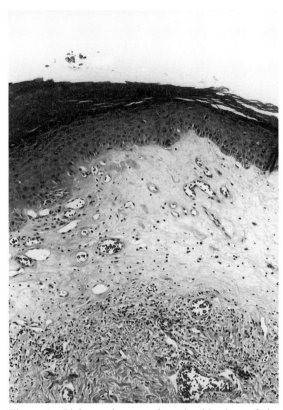

Figure 1 Lichen sclerosus: there is thinning of the epithelium, with dermal edema and homogenization; hyperkeratosis and dermal inflammation are variable

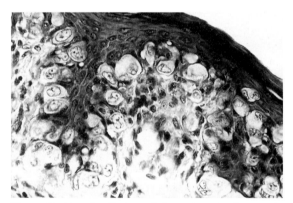

Figure 3 Paget's disease of the vulva: the large pale Paget cells are seen at the dermal-epidermal junction, and percolating up the epithelium

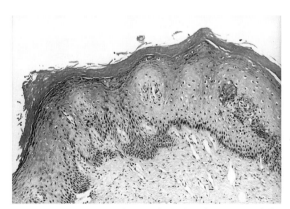

Figure 2 Squamous hyperplasia is characterized by hyperkeratosis, acanthosis (widening and fusing of the rete pegs) and chronic inflammation

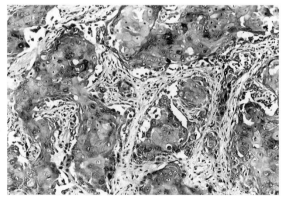

Figure 4 Squamous cell carcinoma of the vulva: this keratinizing tumor infiltrates in characteristic nests

Vagina

With estrogen deficiency the vagina shortens, with loss of rugae, and becomes pale and friable. There is loss of elasticity. Atrophy of the Bartholin's glands contributes to decreased lubrication. Dyspareunia may be a problem. Histologically, loss of glycogen and flattening of the epithelium can be noted. The loss of glycogen leads to decreased Doderlein bacilli with their production of lactic acid. This leads to an alkaline pH, which predisposes to atrophic vaginitis (Figure 5)[5]. Overgrowth of enteric bacteria at this pH predisposes also to urinary tract infections[6]. Although no longer much utilized in clinical practice, with sensitive blood tests available, some indication of estrogen deficiency in the region can be obtained by determining a maturation index. Vaginal symptoms do not necessarily correlate with the index. A swab taken from the lateral vaginal wall is examined in the cytology laboratory, and the maturation of the cells is evaluated. There are three types of squamous cells potentially present in the vagina: superficial cells, intermediate cells and parabasal cells. In cycling women, the superficial and intermediate cells predominate. With estrogen deficiency, there is a shift towards intermediate and parabasal cells. The index is reported as the proportions of 100 cells counted in terms of parabasal : intermediate : superficial. Smears of cycling women will have superficial and intermediate cells in varying proportions, while postmenopausal smears are more likely to contain intermediate and parabasal cells (Figure 6). It should be noted that the ratios are variable for all age groups, and cannot be relied upon in the face of inflammation.

Loss of pelvic fascial support is multifactorial, and relates to estrogen, genetics, parity, birth trauma and conditions of excess intra-abdominal pressure such as obesity, chronic obstructive pulmonary disease and constipation. In addition, skeletal muscle is replaced by fat and connective tissue during the aging process, contributing to the loss of pelvic support[5]. Women may experience cystoceles, rectoceles, enteroceles and uterine prolapse. Stress incontinence may accompany these changes. Estrogen therapy may be utilized to prepare the vaginal mucosa for reparative surgery.

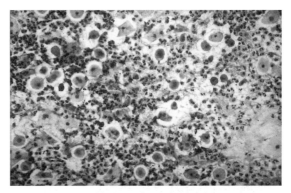

Figure 5 Atrophic vaginitis on Pap smear, characterized by inflammation and a predominance of parabasal cells

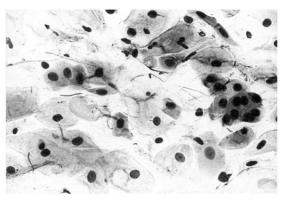

Figure 6 A menopausal Pap smear composed of intermediate cells and smaller parabasal cells

Primary vaginal squamous cell carcinoma does occur in postmenopausal women; however, a primary vulvar or cervical carcinoma with vaginal spread must be considered first.

Cervix

With menopause the cervix decreases in size, with decreased stroma and epithelial atrophy, and may become flush with the vaginal vault[5]. The squamocolumnar junction (Figure 7) tends to move upwards, making colposcopic evaluation for neoplastic and preneoplastic disease more difficult. Cervical stenosis may occur, and may lead to pyometra or hematometra. The cervix may show erosion: the loss of superficial epithelial layers, or true ulceration with loss of epithelium and formation of granulation tissue. Cervical ectropion, the presence of endocervix on the portio, may be seen secondary to bilateral lacerations at childbirth[5].

Many squamous cell carcinomas that occur in the cervix are seen in postmenopausal women. Many women with cervical cancer have not received a Pap smear for several years prior to diagnosis. It is critical for postmenopausal women to continue to receive gynecological care. Although grading of cervical carcinoma is performed, the prognosis relates better to the stage of the lesion. Grossly, squamous cell carcinoma of the cervix may be exophytic or endophytic. Histological appearance is similar to squamous cell carcinomas arising elsewhere (see Figure 4). Adenocarcinomas of the endocervix may also be seen in perimenopausal women.

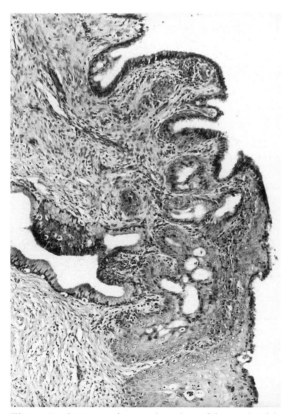

Figure 7 Squamocolumnar junction of the cervix: this migrates upwards as a woman ages; the interface between the two types of epithelium often shows squamous metaplasia

Endometrium

In one study of 801 perimenopausal and postmenopausal women[7] screened prior to estrogen replacement therapy, there was one carcinoma (0.13%), four atypias (total 0.63%), 373 cases of atrophic endometrium (46.9%), 133 proliferative endometria (16.7%), 54 secretory endometria (6.8%), 41 hyperplasias (5.2%) and 195 specimens of tissue insufficient for diagnosis (24.5%). The sampling instrument was not described. These authors concluded that screening biopsy of asymptomatic women was not justifiable. In another study[8], 68% of endometrial samples prior to hormone replacement therapy were atrophic, 23.5% proliferative, 0.5% secretory, 0.6% hyperplastic, 0.07% carcinoma and 6.6% insufficient tissue. Biopsies were performed with a Vabra aspirator. Forty-six cases (1.6%) had polyps, which may be missed by in-office sampling. The authors felt that the low cancer yield reflected the younger patients in this group: most were 45–55 years. They also concluded that a biopsy was not necessary in asymptomatic women prior to instituting hormone replacement therapy.

In the untreated menopausal woman, the endometrium is often thin and inactive. It is easily inflamed, and this may lead to bleeding. All postmenopausal bleeding must be investigated to rule out carcinoma; however, in many cases the bleeding is due to atrophy. In a literature review[4], the most common pathological diagnoses on endometrial sampling performed for postmenopausal bleeding were carcinoma, polyp, pyometra, atrophy, proliferative endometrium, secretory endometrium, hyperplasia and insufficient tissue.

A large number of postmenopausal women will be treated with tamoxifen for breast cancer. Tamoxifen, while utilized for its antiestrogenic activity in the breast, exerts a weak estrogenic effect on the postmenopausal uterus. Endometrial polyps, hyperplasias, carcinomas and other conditions associated with estrogen may be seen in the uterus. The literature has been somewhat controversial as to whether tamoxifen-associated uterine malignancies are of low- or high-risk types. Screening for uterine disease in women taking tamoxifen has included transvaginal ultrasound and biopsy. Many women are currently followed with ultrasound, with biopsy reserved for bleeding[9].

Endometrial sampling performed in-office often produces a scant specimen in postmenopausal women (Figure 8). While the majority of these cases are due to atrophy, it is up to the clinician to determine whether scant tissue in the sample signifies scant tissue in the uterus or insufficient sampling. A normal variant of atrophy, cystic atrophy, can be distinguished from simple hyperplasia by the flattened epithelium of the glands in the former.

Endometrial polyps often occur in the perimenopausal and postmenopausal woman. Endometrial polyps are lined by a surface lining, are polypoid in shape and contain irregular glands in a fibrotic stroma. The stalk contains thick blood vessels (Figure 9). Polyps may be fragmented during removal, and difficult to diagnose histologically with certainty. The polyps seen in association with tamoxifen tend to be large, multiple and with a very fibrotic stroma, although this is not pathognomonic.

Owing to the unopposed estrogen associated with anovulation in the perimenopausal period, endometrial hyperstimulation can occur. Some postmenopausal women also have excess endogenous estrogen, particularly if obese, or in the case of an estrogen-secreting ovarian neoplasm. The endometrium may initially show disordered proliferation, with occasional cystic glands in a proliferative background, insufficient for a diagnosis of hyperplasia. Endometrial hyperplasia is classified by architecture and the presence or absence of cytological atypia. Simple hyperplasia (Figure 10) consists of a mild increase in the gland/stroma ratio, while complex hyperplasia shows greater crowding, still with intervening stroma (Figure 11). Either may occur with or without cytological atypia (Figure 12). Simple hyperplasia with atypia is unusual; as a result, many pathologists shorten the diagnoses to simple, complex or atypical (complex with atypia) hyperplasia. It has been shown[10] that only complex hyperplasia with atypia poses a significant risk of development of endometrial carcinoma. A concurrent unsampled carcinoma may also be present when an endometrial biopsy shows atypical hyperplasia.

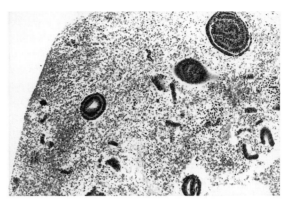

Figure 8 Atrophic endometrium: this biopsy specimen consists of rare detached glandular fragments; while the majority of cases with this appearance can be attributed to atrophy in a postmenopausal woman, it is up to the clinician to determine adequacy of sampling

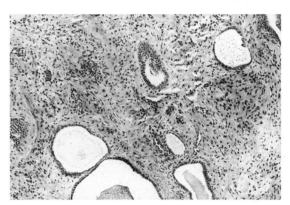

Figure 9 Endometrial polyp: this field from an endometrial polyp shows the irregular glands in a dense stroma

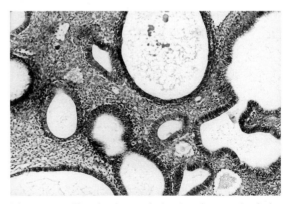

Figure 10 Simple hyperplasia is characterized by dilated glands lined by a proliferative-type epithelium (pseudostratified and mitotically active); there is only a mild increase in the gland/stroma ratio

Endometrial carcinoma may actually arise by two pathogenic disease mechanisms. Estrogen-related neoplasms tend to be well differentiated, less aggressive endometrioid carcinomas (Figure 13), occurring in younger, heavier women, as opposed to the more aggressive non-estrogen-related neoplasms, uterine papillary serous (Figure 14) and clear-cell carcinoma, which are more likely to occur in the older, thinner patient. Malignant mixed mesodermal tumors (Figure 15) also tend to occur in the older postmenopausal patient. For the usual endometrioid endometrial carcinoma confined to the uterus, prognosis relates to tumor grade and depth of invasion, and the pathologist may be called upon to perform an intraoperative

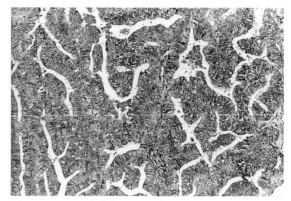

Figure 13 Well-differentiated (FIGO grade 1) endometrial adenocarcinoma, showing back-to-back glands with no intervening stroma

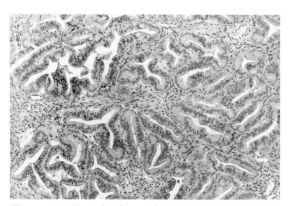

Figure 11 Complex hyperplasia is characterized by a marked increase in the gland/stroma ratio; however, some stroma persists

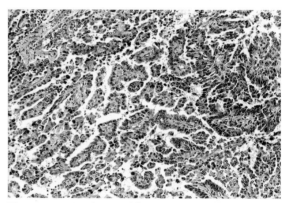

Figure 14 Uterine papillary serous carcinoma: note the papillary configuration and marked cytological atypia

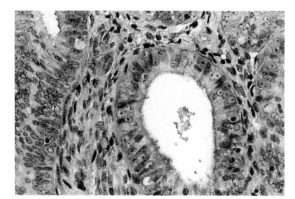

Figure 12 Cytological atypia of endometrial glandular epithelium: the nuclei are larger, rounder, with marginated chromatin, and often prominent nucleoli; the normal oval shape of non-atypical nuclei is also present at the left

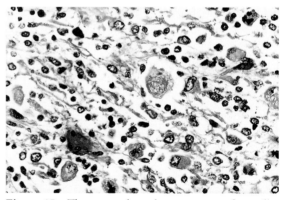

Figure 15 The mesenchymal component of a malignant mixed mesodermal (Müllerian) tumor. Adjacent tumor showed a carcinomatous configuration, not shown. This tumor was heterologous, with rhabdomyosarcomatous differentiation: note the large primitive rhabdomyoblasts

consultation to determine the need for lymph node sampling.

Endometrial biopsies from women experiencing abnormal bleeding while on hormone replacement therapy are often received by the pathology laboratory. Many times, a history of hormonal therapy is not given, and is important for accurate evaluation. Patterns seen reflect the therapy effect as well as the underlying hormonal milieu of the woman. Atrophic, and normal proliferative and secretory patterns are sometimes seen, as are the occasional hyperplasia or carcinoma. Sometimes an irregular pattern of mixed proliferative and secretory changes is seen (Figure 16). If the history is known to the pathologist, the diagnosis can state that the irregular pattern is consistent with hormone replacement therapy. On occasion, these mixed patterns do show worrisome glandular crowding, suggestive of an excess estrogen effect.

Myometrium

The myometrium is also an estrogen target tissue. The size of the uterus decreases with the menopause, bringing the corpus/cervix ratio from 2 : 1 to 1 : 1. Uterine weight decreases from an average of 100 g down to 50-60 g, and may be as low as 25-30 g. Uterine fibroids decrease in size, and may show hyalinization and calcification[5]. Uterine vessels often show atherosclerotic changes.

Fallopian tube

The Fallopian tubes are estrogen target tissues. There is atrophy of epithelium and muscle, with a decrease in tubal length and diameter[5]. It has been shown[11] that Fallopian tube epithelial atrophy mimics endometrial changes in the postmenopausal woman not on hormone replacement therapy.

Ovary

During the fifth month of fetal life, there are approximately 6-7 million oogonia present, with 1-2 million germ cells at birth, and 300 000 at puberty. By 3 years after the menopause, there is virtual depletion of germ cells[12]. The menopausal

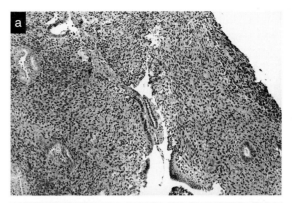
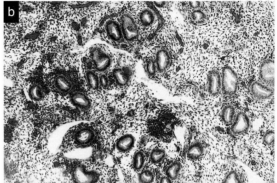
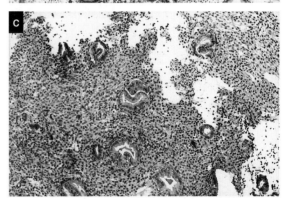

Figure 16 Examples (a, b and c) of endometrial biopsies from women taking hormone replacement therapy showing irregular mixed proliferative and secretory features

ovary decreases in size. The stroma becomes fibrotic, the surface cerebriform. There is depletion of primordial follicles, and the ovary is peppered with corpora albicans (Figure 17). Stromal hyperthecosis, a hyperplastic change consisting of nests of luteinized stromal cells, may occasionally occur in the postmenopausal woman (Figure 18). These ovaries appear enlarged and yellow on cut section, and masculinization of the patient due to hyperandrogenism may lead the clinician to suspect a masculinizing neoplasm.

The risk of ovarian cancer increases with age. Unfortunately, the majority of ovarian carcinomas are diagnosed at an advanced stage, owing to lack of early symptomatology. No efficient mass screening method yet exists. In one study[13], screening was performed initially by transvaginal ultrasound, followed by CA-125, pelvic examination and exploratory laparotomy after two abnormal transvaginal ultrasonic studies. A few early cancers were detected. However, widespread screening for ovarian carcinoma has not been shown to be cost-effective.

Ovarian neoplasms are divided into those of surface epithelial origin, those of stromal origin and those of germ cell origin. Germ cell tumors are usually seen in younger patients, and are not further considered here. Among epithelial neoplasms, the most common are benign serous cystadenomas and cystadenofibromas (Figure 19). The most common type of ovarian carcinoma seen is the papillary serous cystadenocarcinoma, which is histologically similar to uterine papillary serous carcinoma (see Figure 14). Endometrioid carcinoma of the ovary, which resembles endometrial carcinoma histologically (see Figure 13), is almost as common. Stromal tumors of the ovary occurring commonly in the postmenopausal woman

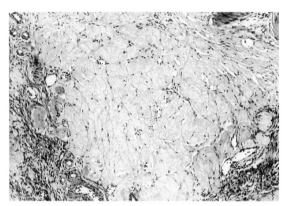

Figure 17 Corpus albicans of the ovary: the shape of a corpus luteum is maintained, as this scar shrinks

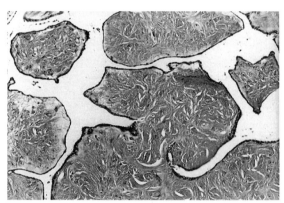

Figure 19 Papillary serous cystadenofibroma of the ovary: the broad papillae are covered by a benign single layer of epithelium that may be flattened, or resemble Fallopian tube epithelium; serous cystadenomas lack the papillae, but have a similar lining

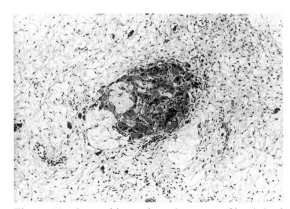

Figure 18 Stromal hyperthecosis: a nest of luteinized stromal cells is seen in the ovarian cortex

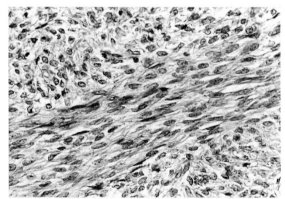

Figure 20 Fibrothecoma of the ovary, composed of uniform spindle cells

include the benign fibrothecoma (Figure 20) and the granulosa cell tumor (Figure 21), which is a slow-growing but malignant neoplasm. Both may produce estrogen, which can lead to endometrial hyperstimulation and subsequent pathology.

Genitourinary system (bladder/urethra)

Urogenital mucosal atrophic changes are due to a combination of age and estrogen deficiency. The proximal urethra, lined by squamous epithelium, undergoes atrophy with estrogen deficiency. Urethral caruncles, ectropion of the mucosa, may occur (Figure 22). The trigone also has estrogen receptors. The risk of urinary outflow obstruction increases with age, because of possible narrowing of the distal urethra. Thus, menopausal women are at increased risk of atrophic trigonitis and the urethral syndrome, with urgency, burning, hesitancy, frequency and nocturia. Stress and urge incontinence can occur. Urinary symptoms may relate to a combination of atrophy, prolapse, susceptibility to infection, decreased bladder capacity, increased intra-abdominal pressure, genetics and superimposed conditions such as congestive heart failure, diabetes and neurological impairment[5,6].

Bone

Approximately 1.5 million fractures per year are attributable to osteoporosis (Figure 23) in the USA. With osteoporosis comes increased risk of vertebral, wrist and hip fractures. Two-thirds of

these patients are women[14]. Bone loss starts at around age 30 years[15] and accelerates after the menopause. There is a ten-fold increase in bone loss for about 10 years after loss of ovarian function. The rate of Colles' fractures increases ten-fold from age 35 to 60. Hip fractures are the 12th leading cause of female death[16], with up to 20% of hip fracture patients dying within a year of the injury[14]. Biochemical markers of bone turnover are increased with menopause[1]. The risk of osteoporosis increases owing to a variety of factors at the

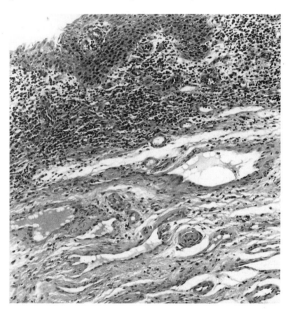

Figure 22 Urethral caruncle: there is chronic inflammation present, and the transitional epithelial lining can be seen at the top of the figure

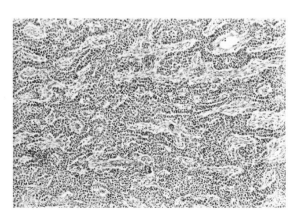

Figure 21 Granulosa cell tumor of the ovary, showing a trabecular configuration

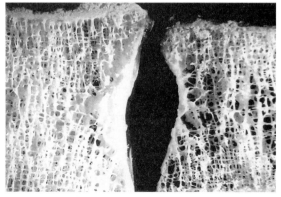

Figure 23 Osteoporosis: note the normal bone on the left, and the decreased bone density of the osteoporotic bone on the right. Photo courtesy of Michael Klein, MD

menopause, some related to estrogen deficiency, some to aging. These include low calcium intake, early menopause, family history, increasing age, lack of exercise, nulliparity, cigarettes and alcohol, thinness and small bones, and White or Asian race[17].

Cardiovascular system

The issue of estrogen's protective effect on the cardiovascular system is complex. Cardiovascular risk after the menopause is associated with less favorable lipid and coagulation profiles, changes in vascular reactivity and other tissue effects[18]. Hormone replacement therapy has been shown to modify cardiac risk[18]. Although many women fear death by cancer the most, the fact is that cardiovascular disease is the leading cause of death in women (Figure 24). Heart disease deaths in women are ten times as frequent as breast cancer deaths[16]. Heart disease accounts for over 50% of postmeno-

pausal deaths, and morbidity and mortality are greater in women[3]. Some evidence suggests that the risk of heart disease is even greater with surgical than with natural menopause[16]. This may be due to the longer hypoestrogenic state. Estrogen replacement therapy may reduce cardiac mortality by as much as 50%[18].

Central nervous system

Studies suggest that estrogen replacement therapy may improve cognition in Alzheimer's disease, and decrease the risk for the disease[19]. The incidence of Alzheimer's disease was reported to be decreased 50% in postmenopausal women on hormone replacement therapy (HRT)[18]. It has been suggested that estrogen may work by improving blood flow and stimulating neurons, and may interact with genetic factors[20]. Alzheimer's disease is characterized histologically by neuritic plaques with deposition of β-amyloid in the plaques and cerebral blood vessels, and the development of neurofibrillary tangles (Figure 25). There are pronounced neurochemical deficits[20].

Skin

Collagen synthesis and maturation are stimulated by estrogen[1]. In one study[21], postmenopausal women taking HRT were shown to have increased skin thickness and sebum production, compared to a group not taking HRT. Pierard and colleagues[22] have also suggested that HRT has

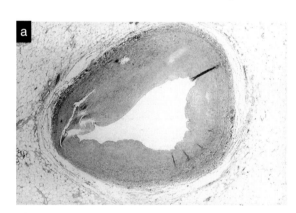

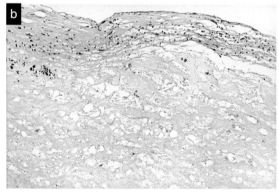

Figure 24 Atherosclerosis: a coronary artery branch shows luminal narrowing (a); an atherosclerotic plaque, showing cholesterol crystals (b)

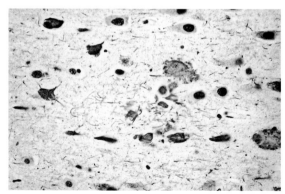

Figure 25 Alzheimer's disease: this section of brain tissue shows the characteristic neurofibrillary tangles (Bodian stain). Photo courtesy of Eun-Sook Cho, MD

beneficial effects on some mechanical properties of skin and may slow intrinsic cutaneous aging.

Breast

There is a decrease in the size of the glands and subcutaneous fat of the breast, as well as a loss of elasticity of Cooper's ligament[5,23] leading to a change of shape, with flattening. Nipples become smaller and flatter, and lose their erectile properties. The risk of breast cancer increases, with most cases occurring after the menopause[24] (Figure 26). There is an 8% overall lifetime risk of breast cancer, which increases with age. There is still debate in the literature regarding the potential risk of estrogen therapy to the breast.

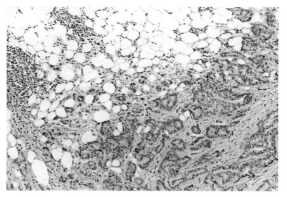

Figure 26 Infiltrating duct carcinoma of the breast

References

1. Greendale GA, Sowers M. The menopause transition. *Endocrinol Metab Clin North Am* 1997;26: 261–77
2. Wich BK, Carnes M. Menopause and the aging female reproductive system [Review]. *Endocrinol Metab Clin North Am* 1995;24:273–95
3. Villablanca A. Coronary heart disease in women. Gender differences and effects of menopause [Review]. *Postgrad Med* 1996;100:191–6
4. Pepe F, Panella M, Pepe G, *et al.* Current aspects of gynecological pathology in postmenopause. *Clin Exp Obstet Gynecol* 1988;15:80–3
5. Brown KH, Hammond CB. Urogenital atrophy. *Obstet Gynecol Clin North Am* 1987;14:13–32
6. Schaffe J, Fantl JA. Urogenital effects of the menopause. *Baillière's Clin Obstet Gynaecol* 1996;10: 401–17
7. Archer DF, McIntyre-Seltman K, Wilborn WW Jr, *et al.* Endometrial morphology in asymptomatic postmenopausal women. *Am J Obstet Gynecol* 1991; 165:317–20
8. Korhonen MO, Symons JP, Hyde BM, *et al.* Histologic classification and pathologic findings for endometrial biopsy specimens obtained from 2964 perimenopausal and postmenopausal women undergoing screening for continuous hormones as replacement therapy. *Am J Obstet Gynecol* 1997;176: 377–80
9. Barakat RR. Tamoxifen and the endometrium. *Cancer Treat Res* 1998;94:195–207

10. Kurman RJ, Kaminski PF, Norris HJ. The behavior of endometrial hyperplasia. A long-term study of 'untreated' hyperplasia in 170 patients. *Cancer* 1985;56:403–12
11. Amso NN, Crow J, Lewin J, *et al.* A comparative morphological and ultrastructural study of endometrial gland and fallopian tube epithelia at different stages of the menstrual cycle and menopause. *Hum Reprod* 1994;9:2234–41
12. Richardson SJ. The biological history of menopause. *Baillière's Clin Endocrinol Metab* 1993;7:1–16
13. DePriest PD, van Nagell JR Jr, Gallion HH, *et al.* Ovarian cancer screening in asymptomatic postmenopausal women. *Gynecol Oncol* 1993;51:205–9
14. Agarwal SK, Judd HL. Menopause. *Curr Ther Endocrinol Metab* 1997;6:624–31
15. Heersche JN, Bellows CG, Ishida Y. The decrease in bone mass associated with aging and menopause [Review]. *J Prosth Dent* 1998;79:14–16
16. Smith RP. Modern menopause management. *Curr Opin Obstet Gynecol* 1994;6:495–8
17. Kain CD, Reilly N, Schultz ED. The older adult. A comparative assessment. *Nurs Clin North Am* 1990; 25:833–48
18. Prelevic GM, Jacobs HS. Menopause and postmenopause. *Baillière's Clin Endocrinol Metab* 1997; 11:311–40
19. Henderson VW. Estrogen, cognition, and a woman's risk of Alzheimer's disease [Review]. *Am J Med* 1997;103:11s–18s

20. van Duijn CM. Menopause and the brain. *J Psychosom Obstet Gynecol* 1997;18:121–5

21. Callens A, Vaillant L, LeCompte P, *et al.* Does hormonal skin aging exist? A study of the influence of different hormone therapy regimens on the skin of postmenopausal women using non-invasive measurement techniques. *Dermatology* 1996;193: 289–94

22. Pierard GE, Letawe C, Dowlati A, *et al.* Effects of hormonal replacement therapy for menopause on the mechanical properties of skin. *J Am Geriatr Soc* 1995;43:662–5

23. Utian WH. The fate of the untreated menopause. *Obstet Gynecol Clin North Am* 1987;14:1–11

24. Wren BG. The breast and the menopause. *Baillière's Clin Obstet Gynaecol* 1996;10:433–47

5

Women's sexual capacities at mid-life

Stephen B. Levine

Introduction

It is difficult to face certain unpleasant aspects of aging. The ultimate difficulty is, of course, death. When reminded of it, we grudgingly acknowledge our ultimate fate, but most of the time we ignore it. The normative processes of aging provide another more humorous motive for denial. When we are young, we designate a portion of the population as 'elderly', and separate ourselves from them. We are less inclined to consider the physiological declines that precede these advanced years until they begin to occur in us. Middle-aged people begin to notice many of the signs of aging: decrements in motor capacity, visual acuity, learning capacity, proper noun retrieval, skin turgor and hair. Despite our assiduous exercise and nutrition programs, we continue to be transformed.

The central hypothesis

This chapter focuses on an unpleasant aspect of the life cycle that our culture has not addressed: the decline of female sexual capacity. The perimenopausal and early menopausal years are marked by a subtle shift in this private sphere of experience for many women. Our medical avoidance of this decline has been so extensive that, as scientists, we still cannot be certain that decline is an absolutely predictable development of the middle years of women's life. The assumption of this chapter is, however, that women's sexual capacity declines during mid-life. This assumption is a hypothesis that awaits further verification. In the meantime, physicians might profit from keeping the hypothesis in mind.

The sexual stages of life

Sex educators like to promulgate the idea that sexuality is an inherent characteristic of humans throughout life. They point to ultrasound evidence of fetal penile erection, and discuss romance and sex among elderly nursing-home residents. This is true enough, but they often fail to emphasize that there are sexual eras during the life cycle. Each of these stages has different biological, social and psychological characteristics and potentials[1]. The stages are:

(1) Childhood: infancy to puberty;

(2) Adolescence: puberty to young adulthood;

(3) Young adulthood: approximately age 20 to mid-forties;

(4) Middle-age: mid-forties to mid-sixties;

(5) Early elderly: mid-sixties to approximately age 80 years;

(6) Advanced elderly: 80 and beyond;

(7) Illness: any time.

Most of what the culture, particularly the commercial, media-making culture, articulates about sexuality is actually only about young adult sexuality. Young adulthood is the era of sexiness, reproduction, orgasmic ecstasy, falling in love, breaking up and new, intensely sexual partnerships, all on a foundation of physical health. This is the era against which all sexuality is measured. For instance, the sexual awakenings of childhood and adolescence, the attempts of the elderly to stave off biological decline and the use of hormone replacement therapy (HRT) to prevent women's sexual involution, each involves a comparison to young adulthood.

Sex and the advanced elderly

Gynecologists are well aware of the anatomical and physiological findings in women over 80 years of age. These include the thin, shortened, dry vagina with a less acid pH, the involuted vulva and uterus, the lax pelvis with various degrees of prolapse, complaints of urge and stress incontinence, atrophied breasts, wrinkled skin, osteopenic skeleton and general frailty. Physicians are much less aware of the sexual implications of these observations in terms of healthy elderly women's drive, motivation to engage in partner sex and masturbation, ease of arousal, orgasmic attainment, and ability to find genital sexual behavior emotionally enhancing. It is difficult to imagine that these women are regularly and intensely sexually active. However, this may be the case, particularly for the exceptionally healthy who, in some survey studies (low response rates), seem to have continued activity[2].

It is a reasonable assumption that, at this phase of life, healthy women's sexual capacity has become a shadow of what it used to be. Many are, for all practical purposes, asexual: no drive, no arousal, no orgasm, no masturbation and no partner activity. They have memory, however, and can evoke it readily by genital self-soothing. They have the capacity pleasantly to give and receive affection, even if their sexual arousal systems have deteriorated. They are like most old elderly men, except that elderly men continue to represent themselves as interested in sexual behavior long after their sexual drive and erectile capacities have vanished[3]. Elderly femininity has little of the ceaseless sexual aspirations of masculinity.

Sex and the early elderly

It is reasonable to assume that even many healthy women over age 65 have limited sexual expression. There is more documentation about this than for the advanced elderly[4,5]. For one thing, women of this age group suffer from unavailability of healthy partners. Even if they have partners, their men are at high risk for erectile dysfunction. These early elderly women rarely raise sexual matters with their gynecologists. Now that there is sildenafil, however, men in this age group sometimes seek sexual rehabilitation[6]. This has implications for their postmenopausal partners, who are now subject to dyspareunia, recurrent urinary tract infection and the need to participate in sexual intercourse long after they had expected to be free of genital intimacies[7].

Youthful male sensibilities

Young physicians of either sex are often shocked to discover that some of their patients, who are two generations older than they are, behave sexually. Young adults generally have a difficult time realizing that the elderly have any sexual expression; they have trouble perceiving women over age 50 as sexually appealing. As women head towards their menopause, they often become more sensitive to the sexual power of younger women, in part because they have already learned about men's taste for younger women. Even men of advanced age see their age mates as relatively sexually uninteresting and typically turn to younger women when they think about sex. The 60-year-old woman, for instance, is more sexually alluring to the 75-year-old than to her male age mates. Both the inability to conceptualize aging women as sexually appealing and men's preference for younger women affect women's adaptation as they age.

The problem of discussing sexual matters explicitly

It is not an easy matter for women, particularly elderly women, to discuss their sexual concerns with their physicians. Not only do many women lack the vocabulary to discuss their sexual function and anatomy clearly, but there is a general fear of being thought of as unladylike if sexual concerns are the focus of the visit to the doctor[8]. The topic is made more difficult for women if the doctor is uncomfortable.

The causes of sexual symptoms

The causes of sexual symptoms of the elderly are immediately clinically focused on biological sources. In this way, the matter appears to be simple. In contrast, the causes of sexual problems in physically healthy young adults are often difficult to understand. If a 30-year-old woman complains to a physician about low sexual desire and less frequent orgasms, the doctor has to be prepared to consider a differential diagnosis that includes physical diseases, ordinary normative physiological variations, personal conflicts about sexual expression, interpersonal dilemmas and cultural factors. In psychiatry, we say that symptoms are multifactorial in origin, meaning we are not certain about their exact cause. If the woman is in her late forties or is already menopausal, we add a new, decidedly biogenic consideration to the search for the causes of her symptoms: changed hormonal milieu. We have to ask ourselves whether her symptoms are the early signs of a genetically programmed dismantling of her sexual physiology that will eventually culminate in a relatively asexual state in her elderly years. This is unless, of course, that we assume that women retain their sexual capacities throughout the life cycle except if they are afflicted with a serious physical or mental illness. There is no reason to think that perimenopausal symptoms in any given woman are either purely psychogenic or purely biogenic[9].

Menopause

Over one million American women become menopausal annually[10]. The USA now contains between 30 and 40 million menopausal women. The average woman can expect to live one-third of her life in menopause. At age 50, many women have already noticed that something is different about themselves sexually.

The time-honored explanation of menopause is estrogen deficiency. Many physiological consequences of this predictable loss of estrogen are well described. The multiple sexual effects on the reproductive tract and on other organ systems are far less well known, however. This is because the topic has not been well studied (medicine studies sexual topics quite haltingly; funding for research is very difficult to obtain). Menopause is not simply estrogen deficiency; its changes are difficult to separate from the inexorable aging process[11], and estrogens are not the only steroid whose production patterns

evolve. It does not seem reasonable to promulgate the idea that all of the menopause-related sexuality changes are reversible with HRT[12]. Estrogen alone, or combinations of estrogen with progesterone or with androgen, may assist some dimensions of the sexual decline. There is, however, a possibility that HRT may worsen some menopausal sexual problems[13].

The missing medical information

Consider these components of sexual function: desire, vaginal lubrication, skin-stimulated arousal, mucosa-stimulated arousal, orgasmic attainment, sense of attractiveness and emotional satisfaction from sexual behavior. Each component may independently improve, worsen or remain unchanged as a woman progresses into the perimenopause and postmenopausal years. At any given assessment point, her sexual function is the profile of these components. Medicine lacks firm, epidemiological prospective data on the percentages of women at particular ages who are in each category. For instance, how many 45- versus 50- versus 55-year-olds with intact pelvic anatomy are improved, worse or the same? Ultimately, we want to know the mechanisms of these changes.

The sexual changes: what seems to be known

Some studies have suggested that up to 50% of women[14] notice the following changes as they enter naturally into the menopause[15]. The following list summarizes what patients are overheard discussing:

(1) Slowness of vaginal lubrication;

(2) Diminished volume of vaginal lubrication, occasionally to the point of painful intercourse for the woman or man;

(3) Less erotic response to vulvar, clitoral, breast and nipple stimulation;

(4) More difficulty focusing on the tactile sensations that previously efficiently created a state of sexual arousal: an increasing preference for intercourse without extensive foreplay;

(5) Diminished drive or an increased freedom from the feeling that sex with a partner or masturbation is necessary to restore comfort;

(6) Fewer sexual fantasies and preoccupations.

McCoy has summarized much of the emerging data from cross-sectional, retrospective and longitudinal studies from nine countries[16]. Ten of 11 studies have found a decrement in sexual interest (also called desire, frequency of thoughts and fantasies, motivation). Eight of eight studies found a decrement in the frequency of intercourse. Three of four placebo-controlled studies found a decrement in orgasmic attainment frequency. One longitudinal study found less satisfaction with sex because of their decreased partner interest in them[17].

All research in this area is limited by methodological problems. Nonetheless, these data and clinical impressions point towards biological-based sexual changes of the perimenopausal and early menopausal years. Most are present well *before* the last menstrual period[18]. It is important to emphasize the *biological* basis of these changes, because women themselves tend to explain the earliest manifestations as being because of social or psychological factors. Psychological factors come into play, as they always do, and add to the variability of sexual experience from woman to woman.

These biological changes can be thought of as a loss of sexual efficiency. Orgasmic capacity remains the least affected during the early postmenopausal years, but even some of its physiological characteristics may change. The sensations of genital stimulation by hand, mouth, penis or vibrator may be noticeably different or more difficult to attain, and this may be the source of a lower rate of orgasmic attainment. The loss of sexual efficiency is not a topic, however, that women and their doctors are generally at ease discussing. The sexual losses of women add to their sense that they are getting old. 'Getting old' is often communicated as feeling different in their bodies, noticing changing body contours, a diminished sense of sexual attractiveness and confidence, and becoming invisible to the roving eyes of men[19]. If we speak of women's sense of 'loss', we then should expect that those with a previously good sex life may mourn for their lost capacity. Mourning is always more difficult if the loss cannot be personally acknowledged or recognized by others.

Could these changes have an even higher prevalence?

Not all women mourn their perimenopausal sexual losses. There are numerous matters to consider in understanding this:

(1) Biologically based changes are always variable in their expression, both as to when and to what degree they occur. Some women may have them later or not at all.

(2) Women are reticent to discuss the topic with physicians.

(3) This topic has not been extensively researched. The research that has been done is not widely known by physicians. When studies of HRT and menopausal symptoms are carried out, the usual sexual dimensions that are assessed are vaginal dryness and libido[20]. This limits our awareness of the dimensions of the experience.

(4) Some women may be frightened about admitting the loss of their sexual capacities because of its implications for relationships with partners. Single women looking to participate in a new, lasting relationship might be loathe to consider this change as being due to anything other than psychosocial concerns.

(5) Many women's sex lives have not survived the developmental challenges posed by earlier life. A combination of never-mastered childhood sexual anxieties, sexual adjustment problems with their partner, and failure to adequately negotiate the non-sexual challenges of couplehood have long before created various forms of sexual avoidance or male-oriented sexual servicing. These women's loss of sexual efficiency may not be noticed, because their sexual experience never attained a high level of satisfaction when they were healthy young adults.

(6) The noticed sexual changes may be of no consequence because the women have other more

compelling life problems – physical illness in the family, behavioral troubles with a child, financial difficulties, etc.

By the perimenopausal years, some women have long given up on the aspiration to have a wonderful sex life. These women find relief in their loss of sexual feelings and capacities, and hide behind the belief that 'I'm too old for that now'.

Endocrine physiology

Three types of menopause are recognized[21]:

(1) Natural;

(2) Premature: definitions vary between less than 40 and less than 45 years old for this apparently normal occurrence; cigarette smoking may play a role in the genesis of premature menopause[22];

(3) Artificial: induced by surgery, illness, medication or radiation[23].

In natural menopause, the process is gradual and probably begins to occur over a decade before the last menstrual period[24]. Estradiol and progesterone gradually diminish and follicle stimulating hormone (FSH) levels increase. Ovarian granulosa cell production of inhibin, a hormone which limits the production of FSH, slowly diminishes. As a consequence, FSH levels remain high. Levels above 40 IU/l are the accepted standard indication of ovarian failure.

Between the phase of regular menstruation and menopause, ovarian production rates of individual hormones diminish by differing degrees. Estradiol production diminishes by approximately 85% and estrone by approximately 58% (estrone is the weaker estrogen, which menopausal women convert in small amounts to estradiol). Ovarian production rates of the androgens diminish less than those of the estrogens. The androstenedione rates fall by approximately 67% while testosterone production diminishes by only approximately 29%. Progesterone diminishes by 99%[25]. Estrogen levels can be quite variable from woman to woman, because the ovaries may still periodically secrete estrogens in the first few years after the last menses[26].

Many consider the menopause to result not only from a relative ovarian failure but from changes in the pituitary gland. Luteinizing hormone (LH) continues to stimulate the ovarian stroma's production of testosterone, but not as efficiently. Adrenal cortical androgens, such as dehydroepiandrosterone sulfate (DHEAS), which are stimulated by adrenocorticotropic hormone (ACTH), also reach a low point around the menopause. DHEAS is the most abundant androgen in circulation. It declines throughout adulthood until menopause, when it stabilizes.

Sexual anatomical, physiological and behavioral changes

The major underlying consequence of ovarian failure is a decrease in pelvic blood flow. Pubic hair become less numerous and coarser. The labia majora shrink, as do the labia minora and clitoris. Progressively fewer women exhibit expansion and color changes of the labia as they pass into their sixties[27]. The tumescent responses of the clitoris occur in only about 20% of women over age 50. The vagina bears the most significant impact of the menopause. Its changes are more apparent than those of the external genital structures. Its surface flattens, losing its rough, ridged appearance. The surface initially thins to just a few cell layers, making capillaries visible, but with further atrophy the surface becomes smooth, shiny and pale. The depth decreases and the walls lose their elasticity because fibrous connective tissue replaces muscle cells. The biochemical environment becomes less acidic, which creates a shift in vaginal flora. The uterus gradually returns to its prepubertal size. The dramatic decrease in blood flow to the vulva and vaginal areas of approximately 60% and the histological effects of this process explain the slower and less copious vaginal lubrication. Orgasmic contractions of the vagina still occur at age 60, but contraction of the rectum does not seem to occur as it does in menstruating women. Several common symptoms of this phase seem to be related to these changes: dyspareunia, post-intercourse spotting, post-intercourse urinary tract infections, vaginitis and vulvadynia.

Rates of masturbation and of marital sexual behavior decline. Women evidence more sexual disinterest and absence of sex than men of the same age[28]. In studies of the sexual patterns of menopausal women performed in the 1970s, the sexual changes were almost entirely explained by the partners' diminishing interest, ability, health or availability. This conclusion no longer seems tenable[29].

In the late 1970s, Hallström looked carefully at the issue of women's sexual changes with a physically healthy large sample, and demonstrated that first, the climacteric brought reduction in sexual interest, capacity for orgasm and coital frequency, and second, this was not simply a response to men's declining interest[30]. These findings were confirmed in a prospective study[18].

Much of the literature for the lay public minimizes the sexual consequences of the menopause, except to suggest that they are correctable with estrogen and sex counselling[31, 32]. Today, there is a new social phenomenon apparent: the growing belief that the administration of testosterone can completely sexually restore women.

The hormonal fix of menopausal sexual deficits?

There are three typical indications for HRT: stopping hot flushes; delaying osteoporosis; and preventing coronary artery disease. When women bring up their new sexual deficits, physicians may add sexual dysfunction to the list of indications, with some justification[33]. A controlled study has shown that the use of estrogens positively correlates with most parameters of sexual function[34]. Much clinical experience and many studies, however, suggest that estrogens alone do not correct most of the sexual deficits in menopausal women, even though they are helpful for vaginal dryness and to restore a sense of well-being[35]. A failure to increase sexual desire has been found in five studies using conjugated equine estrogens: Premarin®[36]. Estrogen increases the concentration of sex hormone binding globulin, which decreases the amount of bioavailable testosterone. This raises the possibility that estrogen replacement may diminish some women's sexual drive further by limiting testosterone's effect on the limbic system.

The mechanisms by which androgens create sexual drive are a mystery. Women have three sources of androgens: the ovaries, the adrenals and the peripheral conversion of other sex steroids to testosterone in adipose tissue, muscle and skin. Menstruating women generate about 7 mg of testosterone a month from three sources: 25% from the ovaries, 25% from the adrenals and 50% from peripheral conversion[37]. Androgens circulate both bound to carrier proteins and in a free or unbound state. Sexual drive may be a result of androgen effects within the brain as well as many other places in the body. Receptors for sex steroids exist in many tissues including the breast, vagina, skin, vulva, urethra, bladder trigone, uterus, oviducts, blood vessels, pituitary, hypothalamus, limbic forebrain and cortex. While androgens usually decline in the natural menopause, a minority of women may actually have more for several years. They may have differing sources of androgen: more from peripheral conversion, less from the ovarian stroma. When women's menopausal sexual symptoms are treated with testosterone, the amounts given are usually far greater than 7 mg/month. The physiology of drive must be far more refined and complex than the therapeutic approach of providing supranormal levels of this hormone. The highest doses of androgens are those given by injection; when androgens are given in pill form, poor absorption and first-pass hepatic metabolism limit serum levels. Hormones are regulated by feedback mechanisms so that if exogenous testosterone is given, endogenous production may decline. In addition, the initial high-dose effects of androgens do not necessarily continue as the supranormal levels are maintained[38]. Naturally menopausal women's sexual drive is not merely manipulatable by administration of androgens.

Men in their fifties often experience a decreased sex drive without a dramatic decrement in their androgen production. This raises the possibility that the sexual drive deficits are part of a larger physiological process (aging) that is measured by endocrine changes, loss of cellular receptors for androgen, loss of enzymatic activity that converts testosterone into a form that can be used within the cytoplasm or nucleus of cells, and unknown features. Menopause *per se* may be only a small and relatively unimportant part of the explanation. It is far more sobering to think that sexual drive deficits are part of the genetic programming of human beings and have multiple, complex body-wide determinants involving subcellular, cellular, tissue and organ system changes.

The strongest current evidence that androgen replacement can help with the menopausal sexual symptoms is from studies of ovariectomized women. Only those with testosterone or estrogen-testosterone injections improved sexually; those taking placebo or estrogen alone did not[39]. Left unanswered is the question of how long testosterone can sustain the sexual interest of these women. The data are far less clear about whether administration of androgens to women with a natural menopause reverses their new sexual deficits. There is some concern about testosterone's effect on lipid profiles[40]. Many clinicians claim good results[41], while several placebo-controlled studies using sexual interest or intercourse frequency as an outcome measure show no effect. Typically, an androgen is added to HRT after the patient has not responded to estrogen alone[42]. This area requires more careful study, particularly now that some women are clamoring for testosterone[43].

The results of studies of the effect of estrogen replacement on lubrication adequacy generally consistently point towards improvement. All preparations of estrogens are able to help in this way. What percentage of sexually active women still need external lubricants is not clear. While studies generally cover 6 months or less, one 2-year study demonstrated continual improvement over the study period[44]. Once vaginal lubrication is restored, the issue of diminished interest often remains. When estrogens are perceived to have helped with a diminished sexual drive, the effects are thought to be indirect by helping with other matters that increase the sense of well-being[45], to be slight, to affect only some women[34] or to be related to the specific compound used. Since five double-blind studies using conjugated equine estrogens have failed to demonstrate improved sexual interest, and two of five studies using human estrogen did demonstrate an improvement, more attention needs to be paid to the estrogen compound used and its route of administration[16]. Modern combination preparations (for those with a uterus) contain progestins which, throughout

menstruating life, have been thought to diminish sexual drive.

There are other reasons not to assume that there is a ready hormone fix for menopausal sexual difficulties. A carefully performed community-based study of middle-aged women not taking hormone replacement, which used sophisticated statistical analyses, failed to demonstrate any contribution of either serum estrogens or androgens to carefully defined parameters of sexual adjustment[46]. Approximately 10% of women have a medical contraindication to the use of HRT. (Anecdotally, significant sexual deficits are brought about by menopause resulting from breast cancer treatments, including tamoxifen, in young women. In this natural experiment, women in their twenties and thirties seem to have similar sexual complaints to those in women undergoing natural menopause decades later. At this point, there is little endocrine help for them.) While the acceptance rate of HRT in studies carried out by academic investigators is high – approximately 80% of women maintain their treatment during the study protocols – in community studies, after 3 years three-quarters are no longer using HRT[47]. The reasons for this include: wishing no longer to have periods; dislike of premenstrual-like discomfort; episodes of breakthrough bleeding that require a work-up for uterine cancer; fear of breast or uterine cancer; and the wish to live naturally. The highest estimate of eligible American women taking HRT is 34%, and in some subgroups it is 10%[48]. A study of British physicians starting HRT found that 50% were still taking it after several years[49]. Even among women who are some of the most highly informed about the short- and long-term benefits of HRT, the drop-out rate is high.

Among the encouraging information about sexual function in this age group is the confirmation of an older clinical impression: in a study of 52 women between ages 50 and 67 years, those who had intercourse at least three times a month had less vaginal atrophy than those who had intercourse less than ten times a year[50]. Similarly, in a study of perimenopausal women, weekly intercourse was associated with less urogenital atrophy[51]. Here is another reason to be encouraging from my practice:

A 59-year-old business woman who is highly motivated to look young and beautiful by all means available from modern medicine has spent her adult sexual life in a series of affairs. She considers herself sexually gifted in her capacities to give and receive sexual pleasures. Her lubrication capacities did not seem to abate as she went through menopause at age 50 and she still has no need for a lubricant. She has been on sequential HRT. Now with a new 15-year-older partner, she is having the best sexual experiences of her life. The couple has sildenafil-assisted intercourse at least four times a week.

There are two compelling reasons to be less than optimistic about HRT as the solution to the problem of menopausal sexual deficits: it is not clear to what extent and for what duration it actually reverses the array of sexual deficits, and most women will not persist in using HRT. The use of non-oral clinical estrogen is encouraging. In the meantime, women age, and perhaps inexorably move towards the time that they become relatively asexual, and the culture remains silent about that which we cannot change. We ought seriously to consider reversing this silence through more epidemiological, physiological and pharmacological research.

References

1. Levine SB. *Sexuality in Mid-Life*. New York: Plenum, 1998
2. Bretschneider JG, McCoy NL. Sexual interest and behavior in healthy 80 to 102 year olds. *Arch Sex Behav* 1988;17:109–29
3. Mulligan T, Moss CR. Sexuality and aging in male veterans: a cross-sectional study of interest, ability, and activity. *Arch Sex Behav* 1991;20:17–26
4. Starr BD, Weiner MB. *Sex and Sexuality in the Mature Years*. Briarcliff Manor, NY: Stein and Day, 1981
5. Verwoerdt A, Pfeiffer E, Wang HS. Sexual behavior in senescence: patterns of sexual activity and interest. *Geriatrics* 1969;24:137–54
6. Goldstein I, Rosen R, Padma-Nathan H, *et al.* Sildenafil in the treatment of erectile dysfunction. *N Engl J Med* 1998;338:1397–404
7. [Letters to the editor.] *N Engl J Med* 1998;339:700–2
8. Levine SB. *Sex is not Simple*. Columbus, OH: Ohio Psychology Publications, 1989
9. Kingsberg SA. Postmenopausal sexual functioning: a case study. *Int J Fertil* 1998;43:122–8
10. US Congress. US Office of Technology Assessment 3, Washington, DC, 1992
11. Wise PM, Krajnak KM, Kashon ML. Menopause: the aging of multiple pacemakers. *Science* 1996;273: 7–70
12. Walling M, Andersen BL, Johnson SR. Hormonal replacement therapy for postmenopausal women: a review of sexual outcomes and related gynecologic effects. *Arch Sex Behav* 1990;19:119–37
13. Sherwin BB. Use of combined estrogen–androgen preparations in the postmenopause: evidence from clinical studies. *Int J Fertil* 1998;43:98–103
14. Sherwin BB. Sexuality and the menopause. In Berg G, Hammar M, eds. *The Modern Management of the Menopause*. Carnforth, UK: Parthenon Publishing, 1993:617–20
15. Bachman GA. Influence of menopause on sexuality. *Int J Fertil Menopausal Stud* 1995;40(Suppl): 16–22
16. McCoy NL. Sexual issues for postmenopausal women. *Top Geriatr Rehab* 1997;12:28–39
17. Hasselquist MB, Goldberg N, Schroeter A, Spelsberg TC. Isolation and characterization of the estrogen receptor in human skin. *J Clin Endocrinol Metab* 1980;50:76–82
18. McCoy NL, Davidson JM. A longitudinal study of the effects of menopause on sexuality. *Maturitas* 1985;7:203–10
19. Greer G. *The Change: Women, Aging, and the Menopause*. New York: Knopf, 1992
20. Wiklund I, Hoist J, Karlberg J, *et al.* A new methodologic approach to the evaluation of quality of life in post-menopausal women. *Maturitas* 1992;14:211–24
21. Special Advisory Committee on Reproductive Physiology. *Menopause*. Ministry of Supply and Services Canada, Ottawa, 1995
22. Brambilla DK, McKinlay SJ. A prospective study of factors affecting age at menopause. *J Clin Epidemiol* 1989;42:1031–9

23. McCoy NL. The menopause and sexuality. In Sitruk-Ware R, Utian WH, eds. *The Menopause and Hormone Replacement Therapy: Facts and Controversies.* New York: Marcel Dekker, 1900:73–100

24. Longcope C. The endocrinology of the menopause. In Lobo RA, ed. *Treatment of Menopausal Women: Basic and Clinical Aspects.* New York: Raven Press, 1994:47–56

25. Orentreich N, Brind JL, Rizer RL, Vogelman JH. Age changes and sex differences in serum dehydroepiandrosterone sulfate concentrations throughout adulthood. *J Clin Endocrinol Metab* 1984;59:551–5

26. Longcope C, Jaffe W, Griffing G. Production rates of androgens and oestrogens in post-menopausal women. *Maturitas* 1981;3:215–23

27. Masters WH, Johnson V. *Human Sexual Response* Boston, MA: Little Brown, 1966

28. Bretschneider JG, McCoy NL. Sexual behavior and interest in healthy 80- to 102-year olds. *Arch Sex Behav* 1988;17:109–29

29. McCoy NL. Survey research on the menopause and women's sexuality. In Berg G, Hammar M, eds. *The Modern Management of the Menopause.* Carnforth, UK: Parthenon Publishing, 1993:581–8

30. Hallström T. Sexuality of women in middle age: the Gotteborg Study. *J Biosoc Sci* 1979;6(Suppl):165–75

31. American Society for Reproductive Medicine. *Menopause.* Patient Information Series, Birmingham, AL, 1996

32. American College of Obstetrics and Gynecology Patient Education. *The Menopause Years.* Washington, DC, December 1995

33. Sarrel PM. Laser Doppler measurement of peripheral blood flow. In Notelovitz M, van Keep PA, eds. *The Climacteric in Perspective.* Lancaster, UK: MTP Press, 1986:161–73

34. Nathorst-Boos J, Wiklund I, Mattsson LA, *et al.* Is sexual life influenced by transdermal estrogen therapy? A double-blind placebo controlled study in postmenopausal women. *Acta Obstet Gynecol Scand* 1993;72:656–60

35. Studd J. Continuation rates with cyclical and continuous regimes of oral estrogens and progestogens [Editorial]. *Menopause.* 1996;3:181–2

36. Myers LS, Dixen J, Morrissette M, Carmichael M, Davidson JM. Effects of estrogen, androgen, and progesterone on sexual psychophysiology and behavior in post-menopausal women. *J Clin Endocrinol Metab* 1990;70:1124–31

37. Longcope C. Adrenal and gonadal steroid secretion in normal females. *J Clin Endocrinol Metab* 1986;15:215–28

38. Sherwin BB. A comparative analysis of the role of androgen in human male and female sexual behavior: behavioral specificity, critical threshold, and sensitivity. *Psychobiology* 1988;16:416–25

39. Sherwin BB, Gelfand MM, Brender W. Androgen enhances motivation in females: a prospective, cross-over study of sex steroid administration in the surgical menopause. *Psychosom Med* 1985;47:339–51

40. Hickok LR, Toomey C, Speroff L. A comparison of esterified estrogens with and without methyltestosterone: effects on endometrial histology and serum lipoproteins in postmenopausal women. *Obstet Gynecol* 1993;82:919–24

41. Rako S. *The Hormone of Desire: the Truth about Sexuality, Menopause, and Testosterone.* New York: Harmony Books, 1996

42. Plouffe L, Cohen D. The role of androgens in menopausal hormone replacement therapy. In Lorrain J, ed. *Comprehensive Management of Menopause.* New York: Springer-Verlag, 1994:397–408

43. Dopay B, Balos R, Willard N. Improved menopausal symptom relief with estrogen–androgen therapy [Abstr]. *Menopause* 1996;3:233

44. Semmens JP, Tsai CC, Semmens EC, Loadholt CB. Effects of estrogen therapy on vaginal physiology during menopause. *Obstet Gynecol* 1985;66:15–18

45. Special Advisory Committee on Reproductive Physiology to the Drugs Directorate Health Protection Branch Health Canada. *Menopause,* Minister of National Health and Welfare, 1995:43

46. Cawood EHH, Bancroft J. Steroid hormones, the menopause, sexuality, and well-being of women. *Psychol Med* 1996;26:925–36

47. Ettinger B, Li DK, Klein R. Continuation of postmenopausal hormone replacement therapy: comparison of cyclic versus continuous combined schedules. *Menopause* 1966;3:185–9

48. Utian WH, Schiff I. NAMS–Gallup survey of women's knowledge, information sources, and attitudes to menopause and hormone replacement therapy. *Menopause* 1994;1:39–48

49. Isaacs AJ, Britton AR, McPherson K. Utilisation of hormone replacement by women doctors. *Br Med J* 1995;311:1399–401

50. Leiblum S, Bachmann G, Kenmann E, Colburn D, Swartzman L. Vaginal atrophy in the postmenopausal woman: the importance of sexual activity and hormones. *J Am Med Assoc* 1983;249:2195–8

51. Cutler WB, Garcia CR, McCoy N. Peri-menopausal sexuality. *Arch Sex Behav* 1987;16:225–34

Section II
Endocrinology of the menopause

6

The thyroid in the menopause

Bernard A. Eskin

The thyroid gland in adult women normally weighs about 12–20 g and is responsible for extraordinary metabolic activity. The activities of this butterfly-shaped gland vary according to gender, age, reproductive function, climate and nutritional status. The thyroid is essential to women's health with diagnoses of abnormal states occurring five times more often than in men. During the menopause the thyroid gland ages and, while relieved from the modifications caused by sex hormone and reproductive cyclicity, it exhibits the influences of anatomical transformations and physiological conversions of aging. These changes begin in the premenopausal transition, often the result of irregularities in hormone secretions as the ovary wanes.

In general, thyroid disorders increase with aging. They are frequently overlooked because of the symptomatic guises that they may take. Well stated, the clinical presentations of thyroid endocrinopathies may be subtle, non-specific and confusing, with function tests that are misleading. Again, all these may be attributed to normal aging or acute and chronic diseases seen in the mature individual[1]. In this chapter, emphasis is directed towards the perimenopausal and geripausal patient and, where possible, differences from menstruating women that may exist. The essential aspects of thyroid anatomy, physiology, endocrinology, pathology and therapeutics seen in all women are presented and compared.

Anatomy

The thyroid gland is located in the anterior portion of the trachea. It consists of two lobes with a thin isthmus between (Figure 1). The isthmus lies just below the cricothyroid cartilage, which is a convenient clinical landmark on examination. The right lobe is generally larger, more vascular than the left. Both lobes enlarge diffusely with functional disorders.

The thyroid gland is extremely vascular, receiving its blood supply directly from the carotid artery through two major arteries, the superior and inferior thyroid. It is larger in men than in women, although size and weight rely on height and weight of the individual. Reports of an increase in size in aging have been noted; nevertheless, the gland is more nodular with advancing age. Examination and estimation of the size of the thyroid gland in menopausal women is more difficult because arthritic changes in the neck, obesity or pulmonary diseases may be present.

Physiology

Thyroid hormones

The thyroid gland secretes the thyronines, thyroxine (T_4), tri-iodothyronine (T_3) and reverse T_3 (rT_3), which appear to be synthesized from simple substrates of tyrosine and iodine (Figure 2). All of these exist in plasma. T_4 is highest in concentration and appears to be the only one that arises solely from the thyroid gland. Under normal conditions, T_3 is secreted to a slight extent from the thyroid, but most T_3 is obtained from peripheral metabolism by the removal of a single iodine atom from T_4. Present in infants and aging patients, rT_3 and secondary thyronines are derived from peripheral conversion of T_4[2].

Restricted anatomically to the follicles of the thyroid gland is thyroglobulin, a large molecule which contains tyrosyl residues and the amino acid tyrosine (Figure 3). Tyrosyls are proteins which are iodinated directly in the thyroid gland by iodides

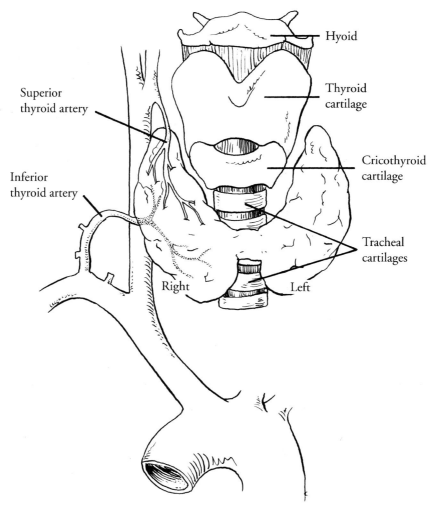

Superior thyroid artery

Inferior thyroid artery

Hyoid

Thyroid cartilage

Cricothyroid cartilage

Tracheal cartilages

Right

Left

Figure 1 Anatomy of the thyroid gland. Note relationship of thyroid gland to trachea and major arterial supply of neck

in the blood. Iodides (designated in Figure 3 as 1) can be generated only from various foods, water supplies and iodine therapies. Generally, the thyroid gland removes most of the iodides from the blood, an important clinical fact. A few non-thyroidal organs accept iodine forms in women: salivary glands, stomach mucosa, mammary tissues (particularly the terminal ducts) and the ovaries[3,4]. The mechanics involved in iodine trapping by these extra-thyroidal organs is unknown[5].

Iodides, upon reaching the thyroid membrane, are introduced into the cell and then converted to iodine by a thyroid peroxidase system (designated in Figure 3 as 2). After the iodine enters the lumen

of the follicle and is oxidized, it is incorporated into organic combinations (designated in Figure 3 as 3). Organic iodinations are generally under the control of thyroid stimulating hormone (TSH) stimulation.

Thus, the formation of tyrosines, monoiodotyrosine (MIT) and di-iodotyrosine (DIT), occurs in approximately equal amounts. Since non-iodinated thyronine has not been demonstrated, the intracellular thyroproteins T_4 and T_3 must arise from iodotyrosines. T_4 would arise from doubling of two DIT molecules, while T_3 would be the result of DIT and MIT moieties (designated in Figure 3 as 4). This is the 'coupling reaction'.

Transport of thyroid hormones: binding proteins

The thyroid hormones T_4 and T_3, as well as other iodinated tyrosyls, are transported in the blood bound firmly although reversibly to the serum proteins: thyroid binding globulin (TBG), thyroid binding prealbumin (TBPA) and albumin. The biological activities, transport through the body as well as degradation of the thyroid hormones, are influenced by the binding affinities of these proteins to the hormones (designated in Figure 3 as 5). The binding procedures are little known; however, many conditions change the concentration of TBG. This, in turn, modifies the final reactions at the target cells. Clinical responses are dependent on the quantity of free thyroid hormones available.

Thyroxine (T_4) is the primary secretory thyronine from the thyroid gland, and is derived only by direct secretion from the thyroid gland. T_3 and rT_3 are present in greater quantities in the blood than can be assigned to thyroid gland secretion only. Peripheral synthesis from T_4 has become apparent quantitatively. Under these circumstances, the formation of T_3 occurs in peripheral locations in such diverse places as nervous tissues (including central nervous system, CNS), liver, kidney and generalized fat.

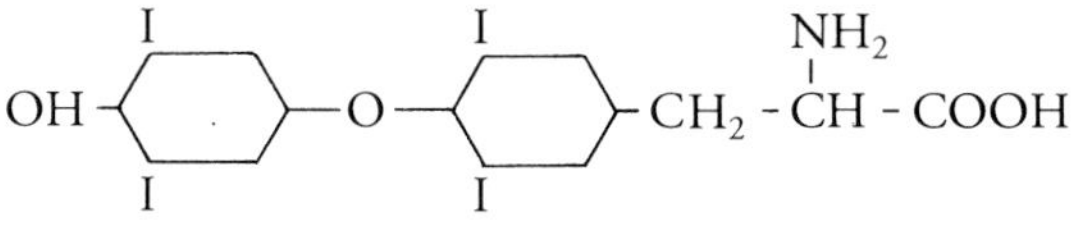

L-thyroxine (T_4)

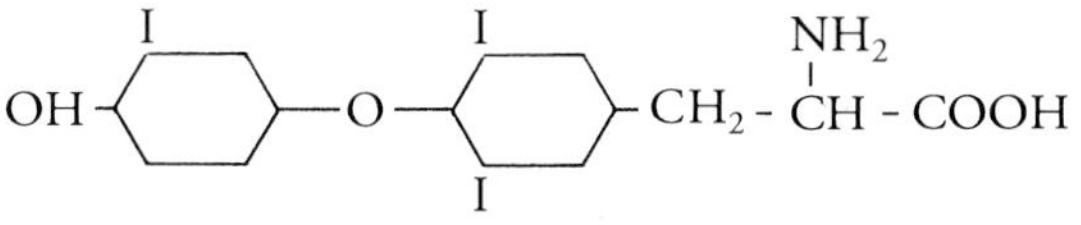

3, 3′, 5-L-tri-iodothyronine (T_3)

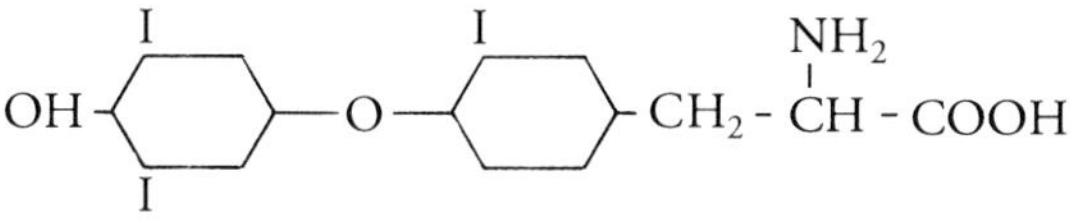

3, 3′, 5′-L-tri-iodothyronine (reverse T_3)

Figure 2 Major thyroid hormones

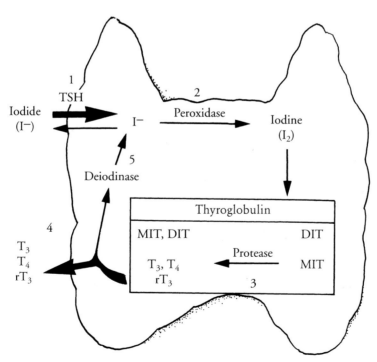

Figure 3 Intrathyroid pathways. Thyroid hormone synthesis as described in text. TSH, thyroid stimulating hormone; DIT, di-iodotyrosine; MIT, monoiodotyrosine; T_3, tri-iodothyronine; T_4, thyroxine; rT_3, reverse T_3

Reverse T_3, found in greater amounts in menopausal and older patients, appears to be biologically inactive[2]. Reverse T_3 may be involved in receptor response in some tissues; thus, when rT_3 is formed, the parent T_4 shares the receptor pool. This reduction in thyroid hormone response decreases thyroid hormone overactivity and may prevent hyperthyroid disease in the tissues, most commonly in the mature patient.

Metabolism and degradation of thyroid hormones

Degradation of T_4 and T_3 is influenced again by binding proteins, TBG, TBPA and albumin. About 10% of the T_4 secreted daily is excreted in the bile as free T_4. In the liver, intracellular breakdown seems to take place in the endoplasmic reticulum of the liver cells. The rest of degradation of the thyroid hormones apparently takes place in liver, kidney and muscle. Cellular degradation, which includes deiodination, takes place in the target organs; deamination, transamination and decarboxylation occur immediately after deiodination.

Endocrinology of thyroid activity

Three major regulatory mechanisms are known to exist for thyroid gland activity. These are: hypothalamic–pituitary–thyroid axis; intrathyroidal autoregulation; and peripheral synthesis and cellular regulation.

Hypothalamic–pituitary–thyroid axis Iodine transport, hormone synthesis and hormone secretion in the thyroid gland are controlled by TSH from the anterior pituitary. Furthermore, it appears that TSH influences both thyroid structure and function, and is involved in the amount and effectiveness of the vascularity, the changes in the epithelial cells, especially their height, and the total amount of stored colloid that occurs in the thyroid gland. It has been well known for many years that TSH is able to control peripherally the intrathyroidal metabolic processes which include glucose oxidation, phospholipid synthesis and RNA synthesis. The release of TSH from the pituitary is caused by the feedback on the pituitary by the free (unbound) forms of both T_4 and T_3 (Figure 4). The specific effect of reverse T_3 remains moot.

Unlike several other endocrine systems, the pituitary secretion (TSH) has the primary control of thyroid metabolism. While the hypothalamus secretes thyrotropin releasing hormone (TRH), it does not appear to be the major regulator of the thyroid through feedback control. The hypothalamus has a modulating influence on the pituitary and resulting TSH secretion. Since there are other factors evident which control pituitary secretions, the final result is often unpredictable (Figure 4). The mechanisms involved have not yet been totally defined. It appears that TRH acts to stimulate first the release and later the synthesis of TSH, while thyroid hormones act to inhibit these functions. Thyroid hormones seem to mediate the feedback regulation of TSH secretion, while TRH determines its set point. Receptor systems for both T_4 and T_3 are present in the pituitary, although binding affinity varies.

Some mechanisms that regulate TSH secretion have been seen to affect TRH receptors which are located on pituitary thyrotropin surfaces. These are modified also by both thyroid and steroid

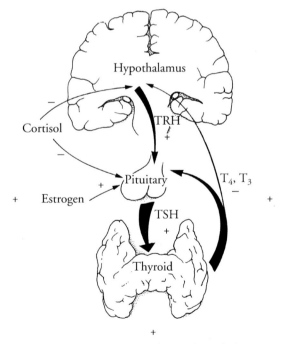

Figure 4 Endocrine control of thyroid hormone secretion. TRH, thyroid releasing hormone; TSH, thyroid stimulating hormone; T_4, thyroxine; T_3, triiodothyronine

hormones (Figure 4). Small doses of thyroid hormone reduce the clinical effectiveness of exogenous TRH on pituitary secretion of TSH. Iodides cause the reverse.

Intrathyroidal autoregulation A basic quantity of hormone must remain stored within the thyroid gland. This constant amount of hormone operates independently of the external secretions and stimulus from the hypothalamus or pituitary. When the synthesis of thyroid hormone decreases, as reflected by a reduction of glandular thyroid hormones, it brings about biochemical changes which increase the synthesis of thyroid hormone. On the other hand, when hormone stores increase there is an inhibition of TSH release with a suppression of the biosynthetic pathways.

Peripheral synthesis and cellular regulation It has become apparent that extrathyroidal metabolism maintains the level and type of thyroid hormone available. Peripheral metabolism consists of first, synthesis of thyroid hormones and second, peripheral action at the target cells.

Metabolic effects of thyroid hormones

The thyroid hormones which are effective (i.e. free T_4 and T_3) stimulate several metabolic functions at the target tissues. The iodine on the T_4 and T_3 structures (Figure 2) is considered a means of stereotypically stabilizing the iodothyronine molecule, since the iodine prevents the free rotation around either oxygen. This configuration is necessary for its attachment to the target receptors.

Thyroid hormones cause:

(1) An increase in oxygen consumption and calorogenesis in the heart, liver, kidney and skeletal muscle;

(2) An increase in the activities of mitachondria;

(3) Conversion of carotene to vitamin A;

(4) An increase in the incorporation of amino acids in the ribosomes;

(5) An increase in bond turnover;

(6) An increase in carbohydrate absorption from the gastrointestinal tract with a decrease in glycogen synthesis;

(7) An increase in RNA plasma flow in glomerular filtration rate;

(8) An increase in the excretion of cholesterol into the biliary tract;

(9) An increase in hepatic cholesterologenesis;

(10) An increase in lipolysis and support actions of catecholamines on this activity.

These biochemical actions result in:

(1) An increase in basal metabolism rate and oxygen consumption (T_3 is three to four times more efficient than T_4 in increasing oxygen consumption while T_4 has a much faster action);

(2) Stimulation and growth processes in various organs and tissues, such as the mammary glands and reproductive system;

(3) Enhanced maturation of the nervous system;

(4) Increased oxygen consumption by the myocardium;

(5) Increased gastrointestinal motility and decreased production of mucoid substance by the mucosa cells;

(6) Increased blood flow to the skin.

Because of these many physiological effects, a remarkable series of clinical responses results.

Clinical aspects of the thyroid

Abnormalities of thyroid function may generate overall abnormal metabolic and hormonal states. As previously stated, thyroid disturbances occur more commonly in women. This is probably due to the repetitive perturbations of reproductive hormone cyclicity and irregularities of menstruation prior to the menopause. During the transitional years, these aberrations can occur when either sex hormone or thyroid hormone homeostasis breaks down[6]. The effect on the other axis is seen when thyroid diseases (both hypo- and hyperthyroidism) cause gynecological irregularities, and, inversely, when irregular ovarian hormone secretions are responsible for thyroid dysfunction. The menopause results when there is reduced estrogen synthesis and release from the ovary and, thus, inadequate endometrial stimuli for menstrual flow. Simultaneously, the thyroid has aged and has been modified throughout reproductive life. In the menopause, the thyroid is associated with a number of morphological and functional changes, such as decreased serum T_3 and mean TSH concentrations, which are to some extent independent of intercurrent non-thyroidal illnesses[7]. The result is an endocrine pattern in the thyroid that is unpredictable[8]. There are specific changes found in menopausal women which are responsible for the increasing morbidity seen (Table 1).

Thyroid diseases in women occur often later in life. Evaluation of function and clinical examination of the thyroid are a priori requirements of the complete evaluation in the pre- and postmenopause. The clinical symptoms manifested are more subtle, because it is anticipated that an aging patient will show energy loss, lethargy, sexual dysfunction, mild depression and other nondefinitive incapacitations brought on by time (a fallacy for this millennium).

Hypothyroidism, hyperthyroidism, thyroid malignancies and the sick euthyroid syndrome are more common in the menopause. While men also have an increased risk for thyroid disease as they age, the resulting numbers characteristically still favor women in the ratio of at least five to one.

Menopausal screening for thyroid disease

In light of the changes occurring, it is advisable to screen perimenopausal women, generally at 35–40, 40–45 and again at 45–50 years of age. Obviously, further tests should be done if thyroid disease is suspected at any time, particularly after the menopause. A number of pathophysiological changes occur in thyroid metabolism at the time of the menopause. While these conditions appear, there is no immediate medical abnormality or concern visible (Table 1). Some geriatricians practice preventive medicine by conducting studies on all patients, men and women, at 65 years of age. However, screening thyroid function tests are not always accurate for patients with acute psychiatric or medical illnesses who are on medications, because of laboratory interference[9].

Table 1 Menopausal changes in thyroid physiology

Decreased
Renal iodide clearance
Thyroid iodide clearance
Total T_4 production
Serum TBG concentration
T_3 concentration
TSH response to TRH
Diurnal variation of TSH
Increased
T_4 degradation
Reverse T_3 concentration
Same
Serum T_4 concentration

T_4, thyroxine; TBG, thyroid binding globulin; T_3, triiodothyronine; TSH, thyroid stimulating hormone; TRH, thyroid releasing hormone

Patients with symptoms of failure to thrive, depression and disability benefit from physical examination and screening for thyroid disease. Subtle evidences of early thyroid problems can be easily treated as needed. The quality of life is greatly improved, and conditions such as elevated cholesterol, apathy and anxiety can be relieved. Screening is easily performed by measuring TSH.

Hypothyroidism

Hypothyroidism is a condition caused by thyroid failure, where there is a deficient supply of thyroid hormone available to peripheral tissues. The range of the thyroid deficiency is extensive; however, it may be only present subclinically[10]. Myxedema is the term applied to the most severe expression of hypothyroidism, and may follow thyroid surgery or radioactive iodine treatment for hyperthyroidism. It occurs spontaneously as so-called idiopathic myxedema (Gull's disease). This is considered the end result of an autoimmune process which is expressed as similar or identical to that in Hashimoto's thyroiditis. Other origins include drug-induction, goiters or hypothalamic and pituitary abnormalities.

Prevalence

The prevalence of hypothyroidism has been reported to increase with age, and up to 10% in menopausal women[11]. Almost one-third of these cases are of iatrogenic origin (Table 2). This disease is infrequently a cause of hospital admissions, since full-blown myxedema is rare. In menopausal women, the pathogenesis seems to be almost entirely explicable on the basis of a chronic auto-immune (Hashimoto's) thyroiditis. However, several causes have been described by thyroido-logists in characterizing the disease (Table 2). Chronic autoimmune thyroiditis is characterized by a focal or diffuse lymphocytic infiltration of thyroid parenchyma, damaged or atrophic folli-cles, and the presence of autoantibodies in the serum. Postmenopausal women have been shown to have an increase in thyroid autoimmunity due to estrogen loss[12].

Diagnosis

Prominent clinical features include a puffy face, a pleasant personality, non-pitting myxedema, marked cold intolerance, and coarse, dry skin and hair[13]. Clinical features of hypothyroidism in the menopause are listed in Table 3. Enlargement of the heart shadow is frequently due to a pericardial effusion. Adrenal function is decreased with 17-ketosteroid and hydroxycorticoid excretion reduced, and serum cortisol and corticoid serum levels lowered. Cardiac output is decreased and the body is less sensitive to catecholamines. Certain signs are readily seen, such as reflex relaxation time, which is markedly prolonged, decreased metabolic rate and increases in blood cholesterol and other lipid fractions.

The signs and symptoms of hypothyroidism in the menopause tend to be non-specific because of the insidious onset of the disease and its long pro-gression[14]. The diagnosis of primary hypo-thyroidism is confirmed by finding an elevation of serum TSH accompanied by a reduced free T_4 level while total T_4 is adequate[9]. The hypothalamic-pituitary axis is so sensitive that it is often possible to detect TSH elevation indicating thyroid damage before the patient notices symptoms. The condi-tion is termed *subclinical hypothyroidism*.

Therapy

Therapy of primary hypothyroidism should be instituted with levothyroxine at a dose that takes

Table 2 Causes of hypothyroidism in the menopause

Primary hypothyroidism
Chronic autoimmune thyroiditis
Radiation
  ^{131}I therapy for hyperthyroidism
  radiation therapy for head and neck cancer
Surgical thyroidectomy
Drugs
  iodine-containing drugs: amiodarone, iodinated glycerol
  antithyroid drugs: propylthiouracil, methimazole
  lithium

Secondary hypothyroidism
Hypothalamic tumors or granuloma
Pituitary tumors
Pituitary surgery
Radiation

Table 3 Clinical features of hypothyroidism in the menopausal woman

Cutaneous
Dry skin
Hair loss
Edema of face and eyelids
Cold intolerance

Neurological
Parasthesia (carpal tunnel syndrome)
Ataxia
Dementia

Psychiatric and behavioral
Depression
Apathy or withdrawal
Psychosis
Cognitive dysfunction

Metabolism
Weight gain
Hypercholesterolemia
Hyperglyceridemia
Peripheral edema

Musculoskeletal
Myopathy
Arthritis/arthralgia

Cardiovascular
Bradycardia
Pericardial effusion
Congestive heart failure

into account the age of the patient, the severity and duration of the hypothyroidism, and the presence of coexisting medical conditions, particularly symptomatic coronary artery disease. Partial substitution of T_3 for T_4 may improve mood and neuropsychological function in older women. This finding suggests a specific effect of T_3 normally secreted by the thyroid gland[15]. An important consideration is whether therapy should be instituted slowly at a lower dose and increasing after treatment observation. In the premenopausal patient, with no complicating illnesses, a starting levothyroxine replacement dose of 0.6–0.7 μg/lb ideal body weight (1.6–1.8 μg/kg) can be given immediately. However, lower doses should be instituted in older menopausal or geripausal patients and those with illnesses that may compromise the capacity of the cardiorespiratory system to respond to an increased metabolic demand[16].

Patients who present with hypothyroidism and symptomatic angina should be evaluated prior to treatment for the presence of a readily treated obstructive lesion of the coronary arteries[17]. The biochemical end-point of therapy is normalization of the serum TSH, and should be done cautiously even if it requires several months to achieve the euthyroid state. Chronic therapy should be monitored at first, at least semiannually by measurements of TSH using a third-generation assay capable of accurately measuring the lower limit of the normal range (usually 0.3–0.5 μIU/l).

Patients with hypothyroidism due to pituitary or hypothalamic causes can be evaluated for deficiencies of other trophic hormones, especially adrenocorticotropic hormone (ACTH). The availability (1999) of thyrotropin-α for injection (Thyrogen®) provides a direct method for testing pituitary release diagnostically. Glucocorticoid replacement may be required prior to instituting levothyroxine treatment to stabilize the condition. Appropriate imaging of the hypothalamic-pituitary region may identify neuroanatomical lesions which require attention first. In these cases, the biochemical end-point of levothyroxine replacement would be a free T_4 level (preferably by radioimmunoassay) or calculations which are in the high normal range.

Malabsorption and old age will increase levothyroxine requirements[18]. Administration of cholesterol or potassium-binding resins, $FeSO_4$, anticonvulsants, certain antacids and amiodarone will decrease the test results. Women who also receive androgens in the menopause (including replacement medications) do not require as much levothyroxine replacement. Appropriate adjustments and more frequent monitoring are necessary when any of these conditions are seen.

A serious complication, myxedema coma, represents the ultimate expression of progressively lowered body metabolism due to a severe lack of thyroid hormone. It occurs only in the elderly. Whether massive or minute doses of hormone should be used in the institution of therapy is not clear. Large doses are favored, but the conditions described previously should be considered. Steroids are always given concurrently, and if the circulation and oxygenation are not well maintained, vasopressor drugs with intubation should be used. Ancillary measures include internal re-administration of fluids while keeping in mind the impaired free kidney clearance of the hypothyroid patient.

Hyperthyroidism

The clinical syndrome of hyperthyroidism is usually caused by Graves' disease or diffuse toxic goiter. Thyroiditis is much less common in menopausal than in premenopausal women[19]. Thyrotoxicosis (symptomatic hyperthyroidism) may also be produced by toxic multinodular goiter, toxic adenomas, excessive thyroid hormone ingestion and several rare syndromes. In older patients, toxic multinodular goiter is more common, reaching as many as one-half of these patients, especially in areas of iodine deficiency. Graves' disease includes thyrotoxicosis, goiter, exophthalmos and pretibial myxedema when fully expressed, but can occur with one or more of these features (Table 4).

Graves' disease, a disease of autoimmunity, shows strong hereditary tendency. Inheritance of specific HLA antigens has been shown to predispose to Graves' disease. Psychic trauma, sympathetic nervous system activation, strenuous weight reduction and iodide administration have also been associated with the initiation of hyperthyroidism.

Immune response is characterized by the presence of abnormal antibodies directed against specific thyroid tissue antigens that particularly

Table 4 Clinical features of hyperthyroidism in the menopause

Cardiovascular
Palpitation
Chronic or intermittent atrial fibrillation
Congestive heart failure

Psychiatric and behavioral
Depression
Apathy
Lethargy
Irritability

Gastrointestinal
Decreased appetite
Weight loss
Nausea
Constipation

Musculoskeletal
Proximal muscle weakness
Muscle atrophy

bind with the thyrotropin receptor. These antibodies act either as agonists or antagonists, thus stimulating or blocking TSH. Antibodies of this type can be measured in 80–100% of untreated patients with Graves' disease. The serum factor TSAb (long-acting thyroid stimulator, LATS) is measurable and most commonly involved. Serum TSH is typically suppressed and may be near zero.

The thyroid gland is hyperfunctioning in Graves' disease, and its activity is not suppressed when exogenous T_3 is administered. The pituitary response to TRH is also suppressed. The gland is unusually responsive to iodide, which both blocks further hormone synthesis and inhibits release of hormone from the gland.

Prevalence

In studies, the incidence of Graves' disease varies from 3.4 to 6.8% of menopausal women. Approximately 10–17% of all hyperthyroid patients are over the age of 60 years. The frequency in women is always greater than in men.

Thyrotoxicosis itself is associated with pathological changes including damage to muscles and mild damage to the liver. Graves' disease is associated with thyroid hyperplasia with lymphoid infiltration, generalized lymphoid hyperplasia, and the specific changes of infiltrative ophthalmopathy and pretibial myxedema.

Diagnosis

The classic features of thyrotoxicosis are described as nervousness, diminished sleep, tremulousness, tachycardia, increased appetite, weight loss and increased perspiration[20]. Graves' disease shows specific symptoms and signs which are associated with goiter, occasionally with exophthalmos, and rarely with pretibial myxedema. Physical findings include fine skin and hair, tremulousness, a hyperactive heart, Plummer's nails, muscle weakness, accelerated reflex relaxation, occasional splenomegaly and often peripheral edema. Thyroid changes seen in menopausal Graves' disease are given in Table 4. Skin changes that are seen are probably autoimmune vitiligo or hives. The extent and degree of hyperthyroid bone diseases, particularly osteoporosis, surpass the effects of menopause on the bone mass[21].

Absence of some of the typical manifestations of hyperthyroidism in the menopause and geripause was called 'apathetic hyperthyroidism' because there were only slight evidences of hypermetabolism. The diagnosis of hyperthyroidism may be overlooked because of apathy, or the dominant clinical findings may be weight loss, cardiac or gastrointestinal manifestations. The prevalence of subclinical hyperthyroidism is higher than that of subclinical hypothyroidism in older women, and it might relate to non-autoimmune factors[22].

The disease typically begins gradually in adult (premenopausal) women and progressively worsens unless treated. Muscle weakness is frequent, myasthenia may coexist, and hypokalemic periodic paralysis may be induced by thyrotoxicosis. Hypercalciuria is frequent, but kidney stones rarely occur. Thyrotoxicosis can cause congestive heart failure, mitral valve prolapse, atrial tachycardia and cardiac fibrillation. Other medical findings may include normocytic anemia, diarrhea without malabsorption, minimal liver damage and hyperbilirubinemia.

The laboratory tests that are most effective for evaluating the status of thyroid function are the sensitive TSH assay or any technique measuring free tri-iodothyronine (T_3). As an initial single test, a sensitive TSH assay may be most cost-effective and specific. Although this may range slightly according to the kit or technique, the sensitive TSH test should yield 0–0.1 μIU/ml in thyrotoxicosis. In menopausal women a range of 0.1–0.25 is sometimes seen, especially with the toxic form of multinodular goiters, more common in this group.

A variety of free thyroxine techniques have become available and are often suitable as a single testing system as well. However, if clinical judgment places considerable doubt on a normal result, an additional test may be employed: serum T_3 level determined by radioimmunoassay. It is almost always elevated in thyrotoxicosis. Interpretations can be made without correcting for protein binding. The serum T_4 level is elevated in 86% of menopausal hyperthyroid patients, providing a reasonably sensitive alternative for hyperthyroidism. However, there are hyperthyroxinemic patients without hyperthyroidism, indicating low specificity of the serum total T_4 assay.

Treatment

In general, the choice of treatment of all forms of thyrotoxicosis requires full patient participation. Thyrotoxicosis in untreated cases leads to cardiovascular damage, bone loss and fractures, or inanition, and can be fatal. The long-term history also includes spontaneous remission in some cases, and eventual spontaneous development of hypothyroidism if autoimmune thyroiditis coexists and destroys the thyroid gland.

Primary treatment of Graves' disease has essentially fallen into three forms: blocking of thyroid hormone synthesis in the thyroid by the use of antithyroid drugs; complete destruction of the thyroid tissues by radioactive iodine; and partial or complete surgical ablation of the thyroid.

In women of child-bearing age, antithyroid drugs are used primarily, unless persistent failure of the medication is apparent. Women in the menopause often do very well on antithyroid medications given for 6 months to a year and then discontinued[23]. This may require longer periods of time or repetitive therapy after an unsuccessful hiatus. The spontaneous successes from medical therapy are satisfying, since both radiation and surgery may induce damage to the thyroids, parathyroids or recurrent nerves. However, side-effects and complications of the medications for the individual must be weighed in each case.

Radioactive ablation, which is commonly used in menopausal women, may cause some damage to the peripheral tissues and most often results in hypothyroidism with a need for treatment. A population-based study (1999) resulted in a decrease in overall cancer incidence and mortality in those treated for hyperthyroidism with radioiodine[24]. The absolute risk of cancers of the small bowel and thyroid remained low, but an increased relative risk was considered a problem requiring long-term vigilance. However, the simplicity of the treatment is useful where the older patient cannot tolerate long-term medical therapy.

Surgery, the usual therapy until 1950, is minimally used for hyperthyroidism. It is generally resorted to when the patient chooses not to have radioactive treatment and is unsuccessful with medical treatment.

Thyroid tumors and malignancy

Adenomas

Thyroid adenomas occur in approximately 2% of the total population. Women have six times as many nodular thyroidal conditions than men. Histological types include embryonal, fetal and follicular adenomas, and colloid nodules. Adenomas are neoplasms and possibly arise from the same types of stimuli that cause carcinomas. There are two types: adenomas which grow slowly and, if non-functioning, produce symptoms because of distortion of local anatomy; and hyperfunctioning adenomas which may suppress the remainder of the gland or induce thyrotoxicosis. Bleeding into an adenoma causes sudden painful enlargement, often with destruction of the lesion. Very rarely, adenomas appear to progress to carcinomas.

Diagnosis

Thyroid nodules are evaluated by a review of features that may suggest malignancy, such as an increase in size, pain, undue firmness or fixation, and the presence of local adenopathy. A basic ultrasound scan of the thyroid is sometimes useful in determining the size of the lesion and the consistency – fluid or solid – of the lesions. Isotope scintiscans and thyroid uptake studies are of some value as well, since the information they provide may suggest an alternative diagnosis, such as multinodular goiter or Hashimoto's thyroiditis, or may show hyperfunction of the adenoma, suggesting that it is a benign lesion[25]. Currently, emphasis is placed upon fine-needle aspiration cytology for evaluation of the possibility of malignancy. This diagnostic procedure appears to be 90–95% accurate in experienced hands[26]. In recent studies, researchers have evaluated the accuracy of molecular diagnosis of residual and recurrent thyroid cancer by amplification of thyroglobulin messenger RNA (mRNA) in peripheral blood[27].

Nodules that, on fine-needle aspiration cytology, are benign may be treated conservatively by administration of thyroid hormone replacement therapy to suppress TSH and prevent further growth. Lesions that have suspicious clinical or physical signs, from which it is impossible to obtain adequate cytological findings, or that have an abnormal cytology should be resected[28]. Hyperfunctioning solitary thyroid nodules can be destroyed by administration of large doses of radioactive iodine or resected.

Carcinoma

Thyroid cancer accounts for 0.6–1.6% of all cancers. Mortality is less than 0.4% of all cancer deaths. An increase in thyroid cancer has been seen in 1999 owing to improved diagnosis; however, mortality has decreased as a result of early detection.

Prevalence

Thyroid carcinomas occur with an incidence of 30–60 new cases per million population per year, and a mortality of approximately 4.5 per million population per year[28]. Thyroid neoplasia has been shown to be caused by prior irradiation of the thyroid. Even small doses such as 7–20 rad have an adverse effect. Doses of several hundred rads may increase the incidence of malignancy over 100-fold. Chronic stimulation by TSH can also produce malignant change in the human thyroid. Occult cancers that are generally less than 0.5 cm in their greatest diameter occur in up to 6% of adult thyroids, but rarely appear to change into clinically significant thyroid tumors.

Papillary thyroid carcinomas grow very slowly, metastasizing primarily to cervical nodes and later to the lungs. Many persons survive for two to four decades with extensive metastatic disease. Follicular carcinomas invade more aggressively, and are prone to metastasize to soft tissues and bones; resulting mortality is 30–50% over 10–20 years. Medullary thyroid carcinomas develop from thyroid C cells and may occur sporadically or as part of familial syndromes associated with multiple endocrine tumors. These tumors secrete calcitonin, which aids in their detection and management. Undifferentiated or anaplastic thyroid carcinomas are extremely malignant. The vast majority cause death within 4 months to 1 year.

Therapy

The basic therapy for thyroid carcinoma remains surgical resection. The minimum desirable operation is a lobectomy on one side complemented by subtotal thyroidectomy on the opposite side. Many surgeons prefer a near-total thyroidectomy for any tumor larger than 1 cm in size. Modified neck dissection is done if local adenopathy is present. In most instances, residual thyroid tissue is destroyed by administration of ^{131}I. Metastatic thyroid disease that can be shown to accumulate isotope is treated by administration of large doses of ^{131}I on one or more occasions.

Radiotherapy is probably advisable in differentiated thyroid carcinoma that is invasive into the tissue of the neck, in menopausal patients and in recurrences resistant to ^{131}I therapy. Radiotherapy to the thyroid bed is probably advisable in all anaplastic thyroid cancers.

Chemotherapy, depending primarily upon adriamycin, is occasionally valuable in some progressive differentiated, medullary and anaplastic thyroid carcinomas.

Conclusions

Women are more subject to thyroid pathology. Particularly prevalent in menopausal women is hypothyroidism. Examination of the patient should include diagnostic examination and testing when even subtle symptoms are described. Treatment of thyroid disease should be personalized. Nodular changes should be carefully followed by ultrasound and palpation. Biopsy is indicated when the findings are confusing or the disease is rapidly changing. Difficulty often arises with diagnosing thyroid cancer, which requires specialized care. Fine-needle aspiration, now available, has made diagnosis somewhat easier, although diagnostic difficulty remains because of the small sample obtained. Several new methods have become available or are in an experimental status.

Menopausal women should be routinely studied for thyroid disease by a screening test (sensitive TSH) and neck palpation annually from the age of 40. Because of the accessibility of the thyroid, an annual or semiannual examination should be routine. Where there is doubt, the woman should be referred for an endocrine evaluation of her thyroid.

References

1. Wong TK, Hershman JM. Changes in thyroid function in nonthyroid illness. *Trends Endocrinol Metab* 1992;3:8
2. Nishikawa M, Inada M, Naito K, *et al.* Age related changes of serum 3,3'-diiodothyronine, 3',5'-diiodothyronine, and 3,5-diiodothyronine concentrations in man. *J Clin Endocrinol Metab* 1981;52:517
3. Ghent WR, Eskin BA, Low DA, Hill LP. Iodine replacement in fibrocystic disease of the breast. *Can J Surg* 1993;36:453
4. Dunn JT. What's happening to our iodine? [Editorial]. *J Clin Endocrinol Metab* 1998;83:3398–400
5. Eskin BA, Grotkowski CE, Connolly CP, Ghent WR. Different tissue responses for iodine and iodide in rat thyroid and mammary glands. *Biol Trace Element Res* 1995;49:9–19
6. Bagchi N. Thyroid dysfunction in adults over age 55 years. *Arch Intern Med* 1990;150:785
7. Chrovato L, Minotti S, Pinchera A. Thyroid diseases in the elderly. *Baillière's Clin Endocrinol Metab* 1997;11:251–70
8. Hershman JM, Pekary AE, Berg L, *et al.* Serum thyrotropin and thyroid hormone levels in elderly and middle-aged euthyroid persons. *J Am Geriatr Soc* 1993;41:823
9. Brent GA, Hershman JM. Effects of nonthyroidal illness on thyroid function tests. In Van Middlesworth L, ed. *The Thyroid Gland.* Chicago: Year Book Medical Publishers, 1986:83
10. Figg J, Lennung M, Goodman AD, *et al.* The clinical evaluation of patients with subclinical hyperthyroidism and free triiodothyronine toxicosis. *Am J Med* 1994;96:229
11. Faughnan M, LePage R, Fugere P, Bissonnette F, Brossard JH, D'Amour P. Screening for thyroid disease at the menopausal clinic. *Clin Invest Med* 1995;18:11–18
12. Lotz H, Salabe GB. Lipoprotein(a) increase associated with thyroid autoimmunity. *Eur J Endocrinol* 1997;136:87–91
13. Doucet J, Travalle C, Chassagne P, *et al.* Does age play a role in clinical presentation of hypothyroidism? *J Am Geriatr Soc* 1994;42:984
14. Bemben DA, Hamm RM, Morgan L, *et al.* Thyroid disease in the elderly: I. Prevalence of undiagnosed hypothyroidism. *J Fam Pract* 1994;38:577
15. Buneorcius R, Kazanavicius G, Zalinkaviciars R, Prange AJ Jr. Effects of T_4 as compared with T_4 and T_3 in patients with hypothyroidism. *N Engl J Med* 1999;340:424–9
16. Biondi B, Fazio S, Carella C, *et al.* Cardiac effects of long term thyrotropin-suppressive therapy with levothyroxine. *J Clin Endocrinol Metab* 1993;77:334
17. Shapiro LE, Sievert R, Ong L, *et al.* Minimal cardiac effects in asymptomatic athyreotic patients chronically treated with thyrotropin-suppressive doses of L-thyroxine. *J Clin Endocrinol Metab* 1997;82:2592
18. Mariotti S, Barbasino G, Caturegli P, *et al.* Complex alteration of thyroid function in healthy centenarians. *J Clin Endocrinol Metab* 1993;77:1130

19. Davis PJ, Davis FB. Hyperthyroidism in patients over the age of 60 years. *Medicine* 1974;53:161

20. Trivalle C, Doucet J, Chassagne P, *et al*. Differences in the signs and symptoms of hyperthyroidism in older and younger patients. *J Am Geriatr Soc* 1996; 44:50

21. Jodar E, Mung-Jones M, Escobar-Jimenez F, Quesada-Charueco M, Lund del Castillo JD. Bone loss in hyperthyroid patients; influence of aetiology and menopause. *Clin Endocrinol* 1997;47:279–85

22. Chuang CC, Wang ST, Wang PW, Yu ML. Prevalence study of thyroid dysfunction in the elderly of Taiwan. *Gerontology* 1998;44:162–7

23. Yamada T, Aizawa T, Koizumi Y, *et al*. Age-related therapeutic response to antithyroid drugs in patients with hyperthyroid Graves' disease. *J Am Geriatr Soc* 1994;42:513

24. Franklyn JA, Maisoneuve P, Sheppard M, Betteridge J, Boyle P. Cancer incidence and mortality after radioiodine treatment for hyperthyroidism: a population-based cohort study. *Lancet* 1999;353:2111–15

25. Belfiore A. Cancer risk in patients with cold thyroid nodules: relevance of iodine intake, sex, age, and multinodularity. *Am J Med* 1990;150: 785

26. Gharib H, Goellner JR. Fine needle aspiration biopsy of the thyroid: an appraisal. *Ann Intern Med* 1993;118:282

27. Ringel MD, Ladenson PW, Levine MA. Molecular diagnosis of residual and recurrent thyroid cancer by amplification of thyroglobulin messenger ribonucleic acid in peripheral blood. *J Clin Endocrinol Metab* 1998;83:4435–42

28. Mazzaferri EL. Management of a solitary thyroid nodule. *N Engl J Med* 1993;328:553

7

Hormonal changes in the perimenopause and clinical consequences

Mason C. Andrews

Introduction

The term 'perimenopause' refers to the phase of the aging process of women preceding the menopause, during which ovarian function changes and diminishes greatly, resulting in a variety of clinical consequences.

This chapter examines the specific hormonal changes, the clinical expressions thereof and management strategies. The average age of menopause is 51 years[1]. Measurable changes in ovarian pathophysiology occur during the preceding decade. Ovarian function as expressed by fecundity decreases gradually from age 19[2]. However, this gradual decrease begins to accelerate at age 37.5 and, by age 40, results in sharply decreased spontaneous fecundity and decreased responsiveness to stimulation by exogenous gonadotropins[3-5]. After age 40 the rate of spontaneous abortions increases greatly[5]. Clinically observable changes generally begin to appear about 5 years before the final menstrual period.

Pathophysiology

Ovarian function from the standpoint of both estrogen support and reproductive function is completely dependent on the oocyte, which, surrounded by a small layer of epithelial cells, forms the primordial follicle[6]. The original seven million oocytes present in the seventh month of pregnancy decrease to two million by the time of birth. These proceed to atresia or ovulation until no more responsive primordial follicles remain. Generally by age 51, the number has been reduced to below 1000[7] and there is cessation of estrogen production. Only four to five hundred will have achieved, during a lifetime, the requisite set of conditions to produce ovulation (pituitary–ovarian sequences).

The rate of atresia monthly is relatively constant until age 37.5, when it accelerates[7]. Changes in ovarian cyclic function can be detected perhaps 5 years before clinical manifestations, as the number and quality of oocytes decline. An elevation in concentration of follicle stimulating hormone (FSH) to or above 20 mIU/ml during the first 3 days of a clinically normal cycle can be detected[4], indicating decreasing ovarian capacity and reserve. Similar results can be found in any of the conditions associated with premature menopause (endometriosis, ovarian resection, removal of a dominant ovary or immunological disease)[8].

This increased FSH level causes a rapid follicular development, probably recruiting a larger cohort of less responsive oocytes, accelerating their rate of depletion, and results in a shorter follicular phase[9,10]. However, sufficient estrogen is still produced by this failing system for a while, to trigger a luteinizing hormone (LH) surge followed by a corpus luteum, as evidenced by normal serum progesterone and a 14-day cycle (Figure 1).

Later in the perimenopause, the estradiol decreases sufficiently to fail to provide enough LH receptor induction and FSH synergy to trigger ovulation or, when ovulation does occur, to provide sufficient support to the granulosa cells necessary to produce a normal luteal phase (Figure 2)[12,13].

The results are, first, frequently unopposed estrogen stimulating the endometrium, various degrees of hyperplasia, and irregular and excessive bleeding and, second, an additional impediment to fertility.

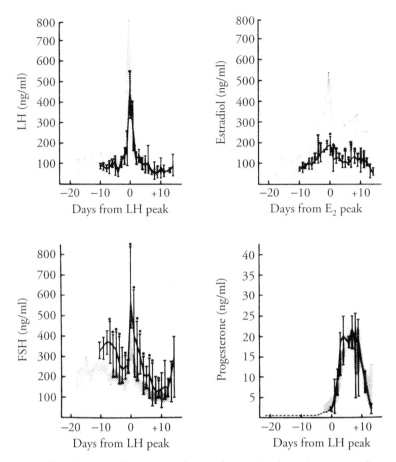

Figure 1 Perimenopausal ovulatory cycles: mean values and range in six perimenopausal women; the follicular phase is shortened to 10 days while the luteal phase remains at 15 days; follicle stimulating hormone (FSH) is higher and estradiol (E_2) is lower than normal for younger ovulatory cycling women. LH, luteinizing hormone. From reference 11, with permission

The sequence of events is quite variable during the 4 years immediately preceding the menopause, fluctuating over months and years, ovulation and regularity appearing and disappearing. Since FSH fluctuates and ovarian responsiveness varies, a single measurement is only partially predictive[14]. FSH measured on day 3 of a cycle gives a most helpful indication of ovarian status. Values of 20 mIU/ml and above with a normal estradiol level on that day are predictive of reduced ovarian capability and responsiveness[5].

The erratic estrogen production is frequently higher during this period, on average, than during years of normal cycling[15], producing clinically abnormal endometrial bleeding, and may be accompanied by vasomotor symptoms, breast soreness and emotional stress-type symptoms. The failure of this increased estrogen to oppose the rising FSH may be explained by consistently decreasing inhibin production[16] by the failing follicular apparatus, which is decreasing in quality and quantity at an accelerated rate.

An example of environmental influence on oocyte longevity may be the observation that smokers experience an earlier menopause than do non-smokers by 1.7 years[17].

An example of genetic influence on oocyte longevity is that a woman having a mother or sister with menopause before age 46 has herself an increased probability of menopause before age 46 from 5 to 25%[18].

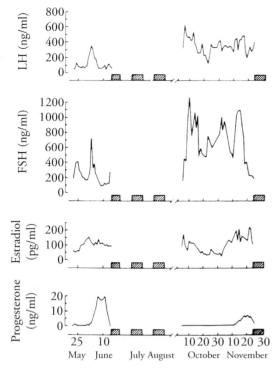

Figure 2 Perimenopausal ovulatory and anovulatory cycles in a 50-year-old woman: hatched areas indicate bleeding episodes; first cycle shows a short follicular phase with a low estradiol and high follicle stimulating hormone (FSH) and luteinizing hormone (LH) level; second cycle which is assayed shows menopausal levels of FSH and LH and an inadequate luteal phase. From reference 11, with permission

Experience with ovulation stimulation and *in vitro* fertilization (IVF) provides useful information about the diminishing ability of the ovary to respond to FSH during the 10 years preceding cessation of ovarian function, as the number and quality of oocytes is phased out. This diminished response results eventually in an inability to increase the number of follicles available for oocyte retrieval with any amount of stimulation. Of the eggs obtained and fertilized, fewer implant, compared to younger IVF patients[19]. Among the reduced number of pregnancies achieved, a much higher rate of pregnancy loss occurs. The rate of miscarriage due to diminishing steroidogenesis, which has been diminishing gradually since age 35, is lower, but that due to the quality of the aging oocytes *in vivo*[15], including a substantial increase in inappropriate chromosomes, is higher.

For these reasons, the ability to achieve a pregnancy and carry it to viability diminishes drastically after age 39[4].

Clinical consequences

Abnormal bleeding

The fluctuating, frequently elevated estrogen levels as cyclic ovarian function diminishes result in irregular and sometimes excessive vaginal bleeding. Also, as ovulatory cycles, and consequent progesterone secretion, decrease in frequency, protracted unopposed estrogen stimulation of the endometrium results in increased endometrial thickness, endometrial hyperplasia and occasionally endometrial carcinoma[20]. Coincidentally, endometrial polyps are most frequently encountered in women between 40 and 55 years of age.[21].

The prevalence of menorrhagia was found by Ballinger and colleagues to be 45% in the early perimenopause and 48% in the late perimenopause[22].

Vasomotor symptoms

It has been generally assumed that hot flushes, which are experienced by 80% of postmenopausal patients, are the result of deficient serum estrogen[23], hypothalamic response thereto by the autonomic system, and catecholamine secretion. Estrogen replacement eliminates them[24]. Sleep disturbance and irritability in estrogen-deficient women respond similarly. Estrogen antagonists (tamoxifen, raloxifene and clomiphene) produce hot flushes in a dose-related manner in varying proportions of women.

A generally accepted bioassay for physiologically adequate estrogen has been considered to be the ability of the endometrium to produce withdrawal bleeding after exposure to and withdrawal from progesterone, endogenous or exogenous. Menstruating women would seem to satisfy this test, and therefore not be at risk of hot flushes. However, Kronenberg[25] found that significant hot flushes occur in 11–60% of menstruating perimenopausal women, but specific estrogen levels in these women are not reported.

Rannevik and associates[26] found no correlation between the severity of vasomotor symptoms and levels of estradiol. However, estrogen levels were found to be lower in premenopausal women having hot flushes than in those without hot flushes[27,28]. Most postmenopausal women have consistently low estrogen levels and have no hot flushes. Prepubertal girls have low estrogen levels and have no hot flushes after the initial transitional years. Postmenopausal women who have never had estrogen levels comparable to those of cycling women (gonadal dysgenesis) do not experience hot flushes unless they are first exposed to estrogen and subsequently withdrawn from it[29]. In view of the above, one must now conclude that a common denominator in the genesis of hot flushes is a diminution in circulating estrogen or its ability to bind to estrogen receptors. The withdrawal phase of erratically fluctuating high levels of estrogen during the perimenopause may explain the rather frequent occurrence of hot flushes and some affective disorders[15] in women who are not yet estrogen deficient.

Affective disorders

The complex personal and social changes prevalent at the time of perimenopause compounded by the endocrine changes result in increased mood disturbances, including depression[30,31]. This is in contrast to previous reports[32,33], but the methodology is now more precise. The mechanism of mood lability during the perimenopause appears to be independent of vasomotor symptoms[30]. The erratic fluctuating levels of estrogen may contribute to affective disorders in the menopause. Mood swings are reported in women with implant-related high estradiol levels and vasomotor symptoms[34]. Estradiol-medicated men show greater chemical evidence of stress than unmedicated men similarly exposed[35]. The perimenopause effect on mood appears to include a different, separate effect from estrogen withdrawal, probably related to fluctuating higher levels of estrogen[30,15].

Sexual function

Perimenopausal and menopausal women remain sexually active but at a lower frequency, and with an increased frequency and severity of sexual dysfunction[36,37]. These are often modifiable by hormone replacement and counselling by generalists or specialists. Prospective and retrospective studies show a gradual decline in sexual arousal and decrease in coital frequency beginning in the perimenopause[36,38]. Lessening of sexual interest and desire, increased time required for arousal and vaginal lubrication, and decreased frequency of orgasm often begin during the perimenopausal years[39]. Loss of lubrication and health of vaginal mucosa can contribute to dyspareunia.

Estrogen deficiency may contribute to changes in sensory perception and central and peripheral nerve function[40]. Androgen reduction is a lesser factor in the perimenopausal years because the ovarian stroma continues its secretion at nearly premenopausal levels. After oophorectomy at any age the loss of testosterone may contribute to impaired libido. Androgens have a role as sex-drive facilitators[41,42]. The contribution to sexual dysfunction resulting from deficient estrogen (dyspareunia, lack of vaginal moisture, thin vaginal mucosa, vulval atrophy) can be easily reversed by administration of systemic or local estrogen. The psychosocial contributions can be reduced by identifying and improving conditions which can be modified, and by cultivating positive, supportive, appreciative interpersonal relationships. Results of serious efforts of this type can be enhanced by simultaneous supraphysiological testosterone administration (intramuscular or transdermal)[42,43].

Osteoporosis

A significant loss of bone density in the hip, vertebrae and forearm in patients experiencing continuing low levels of estrogen (menopausal values) is well documented[44]. This has been demonstrated in premenopausal patients whose serum estrogen level is reduced by medication with gonadotropin releasing hormone (GnRH) agonists or antagonists[45]. Significant and possibly irredeemable bone loss may occur during 6 months of medication. Perimenopausal patients having protracted low estrogen levels may be expected to have similar bone loss, which can be prevented by estrogen replacement. Those having menstrual cycles would be expected not to share this risk, especially in view of the increased estrogen in some[15]. However, a series of studies suggests that, overall, in unmedicated patients the rate of spinal (and sometimes femoral) bone loss in the perimenopause exceeds that found in the early menopause[15,46]. Prior[15] postulated that this difficult to understand, increased rate of bone loss may relate to elevated levels of cortisol, secondary to sleep disruption and emotional stress.

Management

A clear understanding by the patient of the range of symptoms she may encounter during the transition from cyclic ovarian function to actual menopause, and the physiological basis for them, is useful to patients and may be therapeutic. In fact, this is a good time for general assessment of her health status and a plan for the future.

This includes reassurance, information concerning the basis for symptoms as they occur and medication where appropriate. The relationship of affective and vasomotor symptoms to estrogen deficiency can be identified clinically (no menses for more than 2 months, vaginal appearance and cervical mucus) and by laboratory analysis (Pap smear maturation index, FSH > 20 mIU/ml and estradiol < 25 pg/ml), and treated by replacement. Other symptoms include hot flushes, impaired sleep, irritability and depression. Antidepressant therapy has minimal efficacy if estrogen levels are inadequate[47,48].

Estrogen doses equivalent to estradiol 0.05 mg/day transdermally and conjugated estrogens 0.625 mg/day or estradiol 1 mg/day orally are generally appropriate for replacement therapy. For patients younger than 50 years, preparations doubling this dose may be preferred. If the uterus is intact, added progestin is indicated to protect the endometrium against hyperplasia and carcinoma.

Oral synthetic progestins, most commonly medroxyprogesterone acetate 5–10 mg daily for 12 days each month of estrogen medication, achieve this goal with only occasional breakthrough bleeding. The alternative of 2.5 mg every day in the month has attained popularity because of convenience and the usual lack of bleeding after a few months of infrequent unscheduled bleeding. However, clinical trials indicate that the cyclic medication schedule is preferable from the standpoint of reduction of cardiovascular risk factors[49]. Since synthetic progestins oppose, to some extent, the beneficial effect of estrogen on high-density lipoprotein (HDL) and total cholesterol[50] and since pure progesterone does not[51], the use of progesterone for endometrial protection is appealing[52]. Micronized progesterone, 200 mg each night for 12 days each month, is attractive for reducing the cardiovascular risk factors when compared with medroxyprogesterone regimens[53]. Experiments analyzing the coronary arteries of menopausal monkeys show a strong beneficial effect from estrogen, which is reduced by medroxyprogesterone and unimpaired when pure progesterone is used instead[43,54].

The affective and vasomotor symptoms present during the erratic, frequently elevated estrogen fluctuations (usually with some menstrual function) can be modified by estrogen replacement to reduce the depth of estrogen fall, but these are best addressed, in non-smokers, by low-dose estrogen (20 µg)–progestin birth control pills which can suppress the FSH driving the system. This gives an additional benefit by providing contraceptive reassurance. Continuous rather than cyclic estrogen–progestin medication appears to be preferable to prevent mood swings[49]. For patients who must smoke, the standard postmenopausal estrogen–progestin replacement is appropriate.

Excessive and irregular bleeding is the most common symptom of the perimenopause requiring treatment. This is usually the consequence of ovulatory failure resulting in protracted unopposed estrogen, erratic fluctuating estrogen levels and estrogen withdrawal. After excluding anatomical defects and carcinoma of the endometrium, continuous low-dose estrogen–progestin birth control pills are effective. It is here assumed that any polyps will have been discovered and eliminated during the initial search for contributing anatomical defects.

Endometrial ablation or hysterectomy are last resorts, which can frequently be avoided by prophylactic treatment with a progestin-containing estrogen regimen, most conveniently a low-dose contraceptive pill.

Summary and conclusions

For about a decade before the final menstrual period, ovarian function is measurably different, although compensatory mechanisms generally prevent observable clinical changes during the first half of this time, except for a significant decrease in fertility.

The depletion of oocytes, which begins *in utero* and finally terminates ovarian estrogen production at menopause, results in laboratory and finally clinical evidence of dysfunction during the perimenopause. In spite of serum estradiol levels sufficient to produce withdrawal endometrial bleeding with or without ovulation, hot flushes, sleep disorders, affective compromise and even bone loss may occur prior to the menopause.

Unpredictable, irregular and/or heavy vaginal bleeding may occur without skipping periods. Appropriate diagnosis and treatment is important, not only to relieve these symptoms but also to reduce the risk of endometrial hyperplasia and carcinoma. Tissue sampling by office endometrial biopsy and sonographic measurement of endometrial thickness are useful.

The absence of progesterone attenuation of the endometrium due to increasingly frequent ovulation failure is a common contributor. Also, the erratic, fluctuating, frequently higher than normal estradiol serum levels contribute to abnormal bleeding as well as hot flushes, sleep impairment and affective compromise.

Replacing progesterone cyclically is a useful tool to combat abnormal bleeding. Providing a sufficient estrogen base for the endometrium makes intermenstrual bleeding less likely during the ever changing peaks and valleys which characterize estrogen production during this time. Combination estrogen–progestin low-dose contraception (20 μg) is an attractive option for non-smokers. This reduces the risk of bleeding and of endometrial carcinoma. It also eliminates hot flushes and most affective disorders attributable to estrogen fluctuations and provides contraception, reduced though fertility may be.

Elimination of hot flushes in the perimenopause and early menopause may have other important long-term health implications. A part of the beneficial effect of estrogen replacement over all menopausal years is the reduction or delay of Alzheimer's disease. The degree of benefit appears to be related to the length of replacement. In addition, evidence indicates that the replacement of estrogen in the months or years during which hot flushes would otherwise occur is especially important in reducing irreversible damage to brain cells, which would contribute to impaired function during the years ahead[55].

Another long-term health benefit of choosing low-dose estrogen–progestin contraceptive medication during the perimenopause to oppose hot flushes, abnormal bleeding, affective compromise and osteoporosis is the significantly reduced risk of ovarian carcinoma during later years. This reduction, measurable after 6 months of use, is reported to be 40% overall, and reaches 80% reduction of risk of ovarian carcinoma after more than 10 years of use[56].

The sharply reduced fertility during the perimenopause is accompanied by and apparently a result of the decreased quality of the oocytes, in spite of mobilizing larger cohorts by the increased level of FSH. These are more difficult to mobilize by exogenous FSH stimulation. They fertilize and implant less well, have a higher proportion of genetic imperfections and result in a greatly increased proportion of abortions. Supporting the luteal phase may help some patients. However, a far more rewarding health-care goal would be a life-style addressed to earlier reproduction.

References

1. Treloar AE, Boynton RE, Behn BG, Brown BW. Variation of the human menstrual cycle through reproductive life. *Int J Fertil* 1970;12: 77–126
2. Adashi E, Rock J, Rosenwaks Z. *Reproductive Endocrinology, Surgery and Technology.* Philadelphia: Lippincott Raven, 1996;2:1901
3. Muasher SJ, Oehninger S, Simonetti S, *et al.* The value of basal and/or stimulated serum gonadotropin levels in prediction of stimulation response and *in vitro* fertilization outcome. *Fertil Steril* 1988; 50:298
4. Toner JP, Philput CB, Jones GS, Muasher SJ. Basal follicle stimulating hormone level is a better predictor of *in vitro* fertilization performance than age. *Fertil Steril* 1991;55:784
5. Jones GS, Muasher SJ, Rosenwaks Z, Acosta AA, Lie H-C. The perimenopausal patient in *in vitro* fertilization: the use of gonadotropin-releasing hormone. *Fertil Steril* 1986;46:885
6. O'Rahilly R, Muller F. *Developmental Stages in Human Embryos.* Publication 637. Washington, DC: Carnegie Institute, 1987
7. Faddy MJ, Gosden RG, Gougeon A, Richardson SJ, Nelson JF. Accelerated disappearance of ovarian follicles in midlife: implications for forecasting menopause. *Hum Reprod* 1992;7:1342–6
8. Boutteville C, Muasher SJ, Acosta AA, Jones HW Jr, Rosenwaks Z. Results of *in vitro* fertilization attempts in patients with one or two ovaries. *Fertil Steril* 1987;47:821
9. Vollman RF. The menstrual cycle. In Freidman EA, ed. *Major Problems in Obstetrics and Gynecology.* Toronto: WB Saunders, 1977;7:11–193
10. Collett ME, Wertenberger GE, Fiske VM. The effect of age upon the pattern of the menstrual cycle. *Fertil Steril* 1954;5:437–48
11. Sherman BM, Korneman SG. Hormonal characteristics of the human menstrual cycle throughout reproductive life. *J Clin Invest* 1975;55:699
12. Doring GK. The incidence of anovular cycles in women. *J Reprod Fertil* 1969; (Suppl 6): 77–81
13. Metcalf MG, Donald RA. Fluctuating ovarian function in a perimenopausal woman. *NZ Med J* 1979; 89:45–7
14. Santoro N, Brown JR, Adel T, Skurnick JH. Characterization of reproductive hormonal dynamics in the perimenopause. *J Clin Endocrinol Metab* 1996;81:1495–501
15. Prior JC. Perimenopause: the complex endocrinology of the menopausal transition. *Endocr Rev* 1998;1964:417
16. Seifer DB, Gardiner AC, Lambert-Messerlian G, Schneyer AL. Differential secretion of dimeric inhibin in cultured luteinized granulosa cells as a function of ovarian reserve. *J Clin Endocrinol Metab* 1996;81(2):736–9
17. McKinlay SM, Bifano NL, McKinlay JB. Smoking and age at menopause in women. *Ann Intern Med* 1985;103:350–6
18. Cramer DW, Xu H, Harlow BL. Family history as a predictor of early menopause. *Fertil Steril* 1995;64: 740–5
19. van Koold RU, Looman WN, Habbema JDF, Dorland M, te Velde ER. Age dependent decrease in embryo implantation rate after *in vitro* fertilization. *Fertil Steril* 1996;66:769
20. Seltzer VL, Benjamin F, Deutsch S. Perimenopausal bleeding patterns and pathological findings. *J Am Med Women's Assoc* 1990;45:132
21. Jutras ML, Cowan BD. Abnormal bleeding in the climacteric. *J Obstet Gynecol Clin North Am* 1990;17: 409
22. Ballinger CB, Browning NC, Smith AHW. Hormonal profiles and psychological symptoms in perimenopausal women. *Maturitas* 1987;9: 235–51
23. Prior JC. Ovulatory disturbances: they do matter. *Can J Diagn* February 1997:64–80
24. Meldrum DR, Shamonki IM, Freeman AM, Tataryn IV, Chang RJ, Judd HL. Elevations in skin temperature of the finger as an objective index of postmenopausal hot flashes: standardization of the technique. *Am J Obstet Gynecol* 1979;135: 713–17
25. Kronenberg F. Hot flashes: epidemiology and physiology. *Ann NY Acad Sci* 1990;592:52–86
26. Rannevik G, Jeppson S, Johnell O, Bjerre B, Laurell-Borulf Y, Svanberg L. A longitudinal study of the perimenopausal transition: altered profiles of steroid and pituitary hormones, SHBG and bone mineral density. *Maturitas* 1995;21:103–13
27. Abe T, Furvhashi N, Yamaya Y, Wada Y, Hoshiai A, Suzuki M. Correlation between climacteric symptoms and serum levels of estradiol, progesterone, follicle stimulating hormone, and luteinizing hormone. *Am J Obstet Gynecol* 1977;129:65–7
28. Chakravarti S, Collins WP, Thom MH, Studd JW. Relation between plasma hormone profiles, symptoms, and responses to estrogen treatment in women approaching menopause. *Br Med J* 1979;1: 983–5
29. Casper RF, Yen SSC, Wilkes MM. Menopausal flushes: a neuroendocrine link with pulsatile luteinizing hormone secretion. *Science* 1979;205: 823–5
30. Schmidt PJ, Roca CA, Bloc HM, Rubinow DR. *Seminars in Reproductive Endocrinology* 1997;15: 91–100

31. Hay AG, Bancroft J, Johnstone EC. Affective symptoms in women attending a menopause clinic. *Br J Psychiatry* 1994;164:513–16
32. Weissman MM, Leaf PJ, Tischler GL, *et al.* Affective disorders in five United States communities. *Psychol Med* 1988;18:141–53
33. Matthews KA. Myths and realities of the menopause. *Psychosom Med* 1992;54:1–9
34. Gangar KF, Cust MP, Whitehead MI. Symptoms of estrogen deficiency associated with supraphysiological plasma estradiol concentrations in women with estradiol implants. *Br Med J* 1993;299:601–2
35. Kirschbaum C, Schommer N, Federenko I, *et al.* Short-term estradiol treatment enhances pituitary-adrenal axis and sympathetic responses to psychosocial stress in healthy young men. *J Clin Endocrinol Metab* 1996;81:3639–43
36. Bachmann GA. Sexual function in the menopause. *Obstet Gynecol North Am* 1993;20:379
37. Hagstad A. Gynecology and sexuality in middle-aged women. *Women's Health* 1988;13:57–80
38. Cutler WB, Garcia CR, McCoy N. Perimenopausal sexuality. *Arch Sex Behav* 1987;16:225–34
39. Sarrel PM. Sexuality in the middle years. *Obstet Gynecol Clin North Am* 1987;14:49–62
40. Punnonen R. Effect of castration and peroral estrogen therapy on the skin. *Acta Obstet Gynecol Scand* 1972;2(Suppl):1–44
41. Schreiner-Engel P, Schiavi RC, White D, *et al.* Low sexual desire in women: the role of reproductive hormones. *Horm Behav* 1989;23:221–34
42. Sherwin BB. Changes in sexual behavior as a function of plasma sex steroid levels in postmenopausal women. *Maturitas* 1985;7:225–33
43. Andrews MC. Primary care for post reproductive women: further thoughts concerning steroid replacement. *Am J Obstet Gynecol* 1994;170:963
44. Lindsay R, Hart DM, Clark DM. The minimum effect dose of estrogen for prevention of postmenopausal bone loss. *Obstet Gynecol* 1984;63:759–63
45. Adashi E, Rock J, Rosenwaks Z. Philadelphia: Lippincott, 1996:1666
46. Nilas L, Christiansen C. The pathophysiology of peri- and postmenopausal bone loss. *Br J Obstet Gynaecol* 1989;96:580–7
47. Page L. *Menopause and Emotions: Making Sense of your Feelings when your Feelings Make no Sense.* Vancouver: Primavera Press, 1994
48. Schneider LS. Fluoxetine Collaborative Study Group. *Am J Geriatr Psychiatry* 1997;5:97–106
49. Prior JC, Alojado N, McKay DW, Bigna YM. No adverse effects of medroxyprogesterone treatment without estrogen in postmenopausal women: Double-blind, placebo-controlled, crossover trial. *Obstet Gynecol* 1994;83:24–8
50. Hirvonen E, Malkonen M, Manninen V. Effects of different progestogens on lipoproteins during postmenopausal replacement therapy. *N Engl J Med* 1981;304:560–3
51. Kim HJ, Kalkhoff RK. Changes in lipoprotein composition during the menstrual cycle. *Metabolism* 1979;28:663–8
52. The Writing Group for the PEPI Trial. The Postmenopausal Estrogen Progestin Interventions Trial: physical and laboratory measurements (III). *J Controlled Clin Trials* 1995;16(Suppl):36S–53S
53. The Writing Group for the PEPI Trial. Effects of estrogen or estrogen/progestin regimens on heart disease risk factors in postmenopausal women: the Postmenopausal Estrogen/Progestin Intrventions (PEPI) Trial. *J Am Med Assoc* 1995;273:199–208
54. Adams MR, Kaplan JR, Manuck SB, *et al.* Inhibition of coronary artery atherosclerosis by 17-beta estradiol in ovariectomized monkeys. *Atherosclerosis* 1990;10:1051–7
55. Birge S. Hormones and the aging brain. *Geriatrics* 1998;53 (Suppl):S28–S30
56. The Cancer and Steroid Hormone Study of the CDC and NICHD. The reduction in risk of ovarian cancer associated with oral-contraceptive use. *N Engl J Med* 1987;316:650–5

8

Sex steroid hormone metabolism in the climacteric woman

Jesse J. Hade and Alan H. DeCherney

Introduction

Alterations in hormone production, metabolism and efficacy are of critical importance to the homeostasis of the climacteric woman. Imbalances in any of these processes can lead to problems involving irregular vaginal bleeding, osteoporosis, hirsutism and endometrial hyperplasia/cancer.

Menopause is defined by the World Health Organization as the complete cessation of menstruation due to the loss of ovarian follicular activity[1]. It occurs at a median age of 51.3 years and this age does not vary among different cultures or races[2]. Smoking is the only known factor that accelerates the onset of this event[3]. Variation in body size, parity, age of menarche and socioeconomic status do not influence the commencement of menopause. A total of 12 months of amenorrhea needs to elapse prior to establishing this diagnosis and labelling the woman as postmenopausal. Thus, menopause is a retrospective diagnosis.

The climacteric or 'change of life' is the term used to refer to the time interval immediately before the menopause and includes the first year after the menopause. The term climacteric is colloquially known as the perimenopausal period, and is characterized by a change in the endocrine and biological capability of the aging female. It is during this time that the capacity to reproduce fails and hormone production becomes markedly reduced. As a result, women undergo a physiological as well as a psychological transformation.

The ovary

The ovaries contain a maximum number of oocytes during fetal life. At approximately 20 weeks' gestational age the ovaries contain about 7 million germ cells, and by birth only 1–2 million germ cells remain[4]. Upon entry into puberty, the number of oocytes is reduced to 300 000–400 000[5]. A process known as atresia is responsible for this reduction in oocyte number. Although a large number of primary oocytes remain at puberty, only a small fraction mature and undergo ovulation. From menarche to menopause it is estimated that only 300–500 oocytes mature and ovulate.

In a reproductive-age woman the ovary is responsible for secreting the majority of the estrogen found in the circulation. Estrogen, which is secreted by the granulosa cells of the ovary, is predominantly in the form of 17β-estradiol[6]. The production rate of estradiol varies throughout the menstrual cycle. In the early follicular phase the daily production of estradiol can be as low as 20–40 μg/day and as high as 1000 μg/day just prior to ovulation. Estrone, a less biologically active estrogen, is formed by the peripheral conversion of androgens into estrogens[7]. This process produces about 45 μg of estrone per day and has minimal variation throughout the menstrual cycle. An insignificant amount of estradiol is produced by the peripheral conversion of dehydroisoandrosterone and testosterone[8].

Estriol is a low-potency estrogen, and is the predominant estrogen found in the plasma during pregnancy. In non-pregnant women, estriol is derived from the metabolism of estrone and estradiol. During pregnancy, fetal adrenal dehydroepiandrosterone sulfate (DHEAS) is transported to the fetal liver and converted into 16α-OHDHEAS. This hormone then proceeds to the syncytiotrophoblast cells of the placenta where it is transformed into estriol and released into the maternal circulation[9]. Since the direct synthesis of estriol only occurs during pregnancy, the production of estriol and its influence on target organs is insignificant in both the non-pregnant premenopausal and the postmenopausal woman.

The ovaries are also responsible for producing androgens and progesterone. Like estradiol, the production rates of these hormones vary during the menstrual cycle. All of these sex steroids are derived from cholesterol. They share a basic four-ring hydrocarbon skeleton and are differentiated only by their various side-chains. The capacity to convert cholesterol into a progesterone, an androgen or an estrogen depends on the ability of a target cell to accept a cholesterol molecule and then enzymatically alter its chemical configuration.

Variations in the production of these hormones occur as a result of cellular development and proliferation. During the follicular phase of the menstrual cycle, the proliferation of granulosa cells in both the dominant follicle and the cohort of developing follicles causes an increase in estradiol production. Prior to ovulation, the cohort of immature follicles undergoes atresia and provokes a decline in the production of estrogen. Upon ovulation, plasma levels of progesterone increase and the production of estrogen declines. As the corpus luteum forms, the theca interna cells become responsible for the production of estradiol. The cells known as the zona granulosa cells of the corpus luteum are responsible for the production and secretion of progesterone.

Luteinizing hormone (LH) secreted by the cells of the anterior pituitary influences the corpus luteum to continue its production of progesterone. As the level of progesterone rises, the pituitary cells are negatively affected and cause a feedback inhibition of LH production. In the absence of fertilization, the corpus luteum involutes and stops producing both estrogen and progesterone within 14 days after ovulation.

Effect of age on the menstrual cycle

As a woman ages, her bleeding pattern and menstrual cycle length change. Initially, the cycle shortens, then gradually lengthens as anovulation occurs. Eventually, menses ceases completely. Variation in cycle length can begin as early as 26 years of age[10]. However, the shortest menstrual cycles are most commonly observed 3-9 years before the menopause. The reduction in cycle length occurs as a result of a shortening of the follicular phase. These changes in menstrual pattern can last until the menopause, and are a result of follicular atresia and a reduced number of follicles[11].

One of the primary changes associated with advancing age is the loss of regular ovulatory cycles and the reduced ability of maturing follicles to respond to circulating follicle stimulating hormone (FSH)[12]. During the climacteric period, the cyclic secretion of estradiol from granulosa cells diminishes and eventually ceases. Estrone produced from the peripheral conversion of androstenedione quickly becomes the predominant circulating estrogen. It is for this reason that older women have estradiol levels that are lower throughout all parts of the menstrual cycle, when compared with younger women[13]. Just prior to the cessation of bleeding, anovulatory cycles increase in frequency and result in a lengthening of the menstrual cycle. Despite abnormal bleeding patterns during this time, ovulation may infrequently occur and result in a pregnancy.

The source and rate of hormone production change as the number of years beyond the menopause increases. Women who are less than 4 years postmenopausal are capable of secreting testosterone and a small amount of estradiol from their ovaries. Women who are late in the natural menopause (more than 4 years postmenopausal) are unable to produce ovarian estradiol but do continue to secrete testosterone and, to a lesser extent, androstenedione from the ovaries[14]. However, it is important to realize that the major source of plasma estrogens is from extraglandular aromatization of precursors in all postmenopausal women, regardless of the number of years beyond the menopause.

Production of estrogen during the climacteric and postmenopausal period

During the reproductive years there are two major sources of estrogen production. The primary source of circulating estrogen is estradiol, which is produced by the granulosa cells of the developing ovarian follicles. About 95% of circulating estradiol is produced by follicles in the ovary and the remaining 5% is created through the conversion of estrone, testosterone and androstenedione in peripheral tissues[15].

In reproductive-age women, the production of progesterone during the luteal phase of the menstrual cycle induces the enzyme estradiol 17β-hydroxysteroid dehydrogenase[16]. This enzyme is responsible for the conversion of estrone to estradiol and the metabolism of estradiol to estrone[17]. Since progesterone exerts a large influence upon this enzyme, the interconversion between estrone and estradiol is thought to decrease after the menopause. Despite the low progesterone levels during the postmenopausal period, the rate of conversion of estrone to estradiol and the metabolism of estradiol to estrone do not change[18].

DHEAS and its metabolites inhibit the activity of 17β-hydroxysteroid dehydrogenase. Conditions such as liver failure and obesity result in elevated plasma levels of DHEAS and the inhibition of 17β-hydroxysteroid dehydrogenase[19]. Ultimately, this has a profound influence upon the interconversion between estrone and estradiol, and may account for some of the hormonal variation experienced by certain aging women.

The most prominent hormonal change associated with the cessation of ovarian function is the dramatic decline in estradiol production. For the first year after the menopause there is a gradual decline of both estrone and estradiol. After the first year, plasma levels of both estrogen hormones stabilize[20]. The majority of the circulating estradiol in the plasma of postmenopausal women is derived from the peripheral conversion of estrone.

The peripheral conversion of androstenedione and testosterone contributes minimally to the circulating estradiol pool in postmenopausal women[21]. Direct secretion of estradiol from the ovary is negligible. When an oophorectomy is performed on a postmenopausal woman, her circulating level of estradiol does not change[22]. This is further supported by studies which have demonstrated similar estradiol levels in both the ovarian and the peripheral veins of postmenopausal women[23].

Direct glandular secretion of estrone by either the ovary or the adrenal gland is minimal during the postmenopausal years. Peripheral aromatization of androstenedione to estrone increases in women as they become postmenopausal[7]. Half of the estrone that is formed in postmenopausal women is metabolized into estradiol in extraglandular sites[24]. However, the majority of the estradiol that is formed by this process undergoes further metabolic conversion. Thus, only 5% of the original estrone enters the circulation as estradiol[25].

A number of different tissues possess the capability of transforming androstenedione into estrone. These tissues include adipose tissue, bone, brain, breast, hair follicles, muscle, prostate and skin[26-31]. It is speculated that estrone formation can occur in any tissue that is responsive to the actions of estrogen. Nevertheless, adipose tissue is the most important source of peripheral aromatization of androstenedione into estrone[32].

The regulation of extraglandular estrone formation is based on the production rate of androstenedione, and also on the conversion rate of androstenedione to estrone. Since aromatase activity varies with the concentration of androstenedione in the plasma, extraglandular estrone formation is directly proportional to the amount of androstenedione produced[33].

Aromatase activity in adipose tissue is present predominantly in the stromal cells and not in the adipocytes. As an individual gains weight and becomes obese, the number of stromal cells in the adipose tissue increases[34]. In contrast, when an obese individual loses weight, the number of stromal cells does not decrease[35]. The rate of aromatase activity is also controlled by hormonal factors. It has been shown that treatment of adipose tissue with glucocorticosteroids or cyclic adenosine monophosphate (AMP) analogs can increase the rate of aromatase activity as much as 50-fold[36].

With advancing age, there is an increase in the amount of androstenedione converted into estrone[7]. The portion of androstenedione converted to estrone is two to three times greater in postmenopausal woman than it is in premenopausal women. Age and obesity appear to work synergistically in promoting the extraglandular formation of estrone.

Liver disease and failure can also increase extraglandular formation of estrone. The liver is responsible for irreversibly clearing about 90% of the circulating androstenedione[37]. When the liver is incapable of performing this function, a larger fraction of androstenedione continues to circulate in the blood plasma. Thus, a larger amount of precursor (androstenedione) is available for peripheral conversion into estrone. Hyperthyroidism has also been shown to increase the extraglandular formation of estrone[38].

The clearance of estrogen from the cirulation begins in the liver. Estrogen is excreted from the body by hepatic conjugation to glucuronides and sulfates[39]. Nearly 80% of these products are then excreted in the urine and the remaining 20% in the bile. Any process that interferes with the clearance of estrogen could result in elevated levels of circulating estrogen. As a consequence, continuous unopposed estrogen stimulation may cause deleterious end-organ effects and ultimately cancer.

Change in ovarian and adrenal androgen production with advancing age

The ovary

In reproductive-age women, androstenedione is the major androgen produced by the ovary[40]. The mean plasma concentration is approximately 150 ng/dl and rises during mid-cycle by about 15%[41]. After the menopause, the plasma level of androstenedione declines by 50%. This decline in androstenedione in the postmenopausal period is comparable to that observed in younger women after bilateral oophorectomy[42].

Ovarian secretion of androstenedione continues after the menopause but is responsible for only a small fraction of the circulating androstenedione. When a bilateral oophorectomy is performed on a postmenopausal woman, the concentration of androstenedione in the peripheral circulation decreases by only 20%[42]. This is in contrast to a menstruating woman, whose ovaries are responsible for producing 50% of the plasma levels

of androstenedione. Since the metabolic clearance rate for androstenedione is not altered by age or by ovarian function, the 30% difference in androstenedione production between pre- and postmenopausal oaries reflects the declining ability of the aging ovary to produce a androstenedione[43].

During the reproductive years, approximately 50% of the circulating testosterone is derived from the peripheral conversion of androstenedione[44]. The remainder of the circulating testosterone is secreted directly by both the ovaries and the adrenal glands. Each of these glands secretes approximately 25% of the total circulating testosterone. Nearly 14% of the total circulating pool of androstenedione is converted to testosterone in normal premenopausal women.

After the menopause, the levels of androstenedione and testosterone fall, and then stabilize and remain constant[20]. The ovary becomes the major source of testosterone production and secretes more than 60% of the circulating testosterone. Still, the concentration of testosterone in postmenopausal women is 40% less than that found in the circulation of younger women[45].

Although the total plasma concentration of testosterone is decreased in postmenopausal women, the secretion of testosterone by the ovaries may in actuality increase. The increase in testosterone production may be attributed to the elevation of circulating gonadotropins. Elevated levels of gonadotropins can in turn stimulate the hilus cells and luteinized stromal cells of the ovary to secrete more androgens. Ultimately, the increase in testosterone production combined with a markedly reduced estrogen production can cause symptoms of defeminization in some women[46].

The adrenal gland

In normal menstruating women, the ovary and the adrenal cortex contribute nearly equal amounts of testosterone, dihydrotestosterone and androstenedione to the peripheral circulation. Alternatively, DHEAS is almost exclusively produced by the adrenal cortex[47]. In postmenopausal women, androstenedione is secreted almost exclusively by the adrenal glands. Androstenedione levels decrease by almost 45–50% after the menopause, and remain constant even when the ovaries are removed[48].

Plasma levels of dehydroepiandrosterone (DHEA) and DHEAS gradually decline with increasing age[49]. By the time a woman becomes menopausal, her circulating levels of DHEA, DHEAS and adrenal androgens decrease by approximately 20–40%[50]. By age 60, these levels drop by nearly 70% of their peak values[51]. Despite this decline in adrenal androgen production, the secretion of cortisol by the zona fasciculata remains unchanged in elderly women. The central control of cortisol production by both the hypothalamus and anterior pituitary remains unaffected by advancing age. This is reflected by findings of comparable circulating plasma levels of adrenocorticotropic hormone (ACTH) and cortisol in both young and elderly patients. Therefore, the decline of both DHEA and DHEAS production is caused not by a decrease in the central regulatory process of these hormones bur rather by a selective reduction in the number of functional zona reticularis cells in the adrenal cortex[52].

The adrenal glands produce more dihydrotestosterone than do the ovaries in both pre- and postmenopausal women[53]. The adrenal cortex is also the predominant source of 17-hydroxypregnenolone production[45]. The activity of the enzyme 17,20-desmolase is reduced in postmenopausal women. As a result, the adrenal glands' ability to convert C-21 progestins into C-19 androgens is diminished[54].

Progesterone production

In reproductive-age women, the concentration of progesterone rises sharply after ovulation. The granulosa cells or the corpus luteum are responsible for the secretion of progesterone. However, in the follicular phase, the majority of the progesterone is derived from extraglandular conversion of adrenal pregnenolone and pregnenolone sulfate. The contribution of the ovaries to the plasma levels of progesterone is small during this phase of the menstrual cycle.

In postmenopausal women, the site of progesterone production is controversial. Some authorities contend that the ovaries produce a small portion of the total progesterone, while others refute

this notion[55]. Postmenopausal women who have undergone a bilateral oophorectomy will display a sustained progesterone level that is consistent with that of postmenopausal women who have both ovaries. The administration of dexamethasone to postmenopausal women can reduce the level of circulating progesterone to an undetectable concentration. In addition, the administration of ACTH can stimulate progesterone production in these women by as much as 500%[56]. However, human chorionic gonadotropin (hCG) administration does not alter the concentration of progesterone in postmenopausal women with intact ovaries. Therefore, the ability of the ovary to produce progesterone is limited, at best.

In menstruating women, the source of 17-hydroxyprogesterone (17-OHP) is both the ovaries and the adrenal glands. The circulating level of 17-OHP during the follicular phase is low. It rises after ovulation and then peaks during the mid-luteal phase[57]. When measured in the plasma of postmenopausal women, the concentration of 17-OHP is similar to the values observed during the follicular phase of menstruating women. Like progesterone, 17-OHP appears to be secreted predominantly by the adrenal glands in postmenopausal women[58].

Inhibin production

Inhibin is a glycoprotein hormone that is produced by the granulosa cells of a preovulatory follicle. The corpus luteum also produces and secretes inhibin. During the mid-luteal phase, inhibin levels rise and quickly reach its maximum concentration. This mid-luteal rise in circulating inhibin is believed to prevent other follicles from precocious maturation[59].

Inhibin can act directly on the cells of the anterior pituitary and inhibit the synthesis and release of FSH[60]. As the total number of follicles diminishes throughout the span of a woman's life, concentrations of inhibin diminish and cause an elevation in the serum levels of FSH. Elevated levels of FSH may thus be a marker of declining follicular numbers[61].

During the climacteric period, some women will demonstrate regular menstrual periods despite having persistently elevated FSH levels. These FSH levels remain high as a result of reduced inhibin levels. Unlike younger women, perimenopausal women tend to have reduced levels of inhibin in all phases of the menstrual cycle. However, after the menopause, inhibin becomes undetectable in the circulation, and only high levels of FSH can be found[62].

Two forms of inhibin exist: inhibin-b, which is primarily produced by granulosa cells during the early follicular phase and inhibin-a, which is produced late in the follicular phase, and also by the corpus luteum. The rise in the day-3 FSH noted in older women is associated with a decrease in inhibin-b production but not of inhibin-a[63]. As ovaries age, there is a decrease in both inhibin-a and inhibin-b production. This decline of dimeric inhibin production is associated with an elevation of follicular phase FSH levels. In fact, a decline in luteal phase inhibin-a and follicular phase inhibin-b values correlates more consistently with chronological age than does a day-3 FSH value[64].

Hypothalamus and pituitary

In ovulatory women, there is a co-ordinated pulsatile release of both FSH and LH. This pulsatile release is mediated by factors modulating both the hypothalamus and the ovary. In response to the pulsatile release of the gonadotropins, the ovary undergoes monthly synthesis and secretion of estrogen and progesterone, which ultimately feedback and alter the stimulation of the hypothalamus and pituitary.

The hypothalamus is responsible for the pulsatile release of gonadotropin-releasing hormone (GnRH) and the overall regulation of the menstrual cycle in reproductive-age women. Pulsatile release of GnRH is controlled by a combination of neurotransmitters and neuromodulators within the central nervous system. Neuromodulators, such as opioids, influence control over the hypothalamus by decreasing the rate of GnRH pulsation. The hypothalamus is able to communicate with the anterior pituitary via the portal circulation to stimulate the secretion of both LH and FSH. This relationship between the hypothalamus and the pituitary is represented in Figure 1.

Each month, FSH influences a select cohort of primordial follicles to mature into secondary follicles. As these follicles mature, they undergo cellular changes to form a granulosa cell layer. The theca cell layer configures into two layers of cells called the theca interna and the theca externa. The theca externa consists of vascularized connective tissue and has no endocrinological role. The theca interna, which contains LH receptors, allows cholesterol to enter into these cells and then metabolize into androstenedione. This androgen then passes from the theca interna cells into the granulosa cells. The granulosa cells contain the aromatase enzyme and convert androstenedione into estradiol.

As women age and enter into the climacteric period, the levels of FSH and estradiol change. Initially, there is an early rise in both FSH and estradiol in the menstrual cycle, reflecting a decline in the number of functional ovarian follicles. With further aging and follicular depletion, levels of ovarian inhibin decline, resulting in elevated levels of FSH coupled with low estradiol levels. Climacteric women can also have elevated levels of FSH during the luteal phase. This causes premature follicular recruitment and development, and ultimately inadequate estradiol production in the dominant follicle[65]. However, the ovulatory capacity of these women is maintained, and the luteal phase length and secretion of progesterone from the corpus luteum are similar to those of a younger woman.

In the late climacteric period, FSH levels can increase as high as ten to 20-fold above baseline. LH levels, however, do not fluctuate during the climacteric period, and only become elevated after the menopause. Despite a nearly 20-fold rise in FSH levels, LH rises only three to five-fold after the menopause[66]. Women who are 15 or more years postmenopausal experience a decline in LH level to below that of a premenopausal women[67]. Alone, levels of gonadotropins are not useful in determining whether a woman is menopausal or not. Hormonal events are too unpredictable during the climacteric period, and thus cannot be used to determine the true ovulatory status of a woman.

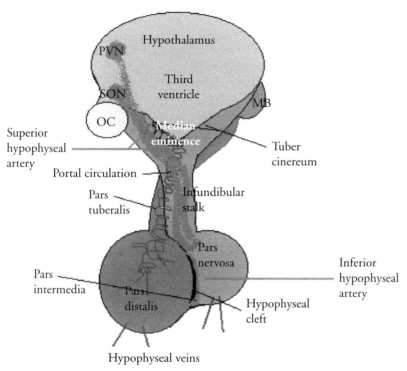

Figure 1 Relationship between the hypothalamus and the pituitary. PVN, paraventricular nucleus; SON, supraoptic nucleus; OC, optic chiasma

Sex hormone transport within the circulation

Sex hormones are transported in the bloodstream either bound to a carrier protein or free in the circulation. Carrier proteins include sex hormone-binding globulin (SHBG) and albumin. These proteins bind to the different sex steroids and make them water-soluble for transport. Only the unbound free-floating hormones can enter the cell and bind to specific receptors on the nuclear membrane. The various tissues, which contain specific estrogen receptors, include the brain, uterus, vagina, vulva, skin, urethra, bladder trigone, bones, breasts, liver and elastic arteries[68].

The main factor that influences the concentration of circulating free hormones is the serum concentration of SHBG. There is a strong negative correlation between body mass index and SHBG levels[69]. As the body mass index increases, the production of SHBG decreases and, therefore, allows more free hormones to circulate within the bloodstream. Older women in general have a higher body mass index than do younger women, and thus lower SHBG levels and more circulating free hormones.

Peripheral hormone conversion

Aromatase in fat tissue is responsible for converting androstenedione to estrone. Other tissues that are capable of doing this include bone, muscle, hair and brain. Factors that increase aromatase activity include obesity, liver disease, hyperthyroidism, compensated congestive heart failure and starvation.

In postmenopausal women, the production of estrogen is almost exclusively from extraglandular aromatization of androstenedione to estrone[43]. Little, if any, estrogen is secreted directly by the adrenals or ovaries. The biologically weaker estrogen, estrone, is produced at a much greater rate than the more potent estrogen, estradiol. The preponderance of circulating estradiol in post-menopausal women is derived from the peripheral conversion of estrone[21]. The metabolic clearance rate of estradiol does not differ between premenopausal and postmenopausal women[21]. In non-obese women, the production of estrone is 40-50 µg/day. However, when the daily production rate of estrone exceeds 70-75 µg/day, uterine bleeding usually occurs[70].

Conclusion

Women go through many biological changes throughout their lives. A delicate balance of hormone production and clearance exists throughout these various stages. When an imbalance occurs, problems may arise. However, exogenous estrogens, progesterones and androgens can correct these imbalances and restore the natural steady state.

References

1. WHO Scientific Group. Research on the menopause. *WHO Tech Rep Ser* 1981:670
2. McKinlay SM, Brambilla DJ, Posner JG. The normal menopause transition. *Maturitas* 1992;14:103-15
3. Richardson SJ. The biological basis of the menopause. *Baillière's Clin Endocrinol Metab* 1993;7:1-16
4. Baker TG. A quantitative and cytological study of germ cells in the human ovaries. *Proc R Soc London B (Biol)* 1963;158:417-33
5. Ohno S, Klinger HP, Atkin NB. Human oogenesis. *Cytogenetics* 1962;1:42
6. Zhang Y, Word A, Fesmire S, *et al.* Human ovarian expression of 17β-hydroxysteroid dehydrogenase types 1, 2, and 3. *J Clin Endocrinol Metab* 1996;81:3594-8
7. Hemsell DL, Grodin JM, Brenner PF, *et al.* Plasma precursors of estrogen. II. Correlation of the extent of conversion of plasma androstenedione to estrone with age. *J Clin Endocrinol Metab* 1974;38:476-9
8. MacDonald PC, Edman CD, Kerber IJ, *et al.* Plasma precursors of estrogen. III. Conversion of plasma dehydroisoandrosterone to estrogen in young non-pregnant women. *Gynecol Invest* 1976;7:165-75
9. Pepe GJ, Albrecht ED. Transutero placental metabolism of cortisol and cortisone during mid and late gestation in the baboon. *Endocrinology* 1984;115:1946-51
10. Treloar AE, Boynton RE, Behn BG, Brown BW. Variation of the human menstrual cycle through reproductive life. *Int J Fertil* 1967;12:77-126
11. Barbo DM. The physiology of the menopause. *Med Clin North Am* 1987;71:11-22
12. Sherman BM, West JH, Korenman SG. The menopause transition: analysis of LH, FSH, estradiol, and progesterone concentrations during menstrual cycles of older women. *J Clin Endocrinol Metab* 1976;42:629-36
13. Sherman BM, Korenman SG. Hormonal characteristics of the human menstrual cycle throughout reproductive life. *J Clin Invest* 1975;55:699-706
14. Vermeulen A. Sex hormone status of the postmenopausal woman. *Maturitas* 1980;2:81-9
15. Hammond CB. Climacteric. In Scott JR, DiaSaia PJ, Hammond CB, *et al.* eds. *Danforth's Obstetrics and Gynecology*, 7th edn. Philadelphia: JB Lippincott, 1994:771-90
16. Tseng L, Gurpide E. Induction of endometrial estradiol dehydrogenase by progestins. *Endocrinology* 1975;97:825
17. Labrie F, Luu-The V, Lin SX, *et al.* The key role of 17β-HSDs in sex steroid biology. *Steroids* 1997;62:148-58
18. Reed MJ, Beranek PA, Ghilchik MW, James HT. Conversion of estrone to estradiol and estradiol to estrone in postmenopausal women. *Obstet Gynecol* 1985;66:361-5
19. Bonney RC, Reed MJ, James VHT. Inhibition of 17β-hydroxysteroid dehydrogenase activity in human endometrium by adrenal androgens. *J Steroid Biochem* 1983;18:59
20. Longcope C, Franz C, Morello C, Baker R, Johnston CC. Steroid and gonadotropin levels in women during the peri-menopausal years. *Maturitas* 1986;8:189-96
21. Judd HL, Shamonki JM, Frumar AM, *et al.* Origin of serum estradiol in postmenopausal women. *Obstet Gynecol* 1982;59:680-6
22. Judd HL, Lucas WE, Yen SSC. Serum 17β-estradiol and estrone levels in postmenopausal women with

and without endometrial cancer. *J Clin Endocrinol Metab* 1976;43:272–8

23. Judd HL, Lucas WE, Yen SSC. Effect of oophorectomy on circulating testosterone and androstenedione levels in patients with endometrial cancer. *Am J Obstet Gynecol* 1974;118:793–8

24. MacDonald PC, Madden JD, Brenner PF, *et al.* Origin of estrogen in normal men and in women with testicular feminization. *J Clin Endocrinol Metab* 1979;49:905–16

25. Gurpide E. Hormones and gynecologic cancer. *Cancer* 1976;38(Suppl 1):503–8

26. Frisch RE, Canick JA, Tulchinsky D. Human fatty marrow aromatizes androgen to estrogen. *J Clin Endocrinol Metab* 1980;51:394–6

27. Naftolin F, Tyan K, Petro Z. Aromatization of androstenedione by the diencephalon. *J Clin Endocrinol Metab* 1971;33:368–70

28. Perel E, Wilkins D, Killinger DW. The conversion of androstenedione to estrone, estradiol and testosterone in breast tissue. *J Steroid Biochem* 1980;13:89–94

29. Schweikert HU, Milewich L, Wilson JD. Aromatization of androstenedione by isolated human hairs. *J Clin Endocrinol Metab* 1975;40:413–17

30. Longcope C, Pratt JH, Schneider SH, *et al.* Aromatization of androgens by muscle and adipose tissue *in vivo*. *J Clin Endocrinol Metab* 1978;46:146–52

31. Schweikert HU. Conversion of androstenedione to estrone in human fibroblasts cultured from prostate, genital and nongenital skin. *Horm Metab Res* 1979;11:635–40

32. Perel E, Killinger DW. The interconversion and aromatization of androgens by human adipose tissue. *J Steroid Biochem* 1979;10:623–7

33. Aiman EJ, Edman CD, Worley RJ, *et al.* Androgen and estrogen formation in women with ovarian hyperthecosis. *Obstet Gynecol* 1978;51:1–9

34. Klyde BJ, Hirsch J. Increased cellular proliferation in adipose tissue of adult rats fed a high fat diet. *J Lipid Res* 1979;20:705–15

35. Siiteri PK, Williams JE, Takaki NK. Steroid abnormalities in endometrial and breast carcinoma: a unifying hypothesis. *J Steroid Biochem* 1976;7:897–903

36. Mendelson CR, Cleland WH, Smith ME, *et al.* Regulation of aromatase activity of stromal cells derived from human adipose tissue. *Endocrinology* 1982:1077–85

37. Rivarola MA, Singleton RT, Mignon CJ. Splanchnic extraction and interconversion of testosterone and androstenedione in man. *J Clin Invest* 1967;46:2096–100

38. Southern AL, Olivo J, Gordon GG, *et al.* The conversion of androgens to estrogens in hyperthyroidism. *J Clin Endocrinol Metab* 1974;38:207–14

39. Stumpf PG. Pharmacokinetics of estrogen. *Obstet Gynecol* 1990;75:9s–14s

40. Bardin CW, Lipsett MB. Testosterone and androstenedione blood production rates in normal women and women with idiopathic hirsutism or polycystic ovaries. *J Clin Invest* 1967;46:891–902

41. Judd HL, Yen SSC. Serum androstenedione and testosterone levels during the menstrual cycle. *J Clin Endocrinol Metab* 1973;36:475–81

42. Judd GE, Lucas WE, Yen SSC. Endocrine function of the postmenopausal ovary: concentrations of androgens and estrogens in ovarian and peripheral vein blood. *J Clin Endocrinol Metab* 1974;39:1020–4

43. Grodin JM, Siiteri PK, MacDonald PC. The source of estrogen production in postmenopausal women. *J Clin Endocrinol Metab* 1973;36:207–14

44. Horton R, Tait JF. Androstenedione production and interconversion rates measured in peripheral blood and studies on the possible site of its conversion to testosterone. *J Clin Invest* 1966;45:301–13

45. Maroulis GB, Abraham GE. Ovarian and adrenal contributions to peripheral steroid levels in postmenopausal women. *Obstet Gynecol* 1976;48:150–4

46. Judd HL, Fournet N. Change of ovarian hormonal function with aging. *Exp Gerontol* 1994;29:285–98

47. Abraham GE. Ovarian and adrenal contribution to peripheral androgens during the menstrual cycle. *J Clin Endocrinol Metab* 1974;39:340

48. Chang RJ, Judd HL. The ovary after menopause. *Clin Obstet Gynecol* 1981;24:181–91

49. Ravaglia G, Forti P, Maidi F. The relationship of dehydroepiandrosterone sulfate (DHEAS) to endocrine-metabolic parameters and functional status in the oldest-old. *J Clin Endocrinol Metab* 1996;81:1173

50. Belanger A, Candas B, Dupont A, *et al.* Changes in serum concentrations of conjugated and unconjugated steroids in 40- to 80-year-old men. *J Clin Endocrinol Metab* 1994;79:1086–90

51. Labrie F, Belanger A, Cusan L, Candas B. Physiological changes in DHEA are not reflected by the serum levels of active androgens and estrogens but of their metabolites: intracrinology. *J Clin Endocrinol Metab* 1997;82:2403–9

52. Herbert J. The age of dehydroepiandrosterone. *Lancet* 1995;345:1193

53. Coyoputa J, Parlow AF, Abraham GE. Simultaneous radioimmunoassay of plasma testosterone and dihydrotestosterone. *Anal Lett* 1972;5:329–40

54. Meldrum DR, Davidson BJ, Tataryn IV, Judd HL. Changes in circulating steroids with aging in postmenopausal women. *Obstet Gynecol* 1981;57:624–8

55. Dennefors BL. Hilus cells from human postmenopausal ovaries: gonadotropin sensitivity, steroid and cyclic AMP production. *Acta Obstet Gynecol Scand* 1982;61:413–16

56. Vermeulen A, Verdonck L. Sex hormone concentration in postmenopausal women. *Clin Endocrinol* 1978;9:59–66

57. Abraham GE, Odell WD, Swerdloff RS, Hopper K. Simultaneous radioimmunoassay of plasma FSH,

LH, progesterone, 17-hydroxyprogesterone, and estradiol-17β during the menstrual cycle. *J Clin Endocr* 1972;34:312–18

58. Vermeulen A. The hormonal activity of the post-menopausal ovary. *J Clin Endocrinol Metab* 1976;42:247–53

59. McLachlan RI, Robertson DM, Healey DL, Burger HD, Kretser DM. Circulating immunoreactive inhibin levels during the normal human menstrual cycle. *J Clin Endocrinol Metab* 1987;65:954–61

60. McLachlan RI, Robertson DM, De Krestser DM, Burger HG. Advances in the physiology of inhibin and inhibin-related peptides. *Clin Endocrinol* 1988;29:77–101

61. Burger HG. Diagnostic role of follicle-stimulating hormone (FSH) measurements during the menopausal transition – an analysis of FSH, estradiol and inhibin. *Eur Endocrinol* 1994;130:38–42

62. Buckler HM, Evans CA, Mamtora H, Burger HG, Anderson DC. Gonadotropin, steroid, and inhibin levels in women with incipient ovarian failure during anovulatory and ovulatory rebound cycles. *J Clin Endocrinol Metab* 1991;72:116–24

63. Klein NA, Illinworth PJ, Groome NP, McNeilly AS, Bataglia DE, Soules MR. Decreased inhibin B secretion is associated with the monotropic FSH rise in older, ovulatory women: a study of serum and follicular fluid levels of dimeric inhibin A and B in spontaneous menstrual cycles. *J Clin Endocrinol Metab* 1996;81:2742–5

64. Danforth DR, Arbogast LK, Mroueh J, *et al.* Dimeric inhibin: a direct marker of ovarian aging. *Fertil Steril* 1998;70:119–23

65. Metcalf MD, Livesey JH. Gonadotropin excretion in fertile women: effect of age and the onset of the menopausal transition. *J Endocrinol* 1985;105:357–62

66. Wide L, Nillus JS, Gemzell C, *et al.* Radioimmunosorbent assay of follicle-stimulating hormone and luteinizing hormone in serum and urine from men and women. *Acta Endocrinol* 1973;174(Suppl):7–58

67. Chakravarti S, Collins WP, Forecast JD, *et al.* Hormonal profiles after the menopause. *Br Med J* 1976;2:281–6

68. Bolognia JL, Braverman IM, Rousseau ME, *et al.* Skin changes in menopause. *Maturitas* 1989;11:295–304

69. Rannevik G, Jeppsson S, Johnell O, Bjerre B, Laurell-Borulf Y, Svanberg L. A longitudinal study of the perimenopausal transition: altered profiles of steroid and pituitary hormones, SHBG and bone mineral density. *Maturitas* 1995;21:103–13

70. MacDonald PC, Grodin JM, Siiteri PK. The utilization of plasma androstenedione for estrone production in women. In *Progress in Endocrinology. Proceedings of the Third International Congress of Endocrinology.* Amsterdam: Excerpta Medica Int Cong Series 184, 1969:770–6

9

Infertility in the older woman

Brian M. Berger

Introduction

A dramatic increase in the numbers of US women with impaired fecundity has occurred over the past decade. This is largely due to the baby-boom cohort of women, many of whom delayed child-bearing, reaching their later and less fecund reproductive years[1]. A recent study projected that the number of women experiencing infertility will range from 5.4 to 7.7 million in 2025, with the most likely number being just under 6.5 million[2]. This is a substantial revision (upwards) in the number of infertile women, largely a result of the increase in the observed percentage of infertile women in 1995[3]. This increase in both rates and numbers has made advanced age the leading cause of infertility in the USA.

Aging, in particular the effect of decreased ovarian reserve and possibly uterine senescence, causes a decreased natural fecundity rate, and adversely affects the success rates of fertility therapy in women over age 35. Pre-stimulation testing has become an important part of infertility management in older women, along with preconceptual counselling on the likelihood of achieving a live birth and the risks of pregnancy at advanced maternal age. Many strategies have been devised in order to improve the chances of achieving a live birth in older women using their own oocytes. In addition, oocyte donation is a highly successful alternative treatment for patients with reduced ovarian function. Finally, new experimental technologies show great promise and may change the spectrum of fertility care in the 21st century.

An overview of fertility

Female life expectancy is higher at birth and at age 65 than the corresponding male life expectancies in the USA – and in most developed countries[4]. Current estimates project that women will live an average of 90 years by the year 2020[5]. However, while women are living longer than ever before, the age of menopause has not changed, occurring at approximately 51 years in the USA[6-8]. The age of menopause and of the preceding reproductive events such as the beginning of subfertility and infertility are likely to be dictated by the process of follicle depletion, leading to loss of oocyte quantity and quality. To some extent this process is influenced by life-style factors such as smoking, and possibly also by the use of oral contraceptives[7,9].

Women can expect to live one-half of their adult lives beyond the menopause, and experience a decline in fertility that precedes the menopause by several years. Therefore, women are infertile for over half of their life expectancy. The advent of assisted reproductive technology (ART) has allowed many women to conceive in situations that were unimaginable only a few years ago. This, in turn, has created numerous medical and ethical dilemmas that we will continue to address well into the next century.

Ovarian function with aging

Whether reproductive aging is an intrinsic ovarian process or the ovary is simply responding to exogenous influences, the ovary in general and its follicles in particular are the primary site of the effects of aging. Ovarian follicles in older ovulatory women have some unique features:

(1) The follicles are the same size as those in younger women, but form more rapidly;

(2) Secretion of estradiol and inhibin is not compromised;

(3) The concentrations of steroids in the follicular fluid are indicative of a healthier follicle, i.e. increased progesterone levels and higher estrogen/androgen ratio;

(4) Serum and follicular fluid levels of insulin-like growth factor-I (IGF-I) are decreased, but there are no differences in IGF-II levels[10].

Older reproductive-age women also have accelerated development of a dominant follicle in the presence of a monotropic follicle stimulating hormone (FSH) rise[11]. This is manifested as a shortened follicular phase and elevated follicular phase estradiol level[12]. The fact that ovarian steroid and inhibin secretion are similar to those in younger women suggests that elevated FSH in women of advanced reproductive age may represent a primary neuroendocrine change, in addition to the ovarian changes associated with reproductive aging.

Female fecundity

Female fertility, in sharp contrast to male fertility[13], is known to decline as early as the third decade of life, with a steep decline after age 35[14]. Age as an independent prognosticator of infertility has been clearly demonstrated[15]. Fertility becomes significantly compromised long before overt clinical signs occur, such as cycle irregularity. The FSH level has been shown to increase sharply with age[16]. Although women are not considered to be menopausal until the cessation of menses for at least 6 months, the FSH level begins to rise at least 5–10 years prior to the menopause. Scott and colleagues[17] showed that FSH measured on the third day of the menstrual cycle was a strong predictor of success rates associated with *in vitro* fertilization (IVF), with levels over 15 mIU/ml predicting poor pregnancy rates. Older women have a significantly shorter follicular phase length associated with an early acute rise in follicular phase estradiol, reflecting accelerated development of a dominant follicle. This is manifested as a shortened follicular phase and elevated FSH and estradiol levels[18]. Investigators have shown that an estradiol measurement on day 3 of the menstrual cycle combined with the day 3 FSH level improves upon the prognostic ability of the measurement of either of these hormones alone[19].

Miscarriage and aneuploidy

Genes and exposures affecting pool size, hormonal homeostasis and interactions between oocytes and their somatic compartment have the potential critically to influence chromosome distribution in female meiosis and affect fertility in humans and other mammals. Much of the decline in fecundity can be attributed to an increasing risk of fetal loss with maternal age[20]. Most of this fetal loss is a result of chromosomal abnormalities: a consequence of aging oocytes. Errors in chromosome segregation are most frequent in meiosis I of oogenesis in mammals, and predominantly predispose specific chromosomes and susceptible chiasmate configurations to maternal age-related non-disjunction[21]. Baseline serum FSH and/or estradiol concentrations may be valuable as predictors of fetal aneuploidy[22]. In morphologically and developmentally normal human embryos, cleavage-stage aneuploidy significantly increases with maternal age[23]. The results suggest that implantation failure in older women is largely due to aneuploidy.

One study analyzed 201 clinical pregnancies in which cardiac activity had been documented by transvaginal ultrasound 35–42 days after ovulation in a previously infertile population treated at a tertiary fertility center[24]. A profound increase in spontaneous abortion rates occurred as a function of maternal age in this population (χ^2 for trend = 15.1). A spontaneous abortion rate of 2.1% was observed for maternal ages ≤35 years, but this rate increased to 16.1% for patients ≥36 years (odds ratio 8.72; 95% confidence interval 2.3–32.9). A five-fold increase in spontaneous abortion rate was observed in women ≥40 years, compared to women 31–35 years (3.8% vs. 20.0%). The incidence of pregnancy loss after confirmation of early fetal cardiac activity by transvaginal ultrasound is substantially greater in infertile patients than previously reported, when considered as a function of maternal age. In particular, patients ≥36 years should be counselled that their risk of spontaneous abortion is significant, even after fetal heart motion is detected on transvaginal ultrasound.

Fertility treatment

The effectiveness of controlled ovarian hyperstimulation together with intrauterine insemination has been established in a meta-analysis[25] and recently in a large prospective study. Guzick and colleagues[26] found that, among infertile couples, treatment with induction of superovulation and intrauterine insemination is three times as likely to result in pregnancy as is intracervical insemination, and twice as likely to result in pregnancy as is treatment with either superovulation and intracervical insemination or intrauterine insemination alone. The treatment, however, appears to be less effective in women over age 40. Pearlstone and co-workers[27] showed, in a prospective analysis of 402 cycles in 85 women age 40 and older, a clinical pregnancy rate of 3.5% per cycle (95% confidence interval (CI) 1.7–5.3%). The live-birth rate was 1.2% per cycle (95% CI 0.1–2.3%). Women with a basal FSH level < 25 mIU/ml and age < 44 years had a clinical pregnancy rate of 5.2% per cycle (95% CI 2.5–7.9%), compared with 0.0% per cycle (95% CI 0.0–2.1%) in cases in which either basal FSH was ≥ 25 mIU/ml or age was ≥ 44 ($p < 0.005$).

The IVF data are slightly better for women over 40; however, the data for women over age 42 are only marginally improved. Lass and colleagues[28] studied 471 women over age 40 undergoing 1087 cycles of IVF. A total of 842 cycles reached oocyte retrieval (77.5%) and 702 had embryos transferred (64.6%). The pregnancy rate was significantly lower in women ≥ 40 years of age than in a control group of women < 40 years of age (11.3% vs. 28.2%). It decreased sharply in women > 42 years of age, and no women > 45 years of age had a child. In addition, women ≥ 40 years of age were more likely to miscarry (27% vs. 12.7%). Yaron and co-workers[29] studied 31 patients over age 45 who underwent 52 treatment cycles in standard IVF. Of the 52 standard IVF cycles, oocytes were retrieved successfully in only 32. Of these, fertilization and embryo transfer were performed in 21 cycles. None of these treatment cycles resulted in a clinical pregnancy.

Strategies to increase response in poor responders undergoing IVF

Poor responders are defined as patients who fail to achieve an estradiol level greater than 500 pg/ml on the day of human chorionic gonadotropin (hCG) administration (luteinizing hormone, LH surge simulation), and in whom no more than three oocytes are obtained. Currently, most IVF cycles are carried out using a long protocol of gonadotropin releasing hormone (GnRH) down-regulation, using GnRH analogs prior to stimulation with gonadotropins[30]. Because pregnancy rates in patients over age 40 have been correlated with the response to gonadotropin stimulation and therefore the number of embryos transferred[31], the standard IVF protocol regimen has been modified to increase the number of oocytes retrieved and thereby increase success rates in poor responders.

One of the most successful regimens uses down-regulation with oral contraceptives combined with microdose GnRH-analog (GnRH-a) administration[32]. Surrey and associates[33] found that a low-dose oral contraceptive (for 21 days) followed by a GnRH-a (leuprolide acetate, 40 µg subcutaneously twice a day) flare and gonadotropin initiated on day 3 of GnRH-a administration statistically increased maximal estradiol levels as well as clinical and ongoing pregnancy rates. Using the same regimen, Scott and Navot[34] found that the patients had a more rapid rise in estradiol levels, much higher peak estradiol levels, the development of more mature follicles, and the recovery of larger numbers of mature oocytes at the time of retrieval. Although these data are encouraging, the effect of this regimen on pregnancy rate and live-birth rate has not conclusively been shown to be statistically different.

Oocyte donation

When oocytes from young women are used to create embryos for transfer to older recipients, implantation and pregnancy rates mimic those seen in younger individuals[35]. Furthermore, following oocyte donation, the number of miscarriages and chromosomal anomalies dramatically decreases. These results strongly suggest that the pregnancy wastage experienced by older women is largely a result of degenerative changes within the aging oocyte. There are data to suggest that pregnancy rates do not depend merely on oocyte age and quality but also on senescent changes in the uterus, for example diminished endometrial receptivity[36]. Whether or not the uterus plays a role in success rates, the poor prognosis for fertility in older women can largely be reversed through oocyte donation from younger individuals.

New technologies

One of the effects of aging is a thickening of the zona pellucida resulting in a failure to hatch and implant. Assisted hatching (AH), probably the most frequently applied clinical embryo micromanipulation procedure, may enhance embryo implantation not only by mechanically facilitating the hatching process but also by allowing earlier embryo–endometrium contact. However, considerable heterogeneity of the studies that have examined the effects of AH does not permit definitive conclusions to be drawn regarding its efficacy. The method usually employed involves the release of acidified Tyrode's medium against the zona pellucida to create an opening approximately 20 μm in diameter. According to one study[37], the outcome of AH is largely dependent on the mode by which the zona pellucida is breached, the size of the artificial gap and the thickness of the zona pellucida, as embryos with zonae thicker than 17 μm rarely implant.

Schoolcraft and colleagues[38] showed that the delivery rate per oocyte retrieval was significantly higher in the AH group (18/38, 48%), compared to the non-hatched controls (3/28, 11%; $p = 0.0003$). Magli and associates[39] showed that with AH, the percentage of clinical pregnancies per cycle was significantly higher in patients over 38 years old than in controls (31% vs. 10% in controls; $p < 0.05$), and in patients with more than three IVF failures than in controls (36% vs. 17% in controls; $p < 0.05$). Tucker and co-workers[40] showed that in female patients aged ≥ 35 years, AH appeared to convey a marginally significant benefit in terms of both the viable pregnancy rate (35.5% AH vs. 11.1% controls) and the embryonic implantation rate (10.3% AH vs. 3.1% controls). Hellebaut and colleagues[41] showed that pregnancy and implantation rates in the groups with and without AH were, respectively, 42.1% vs. 38.1% and 17.9% vs. 17.1%, concluding that AH through partial zona dissection prior to embryo transfer does not improve pregnancy and embryo implantation rates in unselected patients undergoing IVF with or without intracytoplasmic sperm injection (ICSI). Lanzendorf and associates[42] also showed no significant differences in the rates of implantation (11.1% vs. 11.3%), clinical pregnancy (39.0% vs. 41.7%) and ongoing pregnancy (29.3% vs. 35.4%) between the hatched and control groups, respectively. These results suggest that AH may have a significant impact on IVF success rates only in a select subset of older patients.

Experimental technologies

Some oocytes are unable to fertilize and/or develop into normal embryos. It may be possible that the problem is with the machinery of cytoplasm of the oocyte[43]. Therefore, cytoplasmic transfer from a normal oocyte to an abnormal oocyte may overcome the problem. Thus far, only two deliveries have been reported using this technique[44].

Mitochondrial transfer may be another way of enhancing the reproductive potential of older oocytes. Mitochondrial dysfunctions resulting from a variety of intrinsic and extrinsic influences, including genetic abnormalities, hypoxia and oxidative stress, can profoundly influence the level of adenosine triphosphate (ATP) generation in oocytes and early embryos, which in turn may result in aberrant chromosomal segregation or developmental arrest[45]. The developmental competence of mouse and human early embryos appears to be directly related to the metabolic capacity of a finite complement of maternally inherited mitochondria that appear to begin to replicate after implantation. Van Blerkom and co-workers[45] have demonstrated the feasibility of isolating and transferring mitochondria between oocytes, an apparent increase in net ATP production in the recipients, and the persistence of activity in the transferred mitochondria.

Conclusion

Age is the major determinant of female fertility potential. Ovarian aging begins to impact on fecundity rates at age 30, and has a profound effect after age 35, over 10 years before the menopause. Assisted reproductive technology (ART) offers tremendous opportunities for older patients seeking fertility treatment today. The development of new fertility treatment modalities continues to enlarge the armamentarium of reproductive endocrinologists, and will continue to offer new hope well into the next millenium.

References

1. Chandra A, Stephen EH. Impaired fecundity in the United States: 1982-1995. *Fam Plann Perspect* 1998; 30:34-42
2. Stephen EH, Chandra A. Updated projections of infertility in the United States: 1995-2025. *Fertil Steril* 1998;70:30-4
3. Anonymous. Assisted reproductive technology in the United States and Canada: 1995 results generated from the American Society for Reproductive Medicine/Society for Assisted Reproductive Technology Registry. *Fertil Steril* 1998;69:389-98
4. Manton KG. Demographic trends for the aging female population. *J Am Med Women's Assoc* 1997; 52:99-105
5. Murray CJ, Lopez AD. Alternative projections of mortality and disability by cause 1990-2020: Global Burden of Disease Study. *Lancet* 1997;349: 1498-504
6. Brambilla DJ, McKinlay SM. A prospective study of factors affecting age at menopause [Published erratum appears in *J Clin Epidemiol* 1990;43:537]. *J Clin Epidemiol* 1989;42:1031-9
7. McKinlay SM, Bifano NL, McKinlay JB. Smoking and age at menopause in women. *Ann Intern Med* 1985; 103:350-6
8. Bromberger JT, Matthews KA, Kuller LH, Wing RR, Meilahn EN, Plantinga P. Prospective study of the determinants of age at menopause. *Am J Epidemiol* 1997;145:124-33
9. van Noord P, Dubas JS, Dorland M, Boersma H, te VE. Age at natural menopause in a population-based screening cohort: the role of menarche, fecundity, and lifestyle factors. *Fertil Steril* 1997; 68:95-102
10. Klein NA, Battaglia DE, Miller PB, Branigan EF, Giudice LC, Soules MR. Ovarian follicular development and the follicular fluid hormones and growth factors in normal women of advanced reproductive age. *J Clin Endocrinol Metab* 1996;81: 1946-51
11. Klein NA, Battaglia DE, Fujimoto VY, Davis GS, Bremner WJ, Soules MR. Reproductive aging: accelerated ovarian follicular development associated with a monotropic follicle-stimulating hormone rise in normal older women. *J Clin Endocrinol Metab* 1996;81:1038-45
12. Klein NA, Soules MR. Endocrine changes of the perimenopause. *Clin Obstet Gynecol* 1998;41:912-20
13. Gallardo E, Simon C, Levy M, Guanes PP, Remohi J, Pellicer A. Effect of age on sperm fertility potential: oocyte donation as a model. *Fertil Steril* 1996; 66:260-4
14. Hull MG, Fleming CF, Hughes AO, McDermott A. The age-related decline in female fecundity: a quantitative controlled study of implanting capacity and survival of individual embryos after *in vitro* fertilization. *Fertil Steril* 1996;65:783-90
15. van Noord-Zaadstra BM, Looman CW, Alsbach H, Habbema JD, te VE, Karbaat J. Delaying childbearing: effect of age on fecundity and outcome of pregnancy. *Br Med J* 1991;302:1361-5
16. Sherman BM, West JH, Korenman SG. The menopausal transition: analysis of LH, FSH, estradiol, and progesterone concentrations during menstrual cycles of older women. *J Clin Endocrinol Metab* 1976;42:629-36
17. Scott RT, Toner JP, Muasher SJ, Oehninger S, Robinson S, Rosenwaks Z. Follicle-stimulating hormone levels on cycle day 3 are predictive of *in vitro* fertilization outcome. *Fertil Steril* 1989;51: 651-4
18. Toner JP, Philput CB, Jones GS, Muasher SJ. Basal follicle-stimulating hormone level is a better predictor of *in vitro* fertilization performance than age. *Fertil Steril* 1991;55:784-91
19. Licciardi FL, Liu HC, Rosenwaks Z. Day 3 estradiol serum concentrations as prognosticators of ovarian stimulation response and pregnancy outcome in patients undergoing *in vitro* fertilization. *Fertil Steril* 1995;64:991-4

20. O'Connor KA, Holman DJ, Wood JW. Declining fecundity and ovarian ageing in natural fertility populations. *Maturitas* 1998;30:127-36
21. Eichenlaub-Ritter U. Genetics of oocyte ageing. *Maturitas* 1998;30:143-69
22. Nasseri A, Mukherjee T, Grifo JA, Noyes N, Krey L, Copperman AB. Elevated day 3 serum follicle stimulating hormone and/or estradiol may predict fetal aneuploidy [in Process citation]. *Fertil Steril* 1999;71:715-18
23. Munne S, Alikani M, Tomkin G, Grifo J, Cohen J. Embryo morphology, developmental rates, and maternal age are correlated with chromosome abnormalities. *Fertil Steril* 1995;64:382-91
24. Smith KE, Buyalos RP. The profound impact of patient age on pregnancy outcome after early detection of fetal cardiac activity. *Fertil Steril* 1996;65:35-40
25. Hughes EG. The effectiveness of ovulation induction and intrauterine insemination in the treatment of persistent infertility: a meta-analysis. *Hum Reprod* 1997;12:1865-72
26. Guzick DS, Carson SA, Coutifaris C, *et al*. Efficacy of superovulation and intrauterine insemination in the treatment of infertility. National Cooperative Reproductive Medicine Network. *N Eng J Med* 1999;340:177-83
27. Pearlstone AC, Fournet N, Gambone JC, Pang SC, Buyalos RP. Ovulation induction in women age 40 and older: the importance of basal follicle-stimulating hormone level and chronological age. *Fertil Steril* 1992;58:674-9
28. Lass A, Croucher C, Duffy S, Dawson K, Margara R, Winston RM. One thousand initiated cycles of *in vitro* fertilization in women ≥ 40 years of age. *Fertil Steril* 1998;70:1030-4
29. Yaron Y, Amit A, Brenner SM, Peyser MR, David MP, Lessing JB. *In vitro* fertilization and oocyte donation in women 45 years of age and older. *Fertil Steril* 1995;63:71-6
30. Meldrum DR, Wisot A, Hamilton F, Gutlay AL, Kempton WF, Huynh D. Routine pituitary suppression with leuprolide before ovarian stimulation for oocyte retrieval. *Fertil Steril* 1989;51:455-9
31. Widra EA, Gindoff PR, Smotrich DB, Stillman RJ. Achieving multiple-order embryo transfer identifies women over 40 years of age with improved *in vitro* fertilization outcome. *Fertil Steril* 1996;65:103-8
32. Schoolcraft W, Schlenker T, Gee M, Stevens J, Wagley L. Improved controlled ovarian hyperstimulation in poor responder *in vitro* fertilization patients with a microdose follicle-stimulating hormone flare, growth hormone protocol. *Fertil Steril* 1997;67:93-7
33. Surrey ES, Bower J, Hill DM, Ramsey J, Surrey MW. Clinical and endocrine effects of a microdose GnRH agonist flare regimen administered to poor responders who are undergoing *in vitro* fertilization. *Fertil Steril* 1998;69:419-24
34. Scott RT, Navot D. Enhancement of ovarian responsiveness with microdoses of gonadotropin-releasing hormone agonist during ovulation induction for *in vitro* fertilization. *Fertil Steril* 1994;61:880-5
35. Sauer MV, Paulson RJ, Lobo RA. A preliminary report on oocyte donation extending reproductive potential to women over 40. *N Engl J Med* 1990;323:1157-60
36. Borini A, Bianchi L, Violini F, Maccolini A, Cattoli M, Flamigni C. Oocyte donation program: pregnancy and implantation rates in women of different ages sharing oocytes from single donor. *Fertil Steril* 1996;65:94-7
37. Cohen J, Alikani M, Liu HC, Rosenwaks Z. Rescue of human embryos by micromanipulation. *Baillière's Clin Obstet Gynaecol* 1994;8:95-116
38. Schoolcraft WB, Schlenker T, Jones GS, Jones HWJ. *In vitro* fertilization in women age 40 and older: the impact of assisted hatching. *J Assist Reprod Genet* 1995;12:581-4
39. Magli MC, Gianaroli L, Ferraretti AP, Fortini D, Aicardi G, Montanaro N. Rescue of implantation potential in embryos with poor prognosis by assisted zona hatching. *Hum Reprod* 1998;13:1331-5
40. Tucker MJ, Morton PC, Wright G, *et al*. Enhancement of outcome from intracytoplasmic sperm injection: does co-culture or assisted hatching improve implantation rates? *Hum Reprod* 1996;11:2434-7
41. Hellebaut S, De SP, Dozortsev D, Onghena A, Qian C, Dhont M. Does assisted hatching improve implantation rates after *in vitro* fertilization or intracytoplasmic sperm injection in all patients? A prospective randomized study. *J Assist Reprod Genet* 1996;13:19-22
42. Lanzendorf SE, Nehchiri F, Mayer JF, Oehninger S, Muasher SJ. A prospective, randomized, double-blind study for the evaluation of assisted hatching in patients with advanced maternal age. *Hum Reprod* 1998;13:409-13
43. St John J, Barratt CL. Use of anucleate donor oocyte cytoplasm in recipient eggs [Letter; Comment]. *Lancet* 1997;350:961-2
44. Cohen J, Scott R, Alikani M, *et al*. Ooplasmic transfer in mature human oocytes. *Mol Hum Reprod* 1998;4:269-80
45. Van Blerkom J, Sinclair J, Davis P. Mitochondrial transfer between oocytes: potential applications of mitochondrial donation and the issue of heteroplasmy. *Hum Reprod* 1998;13:2857-68

Section III
Clinical problems in the menopause

10

Osteoporosis

Brian M. Berger

Introduction

Osteoporosis is a skeletal disorder characterized by low bone mass and an increased susceptibility to fracture. The past two decades have seen an increase in our understanding of the epidemiology of fractures at the three most frequent sites (the hip, wrist and vertebral body). These new insights have led to the delineation of preventive strategies against these fractures for both the general population and those individuals at highest risk. A new definition of osteoporosis moves this disorder from a disease of fractures to a disease of fracture risks. The goal of osteoporosis therapy is to prevent the morbidity and mortality that arise from the disease. This can be best accomplished by vigorous screening programs and public awareness of the magnitude of the disease.

Prevalence

The incidence of osteoporosis varies from country to country and among different races. In many countries, hip fractures occupy 20% of hospital beds. In England and Wales, the cost of osteoporosis has been estimated at £500 million every year[1]. Osteoporosis affects an enormous number of people, and its prevalence will increase as the population ages. It is estimated that between 13 and 18% of postmenopausal white women in the United States (4–6 million) have osteoporosis, and an additional 30–50% (13–17 million) have low bone density at the hip. Health-care expenditures attributable to osteoporotic fractures in 1995 were estimated at $US13.8 billion, of which $US10.3 billion (75.1%) was for the treatment of white women, $US2.5 billion (18.4%) for white men, $US0.7 billion (5.3%) for non-white women and $US0.2 billion (1.3%) for non-white men[2].

The most common fractures are those of the proximal femur (hip), vertebrae (spine) and distal forearm (wrist), but because osteoporosis is a systemic disease causing bone loss throughout the skeleton, almost all fractures in older adults are due in part to low bone density. Unfortunately, this is a silent epidemic which may present with pain or fractures, or cause damage in an insidious manner until the presentation is far more severe.

Hip fracture can result in up to 10–25% mortality within 1 year. Additionally, up to 25% of hip fracture patients may require long-term nursing-home care, and only a third fully regain their prefracture level of independence. One year after hip fracture, 40% of patients are still unable to walk independently, 60% have difficulty with at least one essential activity of daily living and 80% are restricted in other activities, such as driving and grocery shopping. Moreover, 27% of these patients enter a nursing home for the first time[3]. After adjusting for other factors associated with mortality, women with fractures of the hip or pelvis have a 2.4-fold increase in mortality. Although some of these deaths are undoubtedly the result of chronic conditions that contribute to the hip or pelvic fracture, up to 20% are directly due to the fracture itself[4].

Vertebral fractures also cause significant complications including back pain, height loss and kyphosis. Morbidity and mortality arising from vertebral fracture are less secure than those of the hip and radius[5]. Reasons relate to the uncertain definition of vertebral fracture and its variable clinical expression, and hence its incidence is not known[3]. Using radiological criteria, 50% or more of vertebral fractures may be asymptomatic.

Although the true incidence of vertebral fracture is unknown, there is evidence that it increases exponentially with age in much the same way as for hip fracture. Between the ages of 60 and 90 years, the apparent incidence rises approximately 20-fold in women compared to a 50-fold increase in risk of hip fracture[6]. Postural and height changes associated with kyphosis may limit activity, including bending and reaching, and their cosmetic effects may erode self-esteem, although there does not appear to be any correlation between kyphosis and back pain[7]. Multiple thoracic fractures may result in restrictive lung disease, and lumbar fractures may alter abdominal anatomy, leading to constipation, abdominal pain, distention, reduced appetite and premature satiety.

Physiology of bone

Bone undergoes perpetual remodelling of units aptly named bone remodelling units. These units are continuously changing throughout life in a balance between bone resorption and formation. The two bone types involved in bone remodelling are cortical and trabecular bone. Cortical bone constitutes 80% of total bone, while trabecular bone makes up the remainder. Trabecular bone is the predominant bone type in the spinal column, and is less dense, consisting of a honeycomb structure of marrow and fat. Age-related trabecular bone loss is characterized not simply by a global loss of bone but also by cortical porosity and loss of trabecular connections.

The two main cell types involved are the osteoblasts and osteoclasts, with osteocytes and lining cells performing a supportive role. Osteoblasts are prominent in bone surfaces when bone growth or remodelling is taking place. They secrete collagen to form a non-mineralized matrix which consists of a seam or border of osteoid. The osteoid matures over a period of 1–2 weeks, and lays down a matrix of hydroxyapatite. Among the proteins involved in this process are osteocalcin and alkaline phosphatase, which serve as markers of bone formation (see Table 2).

Osteoclasts are multinucleated giant cells found at the surface of cells undergoing bone resorption. They form pits or lacunae known as the lacunae of Howship. Osteoclasts are responsive to parathyroid hormone (PTH) and are inhibited by calcitonin. They contain lysosomal enzymes which resorb collagen, and markers of collagen resorption such as urinary hydroxyproline and pyridinoline cross-links are used to measure osteoclastic activity.

Parathyroid hormone plays a vital role in the homeostasis of calcium within the blood stream. A decrease in calcium causes an increase in PTH secretion by the parathyroid glands. This stimulates the production of 1,25-vitamin D in the kidneys which, in turn, increases the calcium absorption from the intestines. Parathyroid hormone-related protein (PTHrP), a genetically and structurally distinct hormone which displays similar binding and activation profiles to PTH, has greatly facilitated the effort to establish a structure–biological function relationship by allowing for direct comparisons[8].

Extracellular or plasma calcium ion concentration is held constant at 5 mg/dl through the combined actions of PTH, vitamin D and calcitonin on their target organs, kidney and bone. The thresholds of renal tubular calcium reabsorption and bone resorption and formation are both set at 5 mg/dl. The set point of PTH secretion is also fixed at 5 mg/dl plasma calcium ion. Therefore, the sensing system (parathyroid cell) and the effectors, kidney and bone, are all set to maintain plasma calcium at 5 mg/dl, perhaps through membrane-bound calcium sensor proteins. The effectiveness of this system depends upon the presence of bone remodelling, which allows a swift shift of plasma calcium from and to bone in response to PTH and calcitonin, respectively. In this regard, directing hematopoiesis to bone marrow that provides bone resorbing osteoclasts is critical. It is likely that this shift of hematopoiesis occurred through evolution at the transition from aquatic to terrestrial life, and this event is directed by expression of homing molecule in bone marrow stromal cells.

The recent cloning of receptors for calcitonin and PTH/PTHrP has enabled very rapid progress in understanding the molecular and cell biology of these receptors. In particular, much has been learned about the tissue distribution of these receptors, as well as their mode of interaction with ligands, signal transduction and regulation of expression[9]. A second calcium-regulating hormone (calcitonin) is released by hypercalcemia, and lowers plasma calcium by inhibiting osteolysis. Specifically, it lowers serum calcium by decreasing bone resorption and tubular calcium reabsorption. It is a straight-chain peptide with 32 amino acids and a seven-membered disulfide ring at the N terminal. It is produced by C cells which arise from the neural crest, and is considered a neuropeptide hormone. It is produced in the thyroid of mammals and the ultimobranchial glands of lower vertebrates[10]. An analgesic action, possibly mediated via beta-endorphins, is also evident. Parenteral calcitonin has been shown to stabilize and increase indices of cortical and trabecular bone mass and total body calcium when administered to patients with established osteoporosis. The routine use of this route of administration has been limited by poor patient compliance and tolerability. An intranasal preparation of calcitonin provided a more convenient means of administration[11]. The form most widely used in therapy is salmon calcitonin because of its tremendous potency, compared to human calcitonin[12].

Risk factors

Vertebral bone strength is determined by several factors: cortical thickness, bone size, trabecular bone density and microarchitecture. All these factors change with age as a result of the two dynamic processes: remodelling and modelling. When the changes become pronounced, osteoporotic fractures occur.

Aspects of bone quality to be considered are bone architecture, matrix, mineralization and fatigue damage. The trabecular network becomes progressively disconnected and weaker with age. Death of old osteocytes leads to hypermineralization and brittleness of bone. The stability of bone collagen declines with age, and unremodelled bone accumulates fatigue damage. The lower bone fragility rates in males than in females may be due to a combination of the larger male skeleton, greater cortical bone density after age 60 years, and greater bone turnover which would replace fatigue-damaged bone.

Endowment of skeletal mass

The amount of skeletal mass acquired during adolescence is one of the most important determinants for the risk of postmenopausal and involutional osteoporosis. In both sexes, a large variance in bone mineral density (BMD) and content (BMC) is observed among healthy individuals at the beginning of the third decade. In females, bone mass accumulation occurs predominantly from age 11 to 14, and is drastically reduced by 16 years of age in both lumbar spine and femoral neck[13,14]. A sharp reduction occurs between the second and fourth years after menarche[15]. Although more than 60% of peak bone mineral mass is gained during puberty (mostly at the expense of an increase in bone size while volumetric bone density slightly changes), familial resemblance for most bone traits is already present between daughters and their mothers before puberty[16]. These results indicate that genetic susceptibility to osteoporosis may already be detectable in early childhood. Up to 5% of trabecular bone and 1.5% of total bone will be lost per year after the menopause.

Physical activity has been related to enhanced bone mass and improved physical functioning and, thus, may reduce the risk for osteoporotic fracture. In one study[17], higher levels of leisure time, sport activity and household chores and fewer hours of sitting daily were associated with a significantly reduced relative risk for hip fracture but not wrist or vertebral fracture after adjustment for age, dietary factors, falls at baseline, and functional and health status. Very active women (fourth and fifth quintiles) had a statistically significant 36% reduction in hip fractures (relative risk 0.64; confidence interval 95% 0.45–0.891), compared with the least active women (lowest quintile)[17]. Other studies have arrived at similar conclusions[18,19].

Low serum hormone levels

Women with undetectable serum estradiol concentrations (< 5 pg/ml) have a relative risk of 2.5 for subsequent hip fracture and subsequent vertebral fracture, compared to women with detectable serum estradiol concentrations[20]. Women with both undetectable serum estradiol concentrations and serum sex hormone binding globulin concentrations of 1 μg/dl or more have a relative risk of 6.9 for hip fracture and 7.9 for vertebral fracture[20].

Glucocorticoid use

Glucocorticoids cause bone loss by altering the bone remodelling sequence: bone resorption by osteoclasts is increased, and bone formation by osteoblasts is decreased. Serum levels of osteocalcin are decreased with glucocorticoid therapy, further evidence of decreased osteoblast function. Glucocorticoids decrease calcium absorption by the gastrointestinal tract and increase renal calcium excretion. Several recent studies suggest that low-dose glucocorticoid therapy is not associated with bone loss[21,22].

Thyroid function

Hyperthyroidism and use of thyroid hormone to suppress thyroid-stimulating hormone (TSH) because of thyroid cancer, goiters or nodules seem to have an adverse effect on bone, especially in postmenopausal women; the largest effect is on cortical bone[23]. Although some studies have found that thyroid hormone replacement seems to have a minimal negative clinical effect on bone[24], there is no consistent evidence that low TSH, a sensitive biochemical marker of excess thyroid hormone, is associated with low BMD or accelerated bone loss in older ambulatory women[25].

Smoking

The use of tobacco products is detrimental to the skeleton as well as to overall health. The Framingham Study found that current estrogen use appeared to be protective against bone fractures (adjusted odds ratio, AOR 0.38; confidence interval, CI 0.12–1.21; $p = 0.10$). Among current smokers, however, estrogen use did not protect against fracture (AOR for current use 1.26; CI 0.29–5.45), whereas estrogen was protective in non-smokers (AOR for current or past use 0.37; CI 0.19–0.75; $p = 0.005$). Therefore, smoking may negate the protective skeletal effects of estrogen

replacement therapy[26]. Smokers are at increased risk of hip fracture and their risk rises with greater cigarette consumption. Risk declines among former smokers, but the benefit is not observed until 10 years after cessation[27].

Monitoring bone status

Measuring bone density

Bone mineral density (BMD) measurement (Table 1) can be used to establish or confirm a diagnosis of osteoporosis, predict future fracture risk, and monitor changes in BMD due to medical conditions or therapy. BMD has a continuous, graded, inverse relationship to the risk of fracture: the lower the BMD, the greater the risk.

Measurements of BMD at any skeletal site have value in predicting fracture risk. A variety of densitometers is in clinical use and provides reliable assessment of fracture risk. BMD is expressed as a relationship to two norms: the expected BMD for the patient's age and sex (Z-score), or for young normal adults of the same sex (T-score). The difference between the patient's score and the norm is expressed as a standard deviation (SD) above or below the mean.

Dual-energy X-ray absorptiometry

Dual-energy X-ray absorptiometry (DEXA) is the best method of measuring bone density and, thus, the best available indicator of osteoporotic fracture risk. DEXA can be used to measure bone mineral density in the spine, hip or wrist – the most common sites for osteoporotic fractures. Radiation hazard is small with patient-effective

Table 1 Radiological measurement of bone mineral density (BMD)

Type	Bone type assessed
Dual energy X-ray absorptiometry (DEXA)	trabecular, cortical, whole body
Single-energy X-ray absorptiometry (SXA)	cortical
Radiographic absorptiometry (RA)	trabecular
Quantitative computed tomography (QCT)	trabecular, cortical
Ultrasound densitometry	cortical?

doses of the order of a few microsieverts[28]. *In vivo* measurement precision of the order of 1% is achievable for posteroanterior (PA) scans of the lumbar spine. Lateral scans can achieve measurement precision of the order of 4%[29]. Recent technological developments using X-ray fan beams and multi-element detector arrays on C-arm devices have resulted in faster scan times, higher resolution images, and an ability to perform PA and lateral scanning without the need to reposition the patient. Accuracy of DEXA is dependent upon specific instrumentation and data reduction algorithms, but results generally correlate well with ashed bone measurements[30].

While total-body scans may be precise and offer the advantage of total-body composition determination, BMD values derived from total-body scans cannot currently replace direct measurements. Site-specific measurements are required to assess regional osteopenia. Bone mineral density should be measured only to assist in making a clinical management choice. Measurement of the lumbar spine and femoral neck is standard, but a different site or a single measurement is recommended in specific cases. Unless accelerated bone loss is suspected, DEXA should be repeated every 2–4 years for patients receiving ovarian hormone therapy and 1–2 years for patients undergoing biphosphonate therapy. Measurements and reporting of results must provide actual measurement and its relation to peak bone mass.

Single-energy X-ray absorptiometry

These techniques measure bone density in the forearm, finger and sometimes the heel. Single-energy X-ray absorptiometry (SXA) is a device which incorporates an X-ray tube as a photon source. SXA delivers a radiation exposure of 1.68 mrem, with image quality and spatial resolution comparable to DEXA[31,32].

Radiographic absorptiometry

Radiographic absorptiometry (RA) is a technique that is based on a standard radiograph or computer-generated radiograph of the hand with a metal wedge in the same field. RA is used for bone mass measurement from radiographs of peripheral sites, most commonly the hand or heel. Recently developed new computer-assisted methods have improved RA precision, thus providing a simple and inexpensive technique for screening of bone mineral status of large populations[33].

Quantitative computed tomography

Quantitative computed tomography (QCT) measures trabecular and cortical bone density at several sites in the body, but is most commonly used to measure trabecular bone density in the spine. It may be used as an alternative to DEXA for vertebral measurements[34].

Ultrasound densitometry

Ultrasound assesses bone in the heel, tibia, patella or other peripheral sites where the bones are relatively superficial. Changes in the calcaneal ultrasound parameters in response to treatment of osteoporosis are not a reflection of mineral changes occurring in the lumbar spine and femoral neck in a given individual, and, in this regard, calcaneal ultrasonometry is not a substitute for direct-site DEXA measurement of the lumbar spine and femur, but may be useful in a clinical setting when DEXA access is poor[35].

Serum and urinary measurements of bone turnover

The non-invasive assessment of bone turnover (Table 2) has received increasing attention over the past few years because of the need for sensitive

Table 2 Biochemical measurement of bone mineral turnover

Marker	Source	Marker type
Bone-specific alkaline phosphatase	serum	formation
Osteocalcin	serum	formation
Type I collagen extension peptides	serum	formation
Hydroxyproline	urine	formation
Pyridinium cross-links (Pyr and D-Pyr)	urine	resorption
Deoxypyridinoline	urine	resorption
Pyridinoline	urine	resorption

markers in the clinical investigation of osteoporosis. Markers of bone formation include serum total and bone-specific alkaline phosphatase, serum osteocalcin and serum type I collagen extension peptides. Assessment of bone resorption can be achieved with measurement of urinary hydroxyproline, urinary excretion of the pyridinium cross-links (Pyr and D-Pyr) and plasma tartarate resistant acid phosphatase (TRAP) activity[36]. The immunoassay of human osteocalcin recognizing the intact molecule and its major proteolytic fragment, and that of bone alkaline phosphatase, are currently the most sensitive markers to assess bone formation[37]. For bone resorption, the total urinary excretion of pyridinoline cross-links measured by high pressure liquid chromatography has shown its superiority over all other markers for the clinical assessment of osteoporosis[38]. The recent development of immunoassays recognizing either the free pyridinoline cross-links or pyridinoline cross-linked type I collagen peptides in urine and serum should allow a broad use of this sensitive resorption marker. Programs combining bone mass measurement and assessment of bone turnover in women at the time of the menopause have been developed in an attempt to improve the assessment of the risk for osteoporosis[39].

Treatment (Table 3)

Calcium

A lifelong intake of adequate calcium is necessary for the acquisition of peak bone mass and maintenance of bone health. The skeleton contains 99% of the body's calcium stores; when the exogenous supply is inadequate, calcium is extracted from the skeleton to maintain serum calcium at a constant level.

The recent cloning of an extracellular calcium (Ca^{2+})-sensing receptor (CaR) from the parathyroid gland and the kidney has provided novel insights into the mechanisms that underlie the direct actions of Ca^{2+} on various cells. The receptor is a member of the superfamily of G protein-coupled receptors, activating phospholipase C (PLC) and probably also inhibiting adenylate cyclase in target tissues. In the parathyroid gland it is a key mediator of the inhibition by high Ca^{2+} of PTH secretion and, perhaps, PTH gene expression and parathyroid cellular proliferation. It also appears to represent the major mechanism through which Ca^{2+} stimulates the secretion of calcitonin from the thyroidal C cells. In the kidney, the CaR directly inhibits tubular reabsorption of calcium and magnesium in the thick ascending limb, and may be responsible for the long-recognized, but poorly understood, inhibition of urinary concentrating ability by hypercalcemia[9].

Controlled clinical trials have demonstrated that the combination of supplemental calcium and vitamin D reduces the risk of fracture of the spine, hip and other sites. This positive effect on BMD has been demonstrated, even in a group of early postmenopausal age, with a fairly good initial calcium and vitamin D status[40].

After peak bone mass in women is attained, the benefits of increased dietary calcium or supplemental calcium are uncertain. Some investigators have found that premenopausal women in the fifth decade lose about 1% of spinal trabecular mineral yearly, in spite of a normal serum estradiol level and ample calcium intake[41]. However, calcium supplementation in postmenopausal or oophorectomized women who had been undergoing unopposed estrogen therapy for at least 2 years and whose serum calcium level was suppressed to below the normal range potentiated the effect of estrogen[42].

Long-term administration of calcium supplements to elderly women may partially reverse age-related increases in serum PTH level and bone resorption and decrease bone loss. However, the effects on bone loss are weaker than those reported for estrogen, biphosphonates or calcitonin therapy, indicating that calcium supplements alone cannot substitute for these in treating established osteoporosis[43].

Nonetheless, because of their safety, high tolerance and low expense, increasing daily calcium is a cost-effective way to help reduce fracture risk.

Table 3 Treatments used for prevention of bone loss

Estrogens	Tibolone
Alendronate (Fosamax®)	Calcium
Calcitonin	Exercise
Raloxifene	Parathyroid hormone

Vitamin D

Vitamin D plays a major role in calcium absorption and bone health. Chief dietary sources of vitamin D include vitamin D-fortified milk (400 IU per quart) and cereals (50 IU per serving), egg yolks, salt-water fish and liver. Some calcium supplements and most multivitamin tablets also contain vitamin D. Low-dose vitamin D supplementation has been shown to have only a minor effect in the prevention of osteoporosis in non-osteoporotic, early postmenopausal women, and does not give any benefit additional to that of hormone replacement therapy (HRT) alone[44]. Supplementation with 400 IU vitamin D_3 daily in elderly women has been found to decrease PTH secretion slightly and increase bone mineral density at the femoral neck, but no changes in the biochemical markers of bone turnover were seen[45]. An intake of 400–800 IU of vitamin D per day is recommended for those at risk of deficiency, such as elderly, chronically ill, housebound or institutionalized individuals[46].

Exercise

In postmenopausal women with low bone density, bone loss can be slowed or prevented by exercise plus calcium supplementation or estrogen-progesterone replacement (Table 3). Some studies have found that exercise plus estrogen is more effective than estrogen alone[47]. The amount and type of exercise needed to prevent bone loss is largely unknown. One study found that short-term (7 months) exercise with intensity above the anaerobic threshold is safe and effective in preventing postmenopausal bone loss[48]. A recent meta-analysis of studies on bone loss and the effects of exercise found that the exercise-training programs prevented or reversed almost 1% of bone loss per year in both the lumbar spine and femoral neck for both pre- and postmenopausal women[49]. Another meta-analysis showed a significant effect of physical activity on the bone mineral density at the L2–4 level of the lumbar column in studies published after 1991 (Effect sizes $(ES) = 0.8745$, $p < 0.05$). No effect could be seen, however, on forearm and femoral bone mass[50]. These meta-analyses suggest that exercise programs in a population of post-menopausal women over 50 years of age are effective for preventing spinal bone mineral density loss at the L2–4 level. Further studies are needed to evaluate the effects on the forearm and femoral bone/hip.

Hormone replacement therapy

Estrogen with or without progesterone replacement therapy is the most studied and proven therapy for the prevention of bone loss in estrogen-deficient women. The results of the Postmenopausal Estrogen/Progestin Interventions (PEPI) trial showed significant differences in patients on active treatment, and are worth reviewing[51]. Treatments were: placebo; conjugated equine estrogens (CEEs), 0.625 mg/day; CEEs, 0.625 mg/day plus medroxyprogesterone acetate (MPA), 10 mg/day for 12 days per month; CEEs, 0.625 mg/day plus MPA, 2.5 mg/day daily; or CEEs, 0.625 mg/day plus micronized progesterone 200 mg/day for 12 days per month. Over a time course of 36 months, participants assigned to the placebo group lost an average of 1.8% of spine BMD and 1.7% of hip BMD by the 36-month visit, while those assigned to active regimens gained BMD at both sites, ranging from 3.5 to 5.0% mean total increases in spinal BMD and a mean total increase of 1.7% of BMD in the hip. Women assigned to CEEs plus continuous MPA had significantly greater increases in spinal BMD (increase of 5%) than those assigned to the other three active regimens (average increase, 3.8%). Findings were similar among those adhering to assigned therapy, although, among adherent participants, there were no significant differences in BMD changes among the four active treatment groups[51]. Many other studies have confirmed these results.

In another multicenter study on 9704 ambulatory non-black women 65 years of age or older[52], current estrogen use was associated with a decrease in the risk for wrist fractures (relative risk, RR 0.39; 95% CI 0.24–0.64) and for all non-spinal fractures (RR 0.66; CI 0.54–0.80), when compared with no estrogen use. Results in this study were similar for women using unopposed estrogen or estrogen plus progestin[52]. The potential benefits may be influenced by genotypes of the vitamin D receptor and estrogen receptor. In a study examining BMD differential gains in women of varying receptor status[53], vitamin D receptor and estrogen receptor loci varied from approximately 1.0% (for the total body BMC changes in combined placebo and HRT groups) to approximately 18.7% (for the spine BMD changes in the HRT group)[53]. These results suggest that individual genotypes are important factors in determining changes in bone mass in the elderly with and without HRT, and thus may need to be considered with respect to the treatment to preserve bone mass in elderly Caucasian women.

Another study examined the effect of various doses on BMD[54] and found that esterified estrogens at doses from 0.3 to 1.25 mg/day, administered unopposed by progestin, produce a continuum of positive changes on bone and lipids. Plasma estradiol concentrations increased with esterified estrogens dose and were related to positive bone mineral densities. The 0.3-mg dose resulted in positive bone and lipid changes without inducing endometrial hyperplasia[54]. These benefits appear to be evident in women receiving transdermal estrogen replacement as well[55].

An intriguing study of 65 pairs of twins who were discordant for HRT use[56] showed that among current users of estrogen, BMD was consistently and significantly higher than in non-users at both lumbar spine and femoral neck. Past users of HRT did not, however, show the same benefits. The clinical implications of these findings are that HRT needs to be used continuously to influence BMD and that alternative treatments need to be considered in those who discontinue HRT.

Alendronate

Alendronate is a member of the biphosphonate group of drugs along with etidronate, clodronate, pamidronate, tiludronate and residronate. The biphosphonates bind to bone mineral where they inhibit bone resorption. Well-conducted controlled clinical trials utilizing alendronate sodium indicate that treatment reduces the incidence of fracture at the spine, hip and wrist in patients with osteoporosis. In a large study of 447 women who had recently experienced the menopause, alendronate at 5, 10 and 20 mg/day increased BMD from baseline at the lumbar spine, femoral neck and trochanter by 1-4% and in the total body by 0.3-1.0%[57]. In a study undertaken to determine the response to alendronate therapy in women with postmenopausal osteoporosis who were non-responders to intermittent cyclical etidronate therapy[58], 25 women with postmenopausal osteoporosis (mean $\pm$ SD 65.1 $\pm$ 1.9 years of age), previously treated with intermittent cyclical etidronate with no increase of spine BMD were then changed to alendronate 10 mg/day, which they received for 1.3 $\pm$ 0.1 years. After treatment with alendronate, BMD increased significantly at the lumbar spine (4.4 $\pm$ 0.7% annualized, $p < 0.0001$) and at all hip sites. Bone markers also changed significantly after alendronate treatment: urine deoxypyridinoline fell from 6.8 $\pm$ 0.8 to 5.5 $\pm$ 0.6 μmol/mol creatinine ($p < 0.0001$) and serum bone-specific alkaline phosphatase rose from 4.6 $\pm$ 0.5 to 11.9 $\pm$ 1.0 ng/ml ($p < 0.0001$). This study suggests that alendronate causes more complete suppression of bone resorption and less inhibition (or stimulation) of bone formation.

In a 3-year study of alendronate therapy at three different dosages[59], BMD continued to increase over the entire 3-year study duration in the alendronate-treated groups and, compared with the other dosage groups (5 mg and 20 mg), 10 mg alendronate produced the largest gains in BMD during the third year.

Alendronate therapy is associated with gastrointestinal side-effects. It must therefore be taken on an empty stomach, first thing in the morning, with a large glass of water, at least 30 min before eating or drinking. Patients should remain upright during this interval. The 5-mg dose has been approved by the Food and Drug Administration (FDA) for prevention of osteoporosis, and the 10-mg dose has been approved for treatment. A rare reported complication of alendronate (probably < 1%) is esophageal ulceration.

Calcitonin

Salmon calcitonin, a hormone that inhibits bone resorption, is FDA approved for the treatment of osteoporosis. It is delivered as a single daily intranasal spray that provides 200 IU of the drug.

Epidemiological, retrospective and prospective studies provide a convergent network of evidence that calcitonin administration in osteoporosis contributes to reduce significantly the frequency of subsequent fractures, both in the spine and in the hip. In a randomized controlled study, the rate of patients with new fractures was reduced significantly in the women treated with salcatonin to about one-third of that in the non-salcatonin-treated women (RR 0.23; CI 0.07–0.77)[60]. Nasal calcitonin also possesses a potent analgesic effect, and decreases the number of concomitant analgesic medications[61].

Raloxifene

Raloxifene hydrochloride is a selective estrogen receptor modulator (SERM) with estrogen agonist effects on bone and lipid metabolism and estrogen antagonist effects on reproductive tissues, including the breast. Tissue selectivity of raloxifene may be achieved through several mechanisms: the ligand structure, interaction of the ligand with different estrogen receptor subtypes in various tissues, and intracellular events after ligand binding. Raloxifene, a non-steroidal benzothiophene, cannot be used to treat menopausal symptoms, and it has no beneficial effects on hot flushes or vaginal symptoms. In contrast to estrogen, raloxifene does not induce histopathological evidence of endometrial stimulation in healthy postmenopausal women[62]. In addition, raloxifene lowers serum concentrations of total and low-density lipoprotein cholesterol, and lowers serum lipoprotein(a) levels[63,64]. It also has a favorable, dose-related effect on plasma homocysteine levels in postmenopausal women[65].

The Multiple Outcomes of Raloxifene Evaluation (MORE), a multicenter, randomized, double-blind trial, in which women taking raloxifene or placebo were followed up for a median of 40 months, showed that raloxifene decreased the risk of estrogen receptor-positive breast cancer by 90% (RR 0.10; 95% CI 0.04–0.24), but not estrogen receptor-negative invasive breast cancer (RR 0.88; 95% CI 0.26–3.0). Raloxifene increased the risk of venous thromboembolic disease (RR 3.1; 95% CI

1.5–6.2), but did not increase the risk of endometrial cancer (RR 0.8; 95% CI 0.2–2.7)[66].

Tibolone

Tibolone, a synthetic steroid with estrogenic, androgenic and progestogenic properties, relieves climacteric symptoms and prevents postmenopausal bone loss. Although no studies on fracture risk have been performed, tibolone appears to be at least as efficacious as other forms of HRT with regard to climacteric symptoms. In a randomized controlled trial, tibolone increased bone mass in the spine and prevented bone loss in the forearm in late postmenopausal women, as determined by densitometry and several biochemical parameters of bone turnover. This occurred at two doses (1.25 and 2.5 mg/day), indicating that even lower doses may be efficacious[67]. In a second randomized controlled trial, tibolone induced a significant increase in trabecular (lumbar spine) and cortical (femoral neck) bone mass in postmenopausal osteoporotic women, compared to placebo[68]. Administration of tibolone in association with gonadotropin-releasing hormone analog (GnRH-a) reduced vasomotor symptoms and prevented bone loss, without compromising the therapeutic efficacy of GnRH-a alone[69].

Conclusion

In the 50-year modern history of osteoporosis, advances in therapy and monitoring have given the clinician an enormous armamentarium with which to battle osteoporosis. The challenge for the next 50 years is to reduce bone fracture risk by maintaining and restoring the constituents of BMD. This must be achieved while concomitantly maintaining quality of life and reducing the symptoms of estrogen excess and/or deprivation. Advances in the selective estrogen receptor modulator (SERM) drugs promise to revolutionize the future management of osteoporosis. These innovations will allow clinicians to provide effective prevention of bone fracture morbidity and mortality, while minimizing some of the undesirable effects of estrogen on reproductive tissues.

References

1. Cummings SR, Kelsey JL, Nevitt MC, O'Dowd KJ. Epidemiology of osteoporosis and osteoporotic fractures. *Epidemiol Rev* 1985;7:178–208
2. Ray NF, Chan JK, Thamer M, Melton LJ. Medical expenditures for the treatment of osteoporotic fractures in the United States in 1995; report from the National Osteoporosis Foundation. *J Bone Miner Res* 1997;12:24–35
3. Cooper C. The crippling consequences of fractures and their impact on quality of life. *Am J Med* 1997;103:12S–17S
4. Browner WS, Pressman AR, Nevitt MC, Cummings SR. Mortality following fractures in older women. The study of osteoporotic fractures. *Arch Intern Med* 1996;156:1521–5
5. Nevitt MC, Ettinger B, Black DM, *et al.* The association of radiographically detected vertebral fractures with back pain and function: a prospective study. *Ann Intern Med* 1998;128:793–800
6. Kanis JA, McCloskey EV. Epidemiology of vertebral osteoporosis. *Bone* 1992;13(Suppl 12):S1–10
7. Ettinger B, Black DM, Palermo L, Nevitt MC, Melnikoff S, Cummings SR. Kyphosis in older women and its relation to back pain, disability and osteopenia: the study of osteoporotic fractures. *Osteoporos Int* 1994;4:55–60
8. Mierke DF, Pellegrini M. Parathyroid hormone and parathyroid hormone-related protein: model systems for the development of an osteoporosis therapy. *Curr Pharm Des* 1999;5:21–36
9. Brown EM, Hebert SC. The First Annual Bayard D. Catherwood Memorial Lecture. Ca²⁺-receptor-mediated regulation of parathyroid and renal function. *Am J Med Sci* 1996;312:99–109
10. Copp DH. Calcitonin: discovery, development, and clinical application. *Clin Invest Med* 1994;17:268–77
11. Reginster JY. Calcitonins: newer routes of delivery. *Osteoporos Int* 1993;3(Suppl 2):S3–6, S6–7
12. Gennari C, Agnusdei D, Camporeale A. Long-term treatment with calcitonin in osteoporosis. *Horm Metab Res* 1993;25:484–5
13. Theintz G, Buchs B, Rizzoli R, *et al.* Longitudinal monitoring of bone mass accumulation in healthy adolescents: evidence for a marked reduction after 16 years of age at the levels of lumbar spine and femoral neck in female subjects. *J Clin Endocrinol Metab* 1992;75:1060–5
14. Kroger H, Kotaniemi A, Kroger L, Alhava E. Development of bone mass and bone density of the spine and femoral neck – a prospective study of 65 children and adolescents. *Bone Miner* 1993;23:171–82
15. Bonjour JP, Theintz G, Buchs B, Slosman D, Rizzoli R. Critical years and stages of puberty for spinal and femoral bone mass accumulation during adolescence. *J Clin Endocrinol Metab* 1991; 73:555–63
16. Ferrari S, Rizzoli R, Slosman D, Bonjour JP. Familial resemblance for bone mineral mass is expressed before puberty. *J Clin Endocrinol Metab* 1998;83:358–61
17. Gregg EW, Cauley JA, Seeley DG, Ensrud KE, Bauer DC. Physical activity and osteoporotic fracture risk in older women. Study of Osteoporotic Fractures Research Group. *Ann Intern Med* 1998; 129:81–8
18. Kannus P. Preventing osteoporosis, falls, and fractures among elderly people. Promotion of lifelong physical activity is essential [Editorial]. *Br Med J* 1999;318:205–6
19. Whooley MA, Kip KE, Cauley JA, Ensrud KE, Nevitt MC, Browner WS. Depression, falls, and risk of fracture in older women. Study of Osteoporotic Fractures Research Group. *Arch Intern Med* 1999; 159:484–90
20. Cummings SR, Browner WS, Bauer D, *et al.* Endogenous hormones and the risk of hip and vertebral fractures among older women. Study of Osteoporotic Fractures Research Group. *N Engl J Med* 1998;339:733–8
21. Reid IR. Glucocorticoid effects on bone [Editorial]. *J Clin Endocrinol Metab* 1998;83:1860–2
22. Baylink DJ. Glucocorticoid-induced osteoporosis [Editorial]. *N Engl J Med* 1983;309:306–8
23. Greenspan SL, Greenspan FS. The effect of thyroid hormone on skeletal integrity. *Ann Intern Med* 1999;130:750–8
24. Affinito P, Sorrentino C, Farace MJ, *et al.* Effects of thyroxine therapy on bone metabolism in postmenopausal women with hypothyroidism. *Acta Obstet Gynecol Scand* 1996;75:843–8
25. Bauer DC, Nevitt MC, Ettinger B, Stone K. Low thyrotropin levels are not associated with bone loss in older women: a prospective study. *J Clin Endocrinol Metab* 1997;82:2931–6
26. Kiel DP, Baron JA, Anderson JJ, Hannan MT, Felson DT. Smoking eliminates the protective effect of oral estrogens on the risk for hip fracture among women. *Ann Intern Med* 1992;116:716–21
27. Cornuz J, Feskanich D, Willett WC, Colditz GA. Smoking, smoking cessation, and risk of hip fracture in women. *Am J Med* 1999;106:311–14
28. Huda W, Morin RL. Patient doses in bone mineral densitometry. *Br J Radiol* 1996;69:422–5
29. Seto H, Kageyama M, Nomura K, Kakishita M, Tonami S. Precision of total-body and regional bone mineral measurement by dual-energy X-ray absorptiometry. *Radiat Med* 1991;9:110–13
30. Tothill P, Avenell A. Errors in dual-energy X-ray absorptiometry of the lumbar spine owing to fat

distribution and soft tissue thickness during weight change. *Br J Radiol* 1994;67:71–5

31. Borg J, Mollgaard A, Riis BJ. Single X-ray absorptiometry: performance characteristics and comparison with single photon absorptiometry. *Osteoporos Int* 1995;5:377–81

32. Kelly TL, Crane G, Baran DT. Single X-ray absorptiometry of the forearm: precision, correlation, and reference data. *Calcif Tissue Int* 1994;54:212–18

33. Rossini M, Viapiana O, Adami S. Instrumental diagnosis of osteoporosis. *Aging (Milano)* 1998;10: 240–8

34. Guglielmi G. Quantitative computed tomography (QCT) and dual X-ray absorptiometry (DXA) in the diagnosis of osteoporosis. *Eur J Radiol* 1995;20: 185–7

35. Rosenthall L, Caminis J, Tenehouse A. Calcaneal ultrasonometry: response to treatment in comparison with dual x-ray absorptiometry measurements of the lumbar spine and femur. *Calcif Tissue Int* 1999;64:200–4

36. Christenson RH. Biochemical markers of bone metabolism: an overview. *Clin Biochem* 1997;30: 573–93

37. Adachi JD. The correlation of bone mineral density and biochemical markers to fracture risk. *Calcif Tissue Int* 1996;59(Suppl 1):16–19

38. Garnero P, Delmas PD. New developments in biochemical markers for osteoporosis. *Calcif Tissue Int* 1996;59:2–9

39. Miura H, Yamamoto I, Yuu I, *et al.* Estimation of bone mineral density and bone loss by means of bone metabolic markers in postmenopausal women. *Endocr J* 1995;42:797–802

40. Baeksgaard L, Andersen KP, Hyldstrup L. Calcium and vitamin D supplementation increases spinal BMD in healthy, postmenopausal women. *Osteoporos Int* 1998;8:255–60

41. Citron JT, Ettinger B, Genant HK. Spinal bone mineral loss in estrogen-replete, calcium-replete premenopausal women. *Osteoporos Int* 1995;5: 228–33

42. Mizunuma H, Okano H, Soda M, *et al.* Calcium supplements increase bone mineral density in women with low serum calcium levels during long-term estrogen therapy. *Endocr J* 1996;43:411–15

43. Riggs BL, O'Fallon WM, Muhs J, O'Connor MK, Kumar R, Melton LJ. Long-term effects of calcium supplementation on serum parathyroid hormone level, bone turnover, and bone loss in elderly women. *J Bone Miner Res* 1998;13:168–74

44. Komulainen M, Tuppurainen MT, Kroger H, *et al.* Vitamin D and HRT: no benefit additional to that of HRT alone in prevention of bone loss in early postmenopausal women. A 2.5-year randomized placebo-controlled study. *Osteoporos Int* 1997;7: 126–32

45. Ooms ME, Roos JC, Bezemer PD, van der Vijgh WJ, Bouter LM, Lips P. Prevention of bone loss by vita-min D supplementation in elderly women: a randomized double-blind trial. *J Clin Endocrinol Metab* 1995;80:1052–8

46. Ringe JD. Vitamin D deficiency and osteopathies. *Osteoporos Int* 1998;8(Suppl 2):S35–9

47. Prince RL, Smith M, Dick IM, *et al.* Prevention of postmenopausal osteoporosis. A comparative study of exercise, calcium supplementation, and hormone-replacement therapy. *N Engl J Med* 1991; 325:1189–95

48. Hatori M, Hasegawa A, Adachi H, *et al.* The effects of walking at the anaerobic threshold level on vertebral bone loss in postmenopausal women. *Calcif Tissue Int* 1993;52:411–14

49. Wolff I, van Croonenberg JJ, Kemper HC, Kostense PJ, Twisk JW. The effect of exercise training programs on bone mass: a meta-analysis of published controlled trials in pre- and postmenopausal women. *Osteoporos Int* 1999;9:1–12

50. Berard A, Bravo G, Gauthier P. Meta-analysis of the effectiveness of physical activity for the prevention of bone loss in postmenopausal women. *Osteoporos Int* 1997;7:331–7

51. Anonymous. Effects of hormone therapy on bone mineral density: results from the postmenopausal estrogen/progestin interventions (PEPI) trial. The Writing Group for the PEPI. *J Am Med Assoc* 1996; 276:1389–96

52. Cauley JA, Seeley DG, Ensrud K, Ettinger B, Black D, Cummings SR. Estrogen replacement therapy and fractures in older women. Study of Osteoporotic Fractures Research Group. *Ann Intern Med* 1995;122:9–16

53. Deng HW, Li J, Li JL, *et al.* Change of bone mass in postmenopausal Caucasian women with and without hormone replacement therapy is associated with vitamin D receptor and estrogen receptor genotypes. *Hum Genet* 1998;103:576–85

54. Genant HK, Lucas J, Weiss S, *et al.* Low-dose esterified estrogen therapy: effects on bone, plasma estradiol concentrations, endometrium, and lipid levels. Estratab/Osteoporosis Study Group. *Arch Intern Med* 1997;157: 2609–15

55. Stevenson JC, Cust MP, Gangar KF, Hillard TC, Lees B, Whitehead MI. Effects of transdermal versus oral hormone replacement therapy on bone density in spine and proximal femur in postmenopausal women. *Lancet* 1990;336:265–9

56. George GH, MacGregor AJ, Spector TD. Influence of current and past hormone replacement therapy on bone mineral density: a study of discordant postmenopausal twins. *Osteoporos Int* 1999;9: 158–62

57. McClung M, Clemmesen B, Daifotis A, *et al.* Alendronate prevents postmenopausal bone loss in women without osteoporosis. A double-blind, randomized, controlled trial. Alendronate Osteoporosis Prevention Study Group. *Ann Intern Med* 1998;128:253–61

58. Watts NB, Becker P. Alendronate increases spine and hip bone mineral density in women with postmenopausal osteoporosis who failed to respond to intermittent cyclical etidronate. *Bone* 1999;24:65–8

59. Devogelaer JP, Broll H, Correa-Rotter R, *et al*. Oral alendronate induces progressive increases in bone mass of the spine, hip, and total body over 3 years in postmenopausal women with osteoporosis [Erratum *Bone* 1996;19:78]. *Bone* 1996;18:141–50

60. Overgaard K, Hansen MA, Jensen SB, Christiansen C. Effect of salcatonin given intranasally on bone mass and fracture rates in established osteoporosis: a dose–response study. *Br Med J* 1992;305:556–61

61. Franceschini R, Cataldi A, Cianciosi P, *et al*. Calcitonin and beta-endorphin secretion. *Biomed Pharmacother* 1993;47:305–9

62. Boss SM, Huster WJ, Neild JA, Glant MD, Eisenhut CC, Draper MW. Effects of raloxifene hydrochloride on the endometrium of postmenopausal women. *Am J Obstet Gynecol* 1997;177:1458–64

63. Mijatovic V, van der Mooren MJ, Kenemans P, de Valk-de RG, Netelenbos C. Raloxifene lowers serum lipoprotein(a) in healthy postmenopausal women: a randomized, double-blind, placebo-controlled comparison with conjugated equine estrogens. *Menopause* 1999;6:134–7

64. Delmas PD, Bjarnason NH, Mitlak BH, *et al*. Effects of raloxifene on bone mineral density, serum cholesterol concentrations, and uterine endometrium in postmenopausal women. *N Engl J Med* 1997;337:1641–7

65. Mijatovic V, Netelenbos C, van der Mooren MJ, de Valk-de RG, Jakobs C, Kenemans P. Randomized, double-blind, placebo-controlled study of the effects of raloxifene and conjugated equine estrogen on plasma homocysteine levels in healthy postmenopausal women. *Fertil Steril* 1998;70: 1085–9

66. Cummings SR, Eckert S, Krueger KA, *et al*. The effect of raloxifene on risk of breast cancer in postmenopausal women: results from the MORE randomized trial. Multiple Outcomes of Raloxifene Evaluation. *J Am Med Assoc* 1999;281:2189–97

67. Bjarnason NH, Bjarnason K, Haarbo J, Rosenquist C, Christiansen C. Tibolone: prevention of bone loss in late postmenopausal women [see Comments]. *J Clin Endocrinol Metab* 1996;81:2419–22

68. Bjarnason NH, Bjarnason K, Hassager C, Christiansen C. The response in spinal bone mass to tibolone treatment is related to bone turnover in elderly women. *Bone* 1997;20:151–5

69. Palomba S, Affinito P, Tommaselli GA, Nappi C. A clinical trial of the effects of tibolone administered with gonadotropin-releasing hormone analogues for the treatment of uterine leiomyomata. *Fertil Steril* 1998;70:111–18

11

Menopause and cardiovascular disease

William P. Castelli

Introduction

The number one cause of death in women is a disease related to atherosclerosis such as coronary heart disease, stroke, peripheral vascular disease or other manifestations of vascular disease. Almost twice as many women die from these diseases as from all the cancers put together; in the latest Vital Statistics of the United States it amounted to 45% of deaths in women[1]. As important as the death rates are, the morbidity from vascular disease is even greater considering that, prior to age 65, only about 15% of women die when they develop coronary heart disease; 85% of these women live. Over age 65, the death rate is 20-25% but 75% live. Almost half of the people who live have a lower quality of life; many lose their jobs.

Some 70-75% of the women destined to develop cardiovascular disease could be identified years in advance of their clinical manifestations if their physicians were willing to measure a few simple things on their bodies. These 'things' have come to be known as the risk factors and deal with those well-known items such as cholesterol, blood pressure, smoking, blood sugar, weight and many other variables that are described in this chapter.

Women, more recently, have been involved in trials to lower the risk factor numbers, and these studies have led to clinical strategies to prevent cardiovascular disease in women and offer better treatments for those who have developed the disease. Those health professionals involved with the care of women after the menopause need to recognize the importance of assessing these women for diseases other than just those associated with the reproductive status of women.

Rates of cardiovascular disease

Prior to the menopause, only six women in the Framingham Heart Study developed coronary heart disease[2]. These women can be found in any town in the world. They have familial hypercholesterolemia, familial combined hyperlipoproteinemia or diabetes, and smoke at the same time. Once women pass through the menopause it takes them about 6–10 years to catch up to the same rates of coronary heart disease as occur in men, as indicated by Figure 1 if horizontal lines are drawn onto this. Of course statisticians are taught to draw vertical lines to compare rates at the same age, where women generally run a lower rate of disease until they reach 85 and beyond. The lifetime risk of cardiovascular disease is another way of looking at these rates. In the Framingham Study, the lifetime risk of women, starting at age 40, for coronary disease is 31.7% (95% confidence interval, CI 29.2–34.2), which, when added to the risk of cerebrovascular disease (9%) and other vascular disease (7%), adds up to 47.7% of women developing

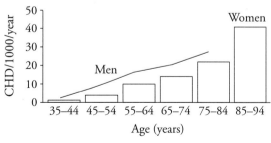

Figure 1 Annual coronary heart disease (CHD) rate for men and women: Framingham Heart Study; National Heart, Lung, and Blood Institute; Boston University School of Medicine. From 30-year database

cardiovascular disease over their lifetime, compared to 54% of men[3].

Blood lipids

Total cholesterol

One of the first lipids to be looked at in the Framingham Heart Study was total cholesterol. As Figure 2 shows, at any age, the higher is the total cholesterol level the higher is the subsequent rate of coronary heart disease. Note that older women do not tolerate cholesterol better than do younger women. The absolute rate in 70-year-old women is double that in 50-year-old women, everything else being equal.

As shown in Figure 3, the total cholesterol level is not sufficient, by itself, to identify 90% of the women at risk, as the bell-shaped curve for all the total cholesterols of the men and women of the Framingham Study who stayed free of coronary heart disease in the first 26 years of the study overlapped the bell-shaped curve for the men and women who developed coronary heart disease, when the total cholesterols were between 150 and 300 mg/dl.

We understand three kinds of risk in medicine: relative, absolute and attributable risk. Relative risk shows that people with a total cholesterol level of 300 mg/dl have five times the rate of disease as people with 150 mg/dl. Absolute risk shows that, for people with a cholesterol level of 300 mg/dl or higher, 90/100 are likely to develop coronary heart disease. It is generally agreed that people with such high cholesterol levels should be treated at any age, because the chance of treating someone who does not need it is low. Attributable risk is more complex. There are several kinds, but that illustrated in

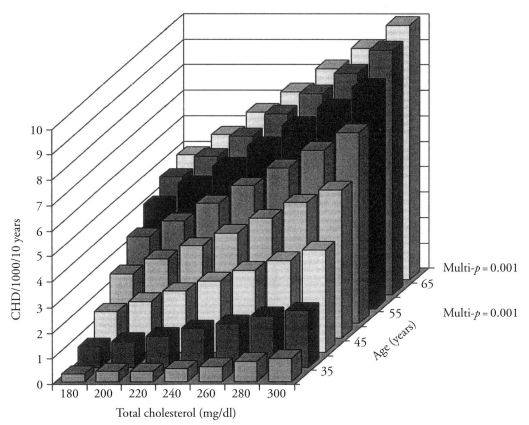

Figure 2 Coronary heart disease (CHD) and total cholesterol in low-risk women: Framingham Heart Study; National Heart, Lung, and Blood Institute; Boston University School of Medicine. Multi-p, after adjustment for systolic blood pressure, cigarettes, diabetes, LVR. From reference 4

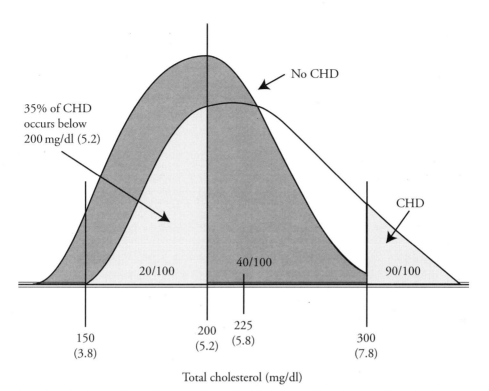

Figure 3 Relative, absolute and population-attributable risk fractions: Framingham Heart Study; National Heart, Lung, and Blood Institute; Boston University School of Medicine. CHD, coronary heart disease. From reference 5

Figure 3 is the population-attributable risk fraction, i.e. the fraction of heart attacks that one would attribute to a particular level of cholesterol. For example, twice as many women with a cholesterol level between 150 and 200 mg/dl all their lives are likely to develop coronary disease as those with a cholesterol level over 300 mg/dl. The National Cholesterol Education Program (NCEP) considered a cholesterol level under 200 mg/dl desirable. Why should this be so, when twice as many women and men develop coronary disease at this level? It is largely because the Education Program ignored attributable risk. They understood absolute risk and, therefore, the rate at cholesterol levels between 150 and 200 mg/dl being 20/100. The reason that there are more heart attacks at 20/100 than at 90/100 is that the incidence of 20/100 relates to 45% of a practice population whereas the incidence of 90/100 relates to just 3% of the practice. If we eliminate all the heart attacks occurring at a cholesterol level over 300 mg/dl, the rate of coronary disease will fall by 10–15%. Eventually we have to find a way to prevent the 35% of

heart attacks that occur at cholesterol levels between 150 and 200 mg/dl. The worst cholesterol level in this regard is between 220 and 225 mg/dl because more coronary disease occurs at that level of cholesterol than at any other, and the rate is 40/100. How does one find just the 20, 40 and 90 out of 100 at these different levels of cholesterol so that one does not treat people who do not need it? This is when one must look at the other kinds of cholesterol found in the blood, of which there are 18 identified to date. One other point: if the total cholesterol level is under 150 mg/dl then the person is like the billions of people on this earth that cannot develop atherosclerotic disease. These people, live in the poorer sections of Asia, Africa and Latin America. Unfortunately, they are now adopting many of the Western dietary practices, for example fast food.

High-density lipoprotein cholesterol

Of the 18 different kinds of cholesterol, the one that needs to be looked at first is high-density lipoprotein (HDL) cholesterol. Figure 4 shows the level of total cholesterol stratified by the HDL cholesterol level in men and women in the Framingham Study. It can be seen that the higher is the HDL level, the lower is the rate of coronary heart disease. The first row of this figure indicates that the high-risk people with a total cholesterol level under 200 mg/dl have a low HDL level. This is true of all the other levels of cholesterol but, the higher the total cholesterol level, the higher the level of HDL cholesterol needed for protection. Rather than memorizing a different HDL level for each total cholesterol level, a simple ratio is sufficient: the total cholesterol divided by the HDL cholesterol. This is the best predictor in the Framingham Study, the Lipid Research Clinics trial, the Physicians' Health Study, the Harvard Nurses' Study, the 4S (Scandinavian Simvastatin Survivors Study) Study, etc.

Figure 5 shows the ratio of total cholesterol/ HDL cholesterol in women. There is another way to think about risk: normal, average and ideal (Dawber TR, personal communication). What is called normal in the United States? 'Average' is

called normal. However, instead of being like the average American, it would be better to be like the average Chinese who cannot develop this disease at 125 mg/dl cholesterol. We need to think about ideal; for now we choose a total cholesterol/ HDL ratio of less than 4.

Low-density lipoprotein cholesterol

Figure 6 shows that the higher the level of low-density lipoprotein (LDL) as measured by the S_f 0–20 lipoproteins, the higher the rate of coronary heart disease. The NCEP guidelines used to evaluate the lipid numbers are not completely followed in clinical practice because of their complexity; most physicians can only remember the three goals of therapy which are the LDL cholesterol levels: 160, 130 and 100 mg/dl. Subjects who have no vascular disease diagnosed to date, and only one other risk factor, should lower their LDL cholesterol level to under 160 mg/dl. Those with two or more other risk factors but no vascular disease should have an LDL cholesterol level under 130 mg/dl. Those with vascular disease should

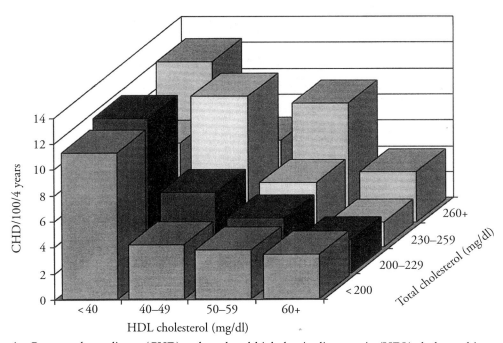

Figure 4 Coronary heart disease (CHD) and total and high-density lipoprotein (HDL) cholesterol in men and women aged 50–59 years: Framingham Heart Study; National Heart, Lung, and Blood Institute; Boston University School of Medicine. From reference 6

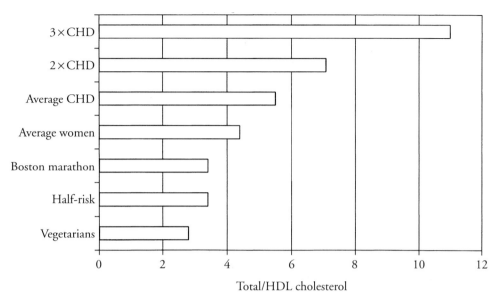

Figure 5 Total/high-density lipoprotein (HDL) cholesterol ratio in women (The goal is < 4): Framingham Heart Study; National Heart, Lung, and Blood Institute; Boston University School of Medicine. CHD, coronary heart disease

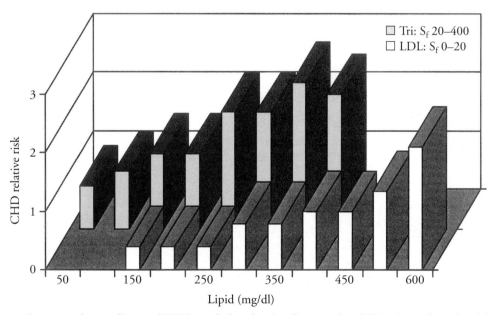

Figure 6 Coronary heart disease (CHD) and low-density lipoprotein (LDL; S_f 0–20) and triglycerides (Tri; S_f 20–400) in women: Framingham Heart Study; National Heart, Lung, and Blood Institute; Boston University School of Medicine. From reference 5

have an LDL cholesterol level under 100 mg/dl. Other risk factors are: family history of vascular disease before the age of 55, hypertension, cigarette smoking, HDL cholesterol level under 35 mg/dl and diabetes. A level of 160 mg/dl LDL seems inappropriate because the average LDL cholesterol level of someone who dies of coronary heart disease in the USA is under 150 mg/dl. The target should be a lot lower than that. For people with the disease, the National Heart, Lung, and Blood Institute post coronary artery bypass graft study has shown that the most reversibility is achieved when the level of LDL cholesterol is under 80 mg/dl (Hunninghake D, personal communication), and the AVERT study showed that reducing levels to an LDL of 77 mg/dl (by giving 80 mg of atorvastatin) produced a significantly lower ischemic event rate in 1.5 years, compared to angioplasty[7].

The seven LDLs

There are seven LDL cholesterols, and the smaller is the LDL particle size, the higher is the heart attack rate[8]. However, similar to total cholesterol, if the total/HDL cholesterol ratio is low, i.e. under 4, then there is enough HDL to protect from the elevated level of LDL. An LDL cholesterol level cannot be interpreted unless the patient's total/HDL ratio is known. As the size of LDL falls, the triglyceride levels rise and the HDL levels fall, as shown in Figure 7. This has led to a new understanding about triglyceride levels in women: namely that, in addition to having atherogenic triglyceride particles, all their LDLs are the more atherogenic, small, dense variety. When a woman's triglyceride level reaches 150 mg/dl, most of her LDL is in the small, dense category.

Triglycerides

As Figure 6 also shows, the higher the triglyceride level in women, the higher the heart attack rate. There are four major classes of triglyceride: two are not atherogenic; one type are the chylomicrons that appear in blood shortly after a high-fat meal; the other type are the larger, very-low-density lipoproteins that come out of the liver after a vegetarian diet, or the intake of estrogen, alcohol or a resin. The two that are atherogenic are the chylomicron remnants and the small, dense, very-low-density lipoproteins. The chylomicron remnants are derived from the chylomicrons after they have had some of their triglyceride fat removed by lipoprotein lipase. The small, dense, very-low-density lipoproteins come out of the liver after diets high in saturated fat and cholesterol. Chylomicrons and chylomicron remnants have been poorly studied because of the use of prolonged fasts prior to measuring blood lipids. The large and small very-low-density lipoproteins constitute the bulk of the triglycerides in fasting blood, with 70% being the small, dense, very atherogenic, very-low-density lipoproteins[10].

However, similar to total cholesterol and LDL cholesterol, triglyceride risk is better ascertained if the HDL cholesterol level is known. As Figure 8 shows, it is particularly the women with high

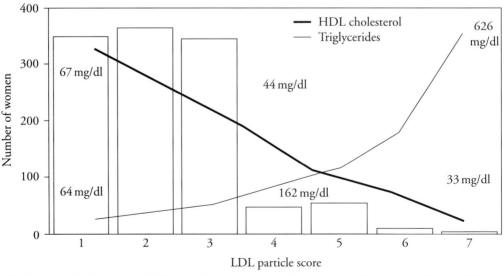

Figure 7 Low-density lipoprotein (LDL) particle size in women: Framingham Heart Study; National Heart, Lung, and Blood Institute; Lipid Metabolism Laboratory, USDA, Tufts University. HDL, high-density lipoprotein. From reference 9

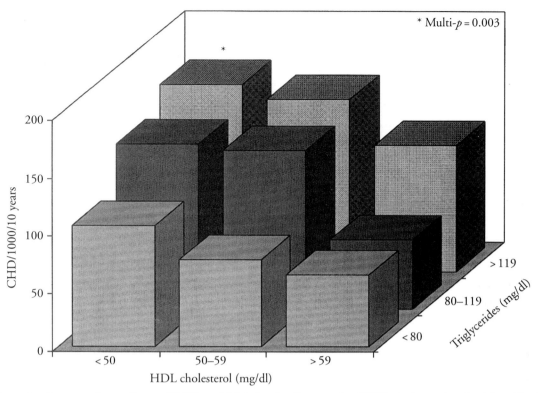

Figure 8 Coronary heart disease (CHD) and high-density lipoprotein (HDL) cholesterol and triglycerides in women: Framingham Heart Study; National Heart, Lung, and Blood Institute; Boston University School of Medicine. From reference 5

triglyceride and low HDL cholesterol levels who incur the highest rate of coronary heart disease. These people have also been found to have other problems. Gerald Reaven showed that they have increased insulin resistance and hypertension, and called this combination syndrome X[11]. Norman Kaplan emphasized the work of Jean Vaque, the French physician who drew attention to the dangers of central obesity[12]. As triglyceride levels rise above 80–90 mg/dl, there is a shift in the size of LDL from larger LDL to smaller, more atherogenic LDL, and when the triglycerides reach 150 mg/dl, all of the LDL has been shifted to the small, dense variety. In addition, women with this syndrome have higher levels of the clotting factors such as fibrinogen and plasminogen activator inhibitor-1 (PAI-1)[16]. They also have higher uric acid levels, which have been associated with higher risk (Figure 9).

The reason that the guidelines have been less stringent with regard to triglycerides is that it has

---

When waist/hip exceeds 0.8
    Glucose 5.5 mmol/l (100 mg/dl)
    Insulin resistance
        insulin > 25 mU/l
        C peptide > 1.3 nmol/l
    BP over 130/85
    Triglycerides 1.7 mmol/l (150 mg/dl)
      small dense β VLDL
    HDL cholesterol 1.17 mmol/l (45 mg/dl)
    LDL
      small dense pattern β
    Uric acid 0.4 mmol/l (7)
    Plasminogen activator inhibitor-1 (PAI-1)
    Microalbuminuria, increased Na/Li
    exchange

Figure 9 Syndrome X (Reaven[11]), deadly quartet (Kaplan[12]), dyslipidemic hypertension (Williams[13]), insulin resistance syndrome[14], metabolic syndrome[15]. BP, blood pressure; VLDL, very-low-density lipoprotein; HDL, high-density lipoprotein; LDL, low-density lipoprotein

only recently been shown that they are an independent risk factor[17].

The most practical way to identify women with a dangerous triglyceride concentration is to find those with a triglyceride level of 150 mg/dl and an HDL level of under 50 mg/dl. As shown in Figure 8, they have a significantly higher heart attack rate, but they are largely ignored in medicine because their total cholesterol levels are frequently under 200 mg/dl and their LDL cholesterol levels are under 130 mg/dl. They have the very atherogenic, small, dense, β very-low-density lipoprotein.

Genetic disorders of lipids

About 5% of postmenopausal women have a very high risk of vascular disease associated with their inherited tendency to have high levels of LDL cholesterol, triglycerides or both. These are generally traits that have run in their families, and many will have a family history of premature vascular disease occurring before the age of 60. Table 1 gives the cut-off points proposed by Levy and Schaefer to identify the women at any age who are most likely to have a 'genetic' tendency to develop high lipids. Those with LDL cholesterol levels at or above that listed for their age are type IIA hyperlipoproteinemic. Those with a triglyceride level at or above that cited for their age are type IV hyperlipoproteinemic. Those who equal or exceed

both numbers for their age are combined type IIB hyperlipoproteinemic[18]. In addition to treating these women more aggressively, it is important to measure the lipids in all of their children. The type IIA's are generally autosomal dominant, and half of their children will inherit this disorder.

Lipoprotein(a)

A new risk factor is lipoprotein(a). It is a combination of an LDL particle with the small 'a' protein, which blocks the conversion of plasminogen to plasmin which, in turn, dissolves the fibrin on endothelial cells. We live in this 'drizzle' of platelets clumping and unclumping, and fibrinogen being converted to fibrin all day long. When the fibrin hits the endothelial cell, it stimulates the cell to send tissue-type plasminogen activator and urokinase to activate plasminogen to plasmin, which will dissolve the fibrin. Figure 10 is the first evidence in women that lipoprotein(a) is associated with increased risk of coronary heart disease[19]. The difficulty with lipoprotein(a) is therapy: to date, only high doses of crystalline niacin have lowered the level to below 30 mg/dl; in most subjects, the solution is to lower their LDL level to under 80 mg/dl and their triglycerides to under 90 mg/dl, to a state at which they cannot develop atherosclerosis.

Lipids and the menopause

When women pass through the menopause, there is a significant rise in LDL cholesterol and a fall in HDL cholesterol. Triglycerides continue to rise. The total cholesterol/HDL ratio and the apolipoprotein B/A ratio rise significantly, as indicated in Table 2.

Estrogen and the menopause

One of the most important events to happen during the menopause is the fall in estrogen. Estrogen is antiatherogenic. The best data come from the work of Clarkson and colleagues in the cynomolgus macaque. These monkeys have 98% of the human genome. They have the same male–female difference in HDL. When they are fed an atherogenic diet, the male total cholesterol/HDL ratio is

Table 1 Low-density lipoprotein (LDL) cholesterol and triglyceride levels (mg/dl) for identifying types of hyperlipoproteinemia. From reference 18

Age (years)	LDL-II	Triglycerides-IV
0–4		96
5–9	125	90
10–14	126	114
15–19	127	107
20–24	136	112
25–29	141	116
30–34	142	123
35–39	161	137
40–44	164	155
45–49	173	171
50–54	192	186
55–59	204	204
60–64	201	202
65–69	208	204
70	189	204

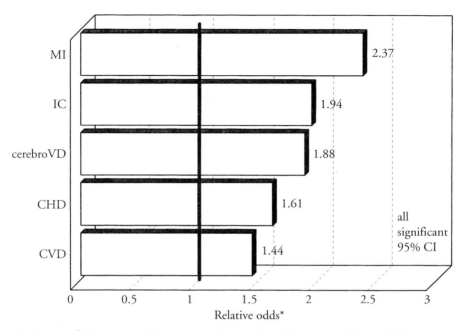

Figure 10 Sinking pre-β lipoprotein(a) in women: Framingham Heart Study; National Heart, Lung, and Blood Institute; Boston University School of Medicine. *Relative odds adjusted for age, body mass index, systolic blood pressure, cigarette use, high-density lipoprotein, low-density lipoprotein, glucose, left ventricular hypertrophy on electrocardiogram. MI, myocardial infarction; IC, intermittent claudication; cerebroVD, cerebrovascular disease; CHD, coronary heart disease; CVD, cardiovascular disease; CI, confidence interval. From reference 19

Table 2 Lipid changes with menopause. From reference 20

	Premenopausal	Postmenopausal	p Value
Total cholesterol (mg/dl)	208	227	0.08
LDL cholesterol (mg/dl)	134	156	0.03
Triglycerides (mg/dl)	87	98	0.30
HDL cholesterol (mg/dl)	56	51	0.10
HDL/total cholesterol	0.27	0.24	0.02
Apo A₁/Apo B	2.41	1.86	0.04

LDL, low-density lipoprotein; HDL, high-density lipoprotein; Apo, apolipoprotein

increased to almost 12. In control females with their higher HDL, the ratio increases to 8; they develop appreciable atherosclerosis but not as much as the males. If the females are given a second-generation progestin which raises LDL and lowers HDL, such as norgestrel, the ratio is increased to 12, but if it is given in the form of a birth-control pill with a high dose of estrogen, the atherosclerosis is greatly diminished. With a second-generation progestin such as levonorgestrel without the estrogen, a high total cholesterol/HDL ratio and increased atherosclerosis result[21]. The same is probably true in human females. In the Harvard Nurses' Study, nurses who took the first generation birth-control pills which caused thrombosis-related deaths produced a 20% lower rate of coronary heart disease if they survived to the menopause, and stopped taking such a high dose of estrogen.

The use of estrogen is a double-edged sword. At any dose it is antiatherogenic. But as the dose rises, the blood starts to clot and this will, at high doses, lead to coronary heart disease and stroke, as it did in the postmenopausal women of the Framingham Study who were taking 2.5 and 3.5 mg of conjugated estrogens[22]. In the Harvard Nurses' Study, postmenopausal women taking estrogen at a dose above 1.25 mg more than doubled their rate of coronary disease[23]. Men given estrogen in the Coronary Drug Project[24] at a dose of 2.5 mg conjugated estrogens died at a significantly higher rate of coronary disease, and this arm of the study was stopped prematurely. The birth-control pill is one of the few medicines in use for which a dose–response curve was never determined. The dose fell in the history of the pill from 150 μg of ethinylestradiol down eventually to 20 μg, but lower doses have never been fully tested. Recently, lower doses have been looked at in the hormone replacement therapy (HRT) field, where 5 and 10 μg of ethinylestradiol with norethindrone provide the same osteoporosis prevention as do higher doses[25].

Epidemiological studies have shown that women taking HRT incur about a 50% lower heart attack rate than those not taking HRT. These are not random trials, and the benefits could have been explained by the healthy cohort effect, namely that the women who self-select to take estrogen are richer and smarter than the women who do not, and do all kinds of other things to improve their risk and that is why they incur such a low heart attack rate[26]. The first random trial, the Heart Estrogen/progestin Replacement Study (HERS), while not in women free of disease, showed only a small fall after several years and even suggested that there was a higher rate of coronary death in the first year, which was probably a statistical artifact due to the very low rate of coronary disease in the first year of the control group compared to years 2, 3, 4 and 5. What the HERS trial did demonstrate is that estrogen therapy is not a substitute for cholesterol therapy. Fewer than 10% of the women had their LDL cholesterols reduced to under 100 mg/dl. The Women's Health Initiative, which is giving estrogen in the primary prevention setting, is still ongoing, and this will be the trial that provides the best evidence of use of HRT in healthy women.

The HERS trial missed an opportunity to study whether the 'old' clotting factors related to risk such as fibrinogen or factor VII, or the 'new' clotting factors which have recently been found to play a role in thrombosis such as Leiden factor V, protein C deficiency, protein S deficiency, prothrombin 20210A, elevated factor VIII and homo-

Table 3 Prevalence of risk factors for thrombosis (%) from reference 27

Risk factor	General population	Patients with thrombosis
Protein C deficiency	0.2–0.4	3
Protein S deficiency	not known	1–2
Antithrombin deficiency	0.02	1
Factor V Leiden	5	20
Prothrombin 20210A	2	6
High factor VIII (> 1500 IU/l)	11	25
Homocysteine > 18.5 μmol/l	5	10

cysteine (Table 3), contribute to the tolerated doses of estrogen or progesterone. Third-generation progestins such as desogestrel, gestodene and norgestimate accelerate the generation of thrombin, which leads to platelet aggregation and generation of fibrin from fibrinogen. Medroxyprogesterone causes vasospasm by itself, but this effect is blunted in animals when estrogen is added.

The Postmenopausal Estrogen/Progestin Interventions (PEPI) study compared the effects of several HRT regimens on lipids, blood pressure and fibrinogen. Compared to estrogen alone, the fall in LDL cholesterol and the rise in HDL cholesterol were only a little less for preparations containing progesterone, with micronized progesterone performing slightly better than medroxyprogesterone. Fibrinogen levels fell with HRT use. Blood pressure, which rises in subjects taking high-dose estrogen such as a 30-μg ethinylestradiol pill or higher, was no greater in women taking HRT than in the control group. Outcome data relating to cardiovascular disease were not measured in this study[28].

The advantages of estrogen, at appropriate doses, continue to be elucidated by new research. Eskin and colleagues have recently proposed a series of new mechanisms by which estrogen provides benefit. In addition to the aforementioned effects on lipids, there are antioxidant effects, including: cardiac estrogen α and β receptors in mice, which could prevent vascular injury and necrosis; stabilization of the norepinephrine release mechanism in the heart; an increase in endothelial-mediated blood flow through enhancement of nitric oxide and improved coronary vasodilatation; a reduction in coronary artery

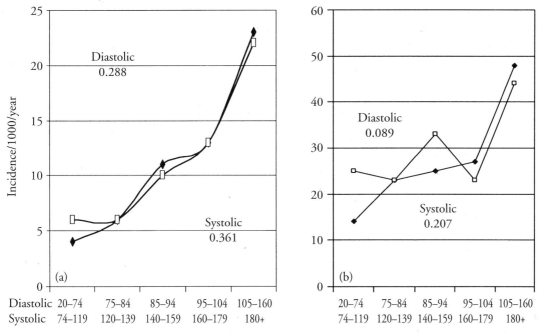

Figure 11 Blood pressure and cardiovascular disease (CVD) in (a) women aged 35–64 years and (b) women aged 65–94 years: Framingham Heart Study; National Heart, Lung, and Blood Institute; Boston University School of Medicine. From reference 30

vasoconstriction via a reduction in endothelin-1; inhibition of platelet aggregation and stimulation of vasodilatation by an increase in prostacyclin production[29].

Hypertension

It is only in those societies that eat a high-salt diet that the blood pressure rises with age. American women live in a society that eats 20 times the amount of salt they need. Blood pressure rises with age in women such that shortly after women pass through the menopause, over half will have high blood pressure defined as 140/90 mmHg or higher.

As diastolic or systolic pressures rise in women, cardiovascular risk, particularly of stroke and heart attack, rises as shown in Figure 11. Of the two measures, systolic pressure is a better predictor than diastolic pressure. Isolated systolic hypertension is also dangerous. The elderly do not tolerate high blood pressure, which is the opposite of what was taught for decades in medicine (Figure 12). Elderly women with isolated systolic hypertension have a

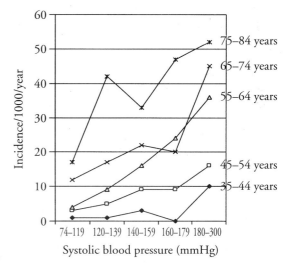

Figure 12 Systolic blood pressure and cardiovascular disease (CVD) in women: Framingham Heart Study; National Heart, Lung, and Blood Institute; Boston University School of Medicine. From reference 30

worse prognosis than do elderly women without hypertension.

Table 4 indicates that half of the coronary disease in women occurs at levels of blood pressure

Table 4 Twelve-year coronary heart disease incidence according to blood pressure category in women

Blood pressure category	Person-years F/U	Events (%)	Relative odds (95% CI)
Normal 120–129/ 80–84 mmHg	20710	29	1
High normal 130–139/ 85–89 mmHg	6043	16	1.31 (0.86–1.99)
Hypertension stage I 140/90 mmHg	7242	32	1.78 (1.19–2.51)
Hypertension stage II–IV	4000	23	2.12 (1.42–3.17)
Total	37995	n = 227	

F/U, follow up; CI, confidence interval

Table 5 Joint National Commission V and VI: classification of blood pressure in adults, 18 years or older. From reference 31

Category	Systolic (mmHg)	Diastolic (mmHg)
Normal	< 130	< 85
High normal	130–139	85–89
Hypertension		
Stage 1 (mild)	140–159	90–99
Stage 2 (moderate)	160–179	100–109
Stage 3 (severe)	180–209	110–119
Stage 4 (very severe)	≥ 210	≥ 120

120–139/80–89 mmHg. The latest Joint National Commission on Hypertension recommendations have tried to address at least half of this risk by setting a new cut-off point at 130/85 mmHg (Table 5).

Cigarette smoking

In 1948, when the first women entered the Framingham Study, of the 35% who said they smoked, virtually none inhaled. Of the major cancers beyond skin cancer, breast cancer was number one in incidence and lung cancer was last. Women learned how to inhale in the 1950s, and by the 1960s they were paying the price for inhaling. The incidences of vascular disease and especially of lung cancer rose, and, in 1987, lung cancer overtook breast cancer and became the number one cancer cause of death in women for the first time in

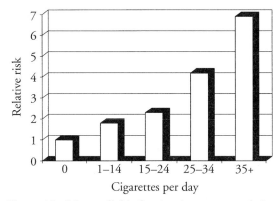

Figure 13 Myocardial infarction in women and cigarette smoking. From reference 32

the history of the USA, as it has been since time immemorial in men. Figure 13 is taken from the work of Rosenberg and her colleagues, and shows that the risk of myocardial infarction is dose-related, rising from a relative risk of 2.0 for 1–14 cigarettes per day to 7.2 for 35 or more[32]. Quitting returns the risk to that of non-smokers within 3 years in this study, but the benefit of quitting may be much quicker. It depends on how people define 'the quitter'. In the Framingham Study, where the smoker had to quit for an entire year to be called a quit-smoker, the risk fell back within 1 year. Women apparently have more difficulty in giving up smoking[33]. Women also tend to smoke 'low-yield' cigarettes, perhaps believing them to be safer, but the evidence shows that these cigarettes are not safer, and lead to just as much coronary heart disease as the old-fashioned high-tar and -nicotine cigarettes[34].

Blood glucose

The higher is the blood glucose, starting at levels even within the normal range, the higher is the rate of cardiovascular disease, in the Framingham Study. Figure 14 shows the hemoglobin A1c levels and prospective risk in this study. Note the bigger jump when the hemoglobin A1c level hits 5.5 mg/dl and above. This is equivalent to a fasting blood sugar level of 100 mg/dl. Subjects whose blood sugar was over 100 mg/dl, but not at the diagnostic level for diabetes at 126 mg/dl, eventually developed diabetes at three times the rate of people with a blood sugar under 100 mg/dl.

The majority of the diabetes in the USA is related to obesity, and getting rid of central obesity would eliminate 80-90% of the diabetes. Female diabetics develop cardiovascular disease at the same rate as men their age. Most diabetics die of cardiovascular disease, and they should be treated as if they already have the disease.

Weight

Weight gain from age 25 in the Framingham Study is a very dangerous risk factor. As people gain weight, their atherogenic lipids rise and their protective lipid HDL falls. Blood pressure, blood sugar, uric acid, the left ventricle size and insulin resistance all rise. Figure 15 shows that incidences

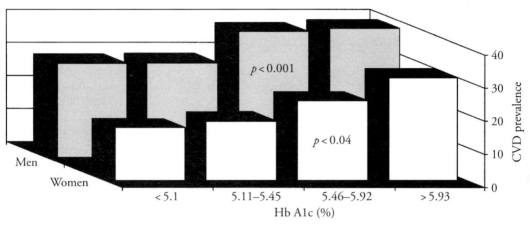

Figure 14 Hemoglobin (Hb) A1c and cardiovascular disease (CVD): Framingham Heart Study; National Heart, Lung, and Blood Institute; Boston University School of Medicine. From reference 35

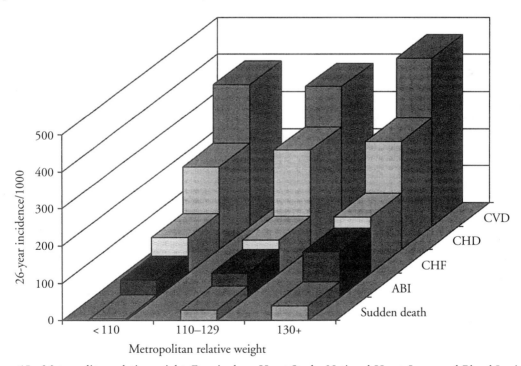

Figure 15 Metropolitan relative weight: Framingham Heart Study; National Heart, Lung, and Blood Institute; Boston University School of Medicine. CVD, cardiovascular disease; CHD, coronary heart disease; CHF, congestive heart failure; ABI, atherothrombotic brain infarction

of cardiovascular disease, coronary disease, congestive heart failure, stroke and sudden death all demonstrate an upward trend. Obesity is an independent risk factor on multivariate analysis for these end-points[36]. The USA is perhaps the 'fattest' country in the world, with food consumption approaching 40% of the food eaten on this earth: not bad for just 7% of the people who live on this earth!

Exercise

As Blair and his colleagues at the Cooper Clinic in Dallas showed, the women of America who exercise the most die at the slowest rate. These women also go on to develop heart attacks at the slowest rate (Figure 16), and incur a lower cancer rate. The low rates in this 8-year study in 3120 women could be achieved with a 30-min/day program[37]. The trade-off of exercise for calories seems unfair. Walking a mile burns off 100 cal; an American candy bar is 2.5 miles; a 'Big Mac' is 5.6 miles; the Burger King 'Whopper' is 6.4 miles. Of course McDonald's is not to be outdone: they are introducing the 'Mega-Burger'. It will have four hamburger patties: as Jay Leno, the late-night comedian commented, 'one burger for each chamber of your heart'. It takes about 35 miles to work off one pound.

Homocysteine

Homocysteine is an amino acid in the blood which is either excreted in the urine or converted back to methionine. Hyperhomocysteinemia is a recessive trait; children who inherited one gene from each parent develop hyperhomocysteinemia with values up at around 100 μmol/l, and they develop atherosclerotic disease as teenagers and occasionally even younger. They have homocysteinuria. Outside of these children it was not thought that homocysteine played a role in medicine until fairly recently. Some 40% of the men and women of the Framingham Study have elevated homocysteine levels with values over 9 μmol/l, where they begin to pay the price. The upper 5% are at 15 μmol/l or higher but, as Figure 17 shows, much lower values over 11 μmol/l lead to significant stenosis in the carotid arteries as seen using ultrasound. These lesions lead to increased stroke, heart attack and death in the Framingham Original and Offspring Cohort. An ideal level would appear to be under 9 μmol/l.

The blood of people with elevated homocysteine levels contains very low levels of folic acid and vitamin B_6. It was imagined at one point that the cure for most Americans would be 1 mg of folic acid per day. For many people this is too little. Then, the recommendation was one B100 capsule per day, with 100 units of all the various vitamin Bs and 400 IU of folic acid. The appropriate method is to measure homocysteine levels and titrate the dose of B100 and folic acid until the ideal < 9 μmol/l is reached. However, it should be pointed out that a prevention trial using folic acid, etc. has not been completed; it has just been started.

Electrocardiographic and echocardiographic findings

First-degree atrioventricular block, atrial premature beats and most isolated, less than one per hour premature ventricular beats, particularly late-cycle, in an electrocardiogram that was otherwise normal did not carry any increased risk. As Table 6 indicates, non-specific ST-T, left ventricular hypertrophy, atrial fibrillation and right and left bundle branch block all carry a statistically significant increased rate of coronary heart disease. Increased left ventricular mass on an echocardiogram is an independent risk factor for coronary heart disease. Using older criteria, the prevalence of mitral valve

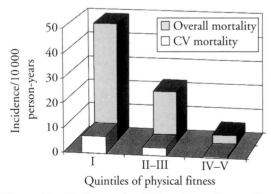

Figure 16 Cardiovascular (CV) and overall mortality in Cooper Clinic women, age-adjusted rate. From reference 37

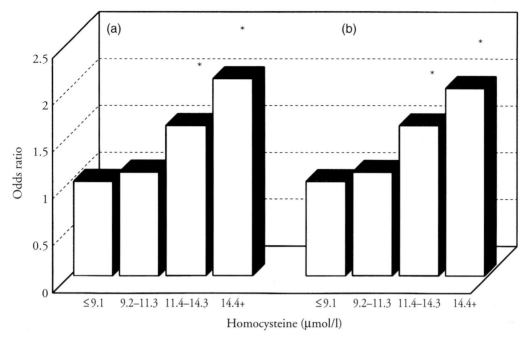

Figure 17 Homocysteine and carotid artery stenosis: (a) adjusted for age and sex; (b) adjusted for sex, age, total cholesterol/high-density lipoprotein, cigarette use, systolic blood pressure. *Significant 95% confidence interval. From reference 38

Table 6 Coronary heart disease and electrocardiogram abnormalities in women: Framingham Heart Study; National Heart, Lung, and Blood Institute; Boston University School of Medicine

	Relative odds
Non-specific ST–T wave	1.92
Left ventricular hypertrophy	3.22
Atrial fibrillation	2.70
Right bundle branch block	3.10
Left bundle branch block	4.20
+ ST segment/ + recovery loop	4.7

prolapse was markedly overstated. Using new criteria, it affects about 2–3% of women.

Stress

The women of the Framingham Study who were bossy, pressed for time, driven to excel or be the best, quick eaters, dissatisfied with their work but unable to take vacations incurred twice the heart attack rate of their easy-going contemporaries. The only categorical job classification that was 'bad' was a clerical–secretarial worker, married to a blue-collar worker, working for an insensitive boss, and with three children. Of course these data were collected for a generation of women who mostly did not work outside the home. It remains for a future study to decide what happens to the home-maker with lots of children who also has a full-time, demanding job, the career-woman of today.

Other risk factors

In past reports it was said that the rise of lipid levels during pregnancy was not a risk factor, but the number of pregnancies is emerging as a modest risk factor. No increase in risk was found for coffee consumption, hours of sleep, marital status or area of town. Fibrinogen, low and very high hemocrit, high pulse rate, low pulse variability, high white blood cell count, C-reactive protein, serum amyloid antigen and positive family history all increase the rate of cardiovascular disease.

Multiple risk factors

As Figure 18 shows, adding one risk factor to another increases the risk of vascular disease. In other renditions of multiple risk, the rate can vary

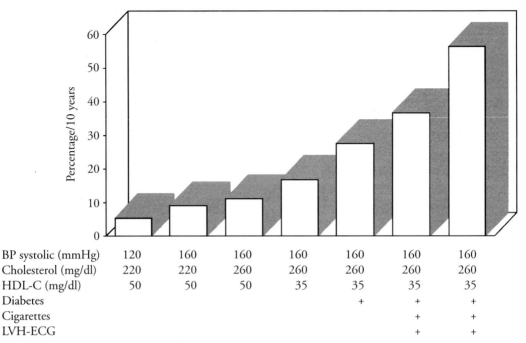

BP systolic (mmHg)	120	160	160	160	160	160	160
Cholesterol (mg/dl)	220	220	260	260	260	260	260
HDL-C (mg/dl)	50	50	50	35	35	35	35
Diabetes					+	+	+
Cigarettes						+	+
LVH-ECG						+	+

Figure 18   Risk of coronary heart disease in women aged 55 years: Framingham Heart Study; National Heart, Lung, and Blood Institute; Boston University School of Medicine. BP, blood pressure; HDL-C, high-density lipoprotein cholesterol; LVH-ECG, left ventricular hypertrophy on electrocardiogram. From reference 39

as much as 70-fold from the lowest to the highest risk. Using a multiple risk factor approach, anyone could go into any town in the world and measure a few simple things on people's bodies and identify 70–75% of the people destined to develop coronary heart disease or cardiovascular disease. Better than that, they could lower these risk factors and prevent the vast majority of vascular disease anywhere in the world. This also indicates that about 25% of the risk factors are still unknown. It remains the work of future generations to solve the rest of this puzzle.

Know your numbers!

Life is a game of numbers. The gift of the people of the Framingham Study was to teach us what the numbers mean. We started with half the men and women in the town in 1948; they were all mostly healthy. We measured all these variables on them and examined them every 2 years to find out who went on to develop cardiovascular and other kinds of disease. They taught us the numbers relating to the people who develop vascular diseases, and these

numbers are the risk factors. They also taught us the numbers relating to the people who stayed free of cardiovascular disease and even a third set of numbers: the numbers which lead to shrinking of the deposits of fat in arteries as shown on repeat angiography.

The numbers needed to sail through life without disease include: if total cholesterol is over 150 mg/dl, essentially a total cholesterol HDL ratio under 4 *and* an LDL level of 110 mg/dl or less and a triglyceride level under 120 mg/dl; blood pressure 120/80 mmHg or less; blood sugar under 100 mg/dl; hemoglobin A_{1c} under 5.5%; zero cigarettes; waist to hip ratio under 0.8; homocysteine under 9 µmol/l; lipoprotein (a) under 20 µg/dl; 2 miles walking per day; less than 20 g of saturated fat per day; less than 300 mg of dietary cholesterol per day. Eliminate white flour and sugar as well, substituting whole grains and vegetables. Keep calories as low as is dictated by exercise performance.

For people trying for reversibility, LDL level should be under 80 mg/dl and triglycerides under 90 mg/dl, then it does not matter what the total cholesterol/HDL ratio is. The other numbers should be as above for primary prevention, except in diet, where the saturated fat consumption must be under 10 g per day and the cholesterol under 100 mg per day.

Treatment

Taking all the diet trials to date, the better they lowered the cholesterol, the better they lowered the heart attack rate. Taking all the drug trials to date, and with the exception of *d*-thyroxine, and probucol used solo, the better they lowered the cholesterol, the lower the heart attack rate. Over 10 000 women have been taking part in cholesterol-lowering trials. They do better than the men with, on average, a 4% fall in coronary heart disease for a 1% fall in cholesterol. With today's powerful statin medications, of which there are currently six different types on the market with more to come, one or fewer tablets of the stronger statins will take most high-risk women to their goal. Of course any adherence to a better diet and exercise lowers the dose of medicine. To achieve triglyceride levels that are really low it is frequently necessary to add a fibrate drug or niacin to the statin to achieve the low triglyceride numbers. In people with any elevation of triglycerides (over 150 mg/dl), fish-oil capsules or ground-up flax-seed oil is used to achieve the same level of omega-3 fatty acids that produced lower coronary heart disease results on the Mediterranean diet.

By the late 1970s, in the USA the Hypertension Detection and Follow-up Program (HDFP)[40]

showed that lowering blood pressure in women improved their outcomes; this was not demonstrated until the early 1980s in the UK with the Medical Research Council (MRC) trial[41]. More recently, the Systolic Hypertension in the Elderly (SHEP) study, treating women with isolated systolic hypertension, has lowered their stroke rate by 38%[42].

Random allocation to exercise, in the Cardiac Rehabilitation trials, lowered the death rate by 37% in the first year, compared to people randomized to the couch[43].

Conclusion

Medical providers who take care of women should realize that they will progress through the menopause and find themselves on an accelerated path to atherosclerotic disease, the number one cause of death and major disability for women. A few simple tests, available virtually everywhere in the world, will allow identification of the women destined to experience cardiovascular disease years in advance of their clinical episodes. Better than that, lowering the cholesterol, blood pressure, blood sugar, cigarette, weight, etc. numbers could prevent these diseases from happening. Women will live longer, but the real benefit is that they will not die when they have a heart attack or stroke; currently 10–15% die under the age of 65, 20–25% die over the age of 65, but 75–90% live and half of them are very chronically ill, and all that could have been prevented.

References

1. Thom TJ, Kannel WB, Siberhshatz H, D'Agostino RB Sr. Incidence, prevalence, and mortality of cardiovascular disease in the United States. In Alexander RW, Schlant RC, Fuster V, eds. *Hurst's The Heart, Arteries and Veins*, 9th edn. New York: McGraw-Hill, 1997:3–17
2. Gordon T, Kannel WB, Hortland MC, McNamara PM. Menopause and coronary heart disease. *Ann Intern Med* 1978;89:157–61
3. Lloyd-Jones DM, Larson MG, Beiser A, Levy D. Lifetime risk of developing coronary heart disease. *Lancet* 1999;353:89–92
4. Anderson KM, Wilson PWF, Odell PM, et *al.* An updated coronary risk profile: a statement for health professionals. *Circulation* 1991;83:357–63
5. Castelli WP. Cholesterol and lipids in the risk of coronary artery disease. The Framington Heart Study. *Can J Cardiol* 1988;4(Suppl A):5A–10A

6. Castelli WP, Garrison RJ, Wilson PWF, Abbott RD, Kalousdian S, Kannel RB. Incidence of coronary heart disease and lipoprotein cholesterol levels. The Framingham Study. *J Am Med Assoc* 1986;256: 2835-8

7. Pitt B, Waters K, Brown W, *et al.* Aggressive lipid-lowering therapy compared with angioplasty in stable coronary artery disease. *N Engl J Med* 1999; 341:70-6

8. Austin MA, Breslow JL, Hennekens CH, Buring JE, Willett WC, Krauss RM. Low-density lipoprotein subclass patterns and risk of myocardial infarction. *J Am Med Assoc* 1988;260:1917-21

9. Campos H. Low density lipoprotein particle size and coronary heart disease. *Arterioscl Thromb* 1992; 12:1410-19

10. Poapst M, Reardon M, Steiner G. Relative contribution of triglyceride-rich lipoprotein size and number to plasma triglyceride concentration. *Arteriosclerosis* 1985;4:381-90

11. Reaven GM. Banting Lecture 1988: Role of insulin resistance in human disease. *Diabetes* 1988;37: 1595-607

12. Kaplan NM. The deadly quartet and the insulin resistance syndrome: an historical overview. *Hypertens Res* 1996;19(Suppl 1):S9-11

13. Williams RR, Hunt SC, Hopkins PN, *et al.* Familial dyslipidemia hypertension: evidence from 58 Utah families for a syndrome present in approximately 12% of patients with essential hypertension. *J Am Med Assoc* 1988;209:3579-86

14. De Franz RA, Ferransini E. Insulin resistance: a multifaceted syndrome responsible for NIDDM, obesity, hypertension, dyslipidemia, and atherosclerotic cardiovascular disease. *Diabetes Care* 1991; 14:173-94

15. Grundy SM. Hypertriglyceridemia, atherogenic dyslipidemia and the metabolic syndrome. *Am J Cardiol* 1998;81:18-25B

16. Juhan-Vague I, Collen D. On the role of coagulation and fibrinolysis in atherosclerosis. *Ann Epidemiol* 1992;2:427

17. Hokanson JE, Austin MA. Plasma triglyceride level is a risk factor for cardiovascular disease independent of high-density lipoprotein cholesterol level: a meta-analysis of population-based prospective studies. *J Cardiovasc Risk* 1996;3:213-19

18. Schaefer EJ, Levy RI. Pathogenesis and management of lipoprotein disorders. *N Engl J Med* 1985; 312:1300

19. Bostom AG, Gagnon DR, Cupples LA, *et al.* A prospective investigation of elevated lipoprotein(a) detected by electrophoresis and cardiovascular disease in women. The Framingham Heart Study. *Circulation* 1994;90:1688

20. Campos H, McNamara JR, Wilson PWF, Ordovas JM, Schaefer EJ. Differences in low density lipoprotein subfractions and apolipoproteins in pre-menopausal and postmenopausal women. *J Clin Endocrinol Metab* 1988;67: 30-5

21. Clarkson TB, Adams MR, Kaplan JR, Shively CA, Koritnik DR. From menarche to menopause: coronary artery atherosclerosis and protection in cynomolgus monkeys. *Am J Obstet Gynecol* 1989;160: 1280-5

22. Wilson PWF, Garrison RJ, Castelli WP. Postmenopausal estrogen use, cigarette smoking, and cardiovascular morbidity in women over 50. The Framingham Study. *N Engl J Med* 1985;313: 1038-43

23. Stampfer MJ, Willett WC, Colditz GA, Speizer FE, Hennekens CH. A prospective study of past use of oral contraceptive agents and risk of cardiovascular diseases - *Engl J Med* 1991;325:756-62

24. Canner PL, Berge KG, Wenger NK, *et al.* Fifteen year mortality in Coronary Drug Project patients: long-term benefit with niacin. *J Am Coll Cardiol* 1986;8:1245-55

25. Speroff L, *et al.* For the CHART group. The comparative effect of bone density, endometrium and lipids of continuous hormones as replacement therapy (CHART study). A randomized control trial. *J Am Med Assoc* 1996;276:1397-408

26. Grodstein F, Stampfer MJ, Colditz GA, *et al.* Postmenopausal hormone therapy and mortality. *N Engl J Med* 1997;336:1769-75

27. Rosendaal FR. Venous thrombosis: a multicausal disease. *Lancet* 1999;353:1167-73

28. The Writing Group of the Pepi Trial. Effects of estrogen or estrogen/progestin regimens on heart disease risk factors in postmenopausal women. *J Am Med Assoc* 1995;273:199-208

29. Eskin BA, Snyder DL, Gayheart P, Roberts J. The protective effect of estrogen on the cardiac adrenergic nervous system. In *Cardiovascular Disease in Women*. Dallas, TX: American Heart Association, 1997:23-30

30. Kannel WB, Wolf PA, Garrison RJ. *Framingham Study, Section 34, 30-year follow-up*. NIH Publication No. 87-2703, 1987

31. Joint National Committee on Detection, Evaluation and Treatment of High Blood Pressure. *The Fifth Report of the Joint National Committee on Detection, Evaluation and Treatment of High Blood Pressure* (JNCV). *Arch Intern Med* 1993;153:154

32. Rosenberg L, Palmer JR, Shapiro S. Decline in the risk of myocardial infarction among women who stop smoking. *N Engl J Med* 1990;322:213-17

33. Fiore MC, Vovotny TE, Pierce JP, Hatzianddreu EJ, Patel KM, Davis RM. Trends in cigarette smoking in the United States: the changing influence of gender and race. *J Am Med Assoc* 1989;261:49-55

34. Palmer JR, Rosenberg L, Shapiro S. 'Low-yield' cigarettes and the risk of non-fatal myocardial infarction in women. *N Engl J Med* 1989;320: 1569-73

35. Singer DE, Nathan DM, Anderson KM, *et al.* Association of HBA_{1c} with prevalent cardiovascular disease in the original cohort of the Framingham Heart Study. *Diabetes* 1992;41:202-8

36. Hubert HB, Feinleib M, McNamara P, Castelli WP. Obesity as an independent risk factor for cardiovascular disease; a 26 year follow-up of participants in the Framingham Heart Study. *Circulation* 1983; 67:768-77

37. Blair SN, Kohl HW III, Paffenbarger RS, Clark DG, Cooper KH, Gibbons LW. Physical fitness and all cause mortality. A prospective study of healthy men and women. *J Am Med Assoc* 1989;262: 2395-401

38. Selhub J, Jacques PF, Bostom AG, *et al.* Association between plasma homocysteine and carotid stenosis. *N Engl J Med* 1995;332:286-91

39. Wilson PWF. Coronary heart disease prediction. *Am J Hypertens* 1994;7:75-125

40. Hypertension Detection and Follow-Up Program Cooperative Group. Five-year findings of the hypertension detection and follow-up program. I Reduction in mortality of persons with high blood pressure, including mild hypertension. *J Am Med Assoc* 1979;242:2562

41. Medical Research Council Working Party. MRC trial of treatment of mild hypertension: principal results. *Br Med J* 1985;291:97

42. SHEP Cooperative Research Group. Prevention of stroke by antihypertensive drug treatment in older persons with isolated systolic hypertension: final results of the Systolic Hypertension in the Elderly Program (SHEP). *J Am Med Assoc* 1991;265:3255

43. O'Connor GT, Buring JE, Yusuf S, *et al.* An overview of randomized trials of rehabilitation with exercise after myocardial infarction. *Circulation* 1989;80:234-44

12

Exercise in the menopause

Laura E. Post

In 1978, the American College of Sports Medicine (ACSM) published its original position statement on exercise. In the two decades since then, the medical community has become increasingly aware of the multiple benefits of regular exercise through numerous studies that document the beneficial effects of activity on overall health. Indeed, this chapter should complement the preceding text by highlighting the effects of exercise on many of the conditions that have already been explored, including osteoporosis, cardiovascular disease, endocrine and neoplastic processes, and depression and cognitive changes with aging. Although the association between exercise and some of these conditions needs much more study, overall, participation in a regular exercise program can be used as a cost-effective intervention for reducing or preventing many of the functional declines associated with aging in women.

Sedentary life-style: a public health threat

Unfortunately, despite growing awareness by both the lay community and medical professionals of the positive effects of exercise in maintaining health, a significant proportion of our population remains physically inactive. Studies have shown that 30–50% of the US population lead sedentary life-styles, defined as no leisure-time physical activity in the past month[1,2]. It has been estimated that as many as 250 000 deaths per year in the USA, approximately 12% of the total, are attributable to lack of regular physical exercise[3]. Because of this significant public health problem, a number of governing bodies, including the Centers for Disease Control and Prevention (CDC), the ACSM and the National Institutes of Health

(NIH) have adopted guidelines for the promotion of regular physical activity in the population.

Healthy People 2000

The ACSM, the CDC and the NIH recommend that every US adult should accumulate 30 min or more of moderate-intensity exercise on most, if not all, days of the week. Moderate-intensity exercise is that performed at an intensity of 3–6 metabolic equivalents of task or METs (work metabolic rate/resting metabolic rate). This would be the equivalent of brisk walking at 3–4 miles per hour for most healthy adults. Only about 22% of Americans are currently active at this level, and the goal of the 'Healthy People 2000' campaign is to increase this number to at least 30% by the year 2000[4]. Among women aged 50–64, a recent survey revealed that less than half of the women interviewed engaged in any regular recreational exercise, and that less than 25% followed the current guidelines[5]. Overall, women over age 65 have one of the lowest levels of physical activity of any demographic group[6,7].

Previous exercise guidelines had advocated 20–60 min of moderate to high-intensity exercise performed three or more times per week. The new recommendations not only emphasize the benefits of moderate-intensity exercise but also encourage the accumulation of activity in short bouts (minimum of 10-min sessions accumulated throughout the day). Evidence suggests that cumulative exercise sessions are as beneficial as longer, sustained periods of training, and they may have the additional benefit of improved patient compliance.

Table 1 gives intensity levels for some common activities. Walking, swimming and aerobics are usually done as dedicated exercise, but daily

Table 1 Exercise intensity

< 3 METs	3–6 METs	> 6 METs
Stroll (1–2 mph)	brisk walk (3–4 mph)	uphill walk
Slow swim	moderate swim	fast swim
Stretches	aerobics	stair climbing

MET, metabolic equivalent of task

activities, such as stair climbing, house cleaning and so on can also be used to achieve 30 min of physical activity. The 1990 National Health Interview Study found that the most commonly reported recreational activities for adults age 65 and older were walking and gardening; other less frequently reported activities included golf, biking and bowling[6].

As the above study illustrates, there are many recreational and daily activities that can be used to fulfil the recommended exercise requirements. The ACSM position papers on exercise make no specific activity recommendations, but do advise aerobic activities in general for the maintenance of health in both young and older adults[8,9]. Clearly, the most effective program is one that a patient will maintain over time, and this is more easily accomplished by emphasizing activities that an individual enjoys doing and that are compatible with their life-style. In approaching the menopausal female, suggesting activities that may have been part of her earlier adult life, such as dancing, walking or swimming, would be reasonable. A beginning exercise prescription for an office worker might include stair climbing; on the other hand, a nature enthusiast may enjoy exploring walking and hiking trails. Whatever the activity, it is important that it will be a program that the patient will incorporate into their daily routine and continue on a regular basis.

Components of an exercise program

The three components of an exercise program are aerobic activities, strength training and flexibility training. Including all of these elements is particularly vital in designing a program for the menopausal female, as maximum cardiovascular function, muscle strength and flexibility all decline with age. Yet, despite these declines, the cardio-

vascular and strengthening responses to exercise by older adults are similar to those of younger adults. Maximal oxygen consumption (VO_2) can be expected to increase by 10–30% with endurance exercise training in both younger and older adults[10,11]. Likewise, two- to three-fold increases in muscle strength can be accomplished in response to resistance training in the older adult – a result similar to findings in a younger cohort[12]. Most studies of regular exercise in the older age group have shown that exercise in general increases the range of motion in multiple joints, even without a planned flexibility training program[13,14]. Thus, the benefits of exercise are achievable by all age groups, and exercise counselling should be an important element in the care of the menopausal woman.

Contraindications to exercise or exercise testing

In a healthy postmenopausal female with no cardiovascular risk factors, there is no indication for exercise stress testing prior to embarking on a graded exercise program. The ACSM lists the following conditions as absolute contraindications to exercise testing or exercise training: new electrocardiogram (ECG) changes or recent myocardial infarction, unstable angina, uncontrolled arrhythmias, third-degree heart block and acute congestive heart failure[15]. Major relative contraindications include uncontrolled hypertension, cardiomyopathies, valvular heart disease, complex ventricular arrhythmias and uncontrolled diabetes, thyroid or other metabolic diseases. The approach to each patient in regard to exercise and exercise testing should be individualized, and in approaching the menopausal female, atypical presentations of cardiac disease should also be kept in mind. The ACSM guidelines for exercise testing[15] can be used as a general schema for evaluating the need for pre-exercise cardiac evaluation and for planning an exercise program.

Writing an exercise prescription

In developing a graded exercise program for a patient, it is important to set reasonable goals based on the baseline level of fitness of each patient. In general, the conditioning intensity of an exercise session is most easily expressed as a percentage of the individual's maximal functional capacity, and the most direct way to do this is through heart rate measurement, with a goal of 60–90% of maximal heart rate achieved (the maximal heart rate is approximately 220 minus the patient's age).

As discussed above, physical activities that use large muscle groups in a continuous, rhythmic manner should be encouraged. Activities such as walking, hiking, swimming, bicycling, rowing, skating, jump roping, skiing and dancing are ideal. Each session should last between 15 and 60 min, with an aerobic component of at least 10 min per session. Ideally, an exercise session should include a 5–10-min warm-up, 10–60 min of aerobic exercise at an appropriate training level (3–6 METs or 60–90% of maximal heart rate) and a cool-down of 5–10 min. The function of the warm-up is to gradually increase the metabolic rate from the resting level to the MET level required for conditioning. Likewise, the cool-down phase should include exercise of diminishing intensity to return the body gradually to the resting state.

Static stretching exercises of the large muscle groups involved in the particular exercise can be used during the warm-up period, and would incorporate one of the three elements of an exercise program: flexibility training. The aerobic training portion can be graded over weeks to months, gradually increasing the session length (with a goal of 30 to no more than 60 min) and, eventually, the intensity as well. Muscle strengthening exercises can be incorporated to complete the triad of strengthening, flexibility and aerobic conditioning.

Exercise counselling

The newly proposed exercise guidelines urge physicians and other health professionals to counsel patients to adopt and maintain regular physical activity. As with counselling on tobacco cessation and other preventive and safety measures, a few studies have shown that counselling on physical inactivity as a modifiable risk factor does seem to be beneficial[16]. The 1990 National Health Interview Study looked at the prevalence of leisure-time physical activity among men and women advised to exercise by their physician as a means of lowering high blood pressure. The patients who received exercise advice from their physicians were 50–60% more likely to exercise than those who had not been counselled in the importance of exercise[17].

As with most behavioral counselling, there are some barriers and misconceptions towards adopting exercise as a life-style change, and these need to be taken into account to obtain most effectively the objective of incorporating physical activity into our patients' daily routine. First, it should be recognized that many patients view exercise as an all-or-nothing venture. Many feel that the inability initially to sustain moderate-intensity exercise for a reasonable length of time makes any attempt at exercise almost futile. Hopefully, emphasizing the recommendations in 'Healthy People 2000' – the accumulation of activity over the course of the day – will decrease this threshold mentality. Second, many patients consider only those activities typically done as dedicated exercise (swimming, jogging, aerobics and so on) to be beneficial to their health. As previously discussed, it is important also to encourage the use of daily activities, such as stair climbing, house cleaning and walking to achieve the 30 min of physical activity recommended in the new guidelines. By doing this, the impact on time management is lessened, as part of the activities are incorporated into the patient's usual routine. Emphasizing the benefits of even modest increases in physical activity, and providing positive reinforcement, is an important element in approaching exercise counselling. Another caveat to share with patients is that the health benefits gained from increased physical activity depend on the patient's initial activity level, with sedentary individuals expected to benefit most from increasing their activity to the recommended level. This steep initial response curve should certainly be a positive message for the more sedentary patient.

In directing exercise counselling efforts towards the groups most at risk, there are several factors that have been shown to correlate with sedentary life-styles. The 1990 Behavioral Risk Factor Surveillance System reported that older age, African-American race, low education, smoking, alcohol use and obesity were all positively correlated with physical inactivity[18]. Conversely, younger age, higher income, lower body mass index and higher education levels have been shown to be associated with more physically active life-styles[19]. Maximal efforts at achieving behavioral changes should probably be focused on African–American women, who meet some of the higher risk criteria for inactive life-styles.

Sedentary life-style: a protean risk factor

The remainder of this chapter is primarily devoted to discussing the role of exercise in reducing the risk of multiple, specific disease processes. Table 2 indicates some of the many correlations that have been studied in relation to exercise and overall health. The aim is to discuss general trends, highlighted by the results of selected studies. For a more comprehensive review of available literature, the reader is directed to other sources, an excellent example of which is the Surgeon General's 'Report on Physical Activity and Health'[20].

Beginning with general effects on health, a large landmark study showed that exercise reduced overall mortality – a very positive message to relay to patients. Several studies have been published over the years documenting the benefits of physical fitness. This study looked at a group of over 10 000 men and 3000 women at the Cooper Clinic, Dallas, Texas and followed them for over 8 years. Physical

fitness was measured by a maximal exercise treadmill test, and patients were assigned to fitness categories based on their age, sex and maximal time on the treadmill. Treadmill time 'quintiles' were determined, and subjects with a treadmill time in the first quintile were assigned to the low-fitness group. Those with scores in the second to the fifth quintiles were assigned to groups two to five, group five being the most fit group.

Overall, this study found a strong, inverse association between fitness and all-cause mortality[21]. Importantly, comparing overall mortality between fitness group one (least fit) and fitness group five (most fit), the major reduction in all-cause death rates was between the first and second fitness levels. This change in fitness would be attainable with only moderate exercise, again emphasizing the fact that even a small change in level of fitness can lead to large health gains.

Obviously, there are multiple variables other than physical activity in a study looking at all-cause mortality. However, the general trends seemed to remain valid after adjustment for age, smoking, cholesterol levels, fasting glucose levels and family history of heart disease. Low physical fitness was an important risk factor for both men and women, and higher levels of physical fitness appeared to delay all-cause mortality. In considering the impact of this study on the population at large, it should be noted that the patient population was generally from middle to upper economic groups, and that most (70%) were college educated. Given the fact that the groups most at risk for sedentary life-style are from the opposite socioeconomic group (low income and less educated), it is clear that additional study needs to be done with at-risk populations, particularly older, low-income African–American women. The primary benefits of enhanced physical fitness for the group studied were in the categories of cardiovascular disease and cancer, issues that are discussed below.

Coronary artery disease and women's health

Coronary artery disease (CAD) is the leading cause of death in women in the USA. In 1991, the age-adjusted death rates per 100 000 from CAD were 197.4 for white women and 129.1 for

Table 2 Effects of exercise on health

Health concern	Correlation with exercise
Overall mortality	inverse association (exercise decreases overall mortality)
Cardiovascular disease	inverse association (decreases the risk of CAD)
Cancer	colon cancer: inverse association; breast cancer: inconsistent findings; endometrial/ovarian cancer: not enough data
Type II diabetes	inverse association (exercise lowers risk of development)
Osteoporosis	probably beneficial but needs more studies (? type of exercise)
Obesity/weight control	may be beneficial
Depression	may be beneficial
Gait stability	may be beneficial

CAD, coronary artery disease

African–American women; this compares to breast cancer rates of 35.5 for white women and 29.3 for African–American women[22]. The incidence of myocardial infarction or death from CAD in premenopausal women is below 1/10 000 per year; one-third of all deaths occur from age 65 to age 74 in women, and a majority of cardiovascular deaths occur after age 75[23]. As noted in the above cited study, the largest reduction in deaths owing to higher levels of physical fitness resulted from a decrease in coronary events. Sedentary life-style is a well-defined cardiovascular risk factor, and it has been estimated that as many as 35% of excess deaths due to CAD could be eliminated by increasing physical activity[24].

There are probably multiple mechanisms by which exercise may contribute to the primary or secondary prevention of CAD. These include delay of progression of coronary atherosclerosis by improving the lipoprotein profile (increasing high-density lipoprotein (HDL)/low-density lipoprotein (LDL) ratio), improving carbohydrate metabolism (increasing insulin sensitivity) and possibly decreasing platelet aggregation. In addition, enhanced physical fitness decreases myocardial work and oxygen demand, and has modest effects on reducing blood pressure.

Exercise may also affect CAD by producing a more favorable overall cardiac risk factor profile. One study examined the effects of fitness levels, again determined by maximal treadmill tests, on multiple cardiac risk factors in healthy women. They found that enhanced physical fitness was associated with lower body weight, a lower incidence of cigarette smoking, lower systolic and diastolic blood pressures and a lower total cholesterol with an improved HDL/LDL ratio[25]. Not surprisingly, the more fit women also had a lower incidence of cardiovascular disease.

Obesity

Along with being a comorbid factor for cardiovascular disease, obesity is at nearly epidemic proportions in the USA. Approximately 33% of US adults are overweight[26], and a tremendous number of health-care dollars are spent on diseases associated with obesity. With estimated health-care expenditures of over $US68 billion per year[27], this problem clearly has economic as well as medical implications. Although an issue in all age groups, progressive weight gain is often a problem in the third to sixth decades of life, and is a common presenting problem in the perimenopausal and postmenopausal female. One contributor to this problem may be an age-related decline in energy expenditure[28], but many other factors probably also contribute, including metabolic and hormonal changes associated with aging.

Obesity is most easily defined in terms of the body mass index (BMI), calculated by dividing the patient's weight (kilograms) by her height (meters) squared. An acceptable BMI for women would be approximately 19–24 or 25. A BMI greater than 27 is associated with a three to four times greater risk of CAD, and is also linked to hypertension, Type II diabetes and some types of cancer[29]. Exercise probably has multiple benefits in weight control, including decreasing appetite and preserving lean body mass. Exercise is also useful in enhancing mood and improving self-image, and these can be useful motivators in maintaining diet programs.

Multiple trials have looked at the relationship of exercise to weight loss. The Minnesota Heart Health Program examined several interventions aimed at increasing physical activity for the purpose of weight loss. These included educational programs and even small financial incentives. Some were effective and others showed no significant change in 1 year of follow-up[30].

Adherence to exercise regimens is an obvious problem; one study that looked at the addition of a walking program for weight loss in obese women reported a 68% drop-out rate[31]. However, those who did continue with the exercise regimen lost significant amounts of fat. Exercise also seems to be an important factor in the maintenance of weight loss over time[32]. Interestingly, adherence to exercise and weight loss and maintenance may be better in programs with low rather than high caloric expenditure[33]. This makes sense in that it is more likely that patients will be able to maintain a low- or moderate-intensity regimen over time, but may become discouraged or burned out with a more strenuous program. Finally, preventing weight gain would eliminate the difficulties involved in treating obesity, and the perimenopausal period appears to be a time frame in which weight control interventions are particularly successful[34].

Type II diabetes: a preventable disease

Recent projections predict that the number of Type II diabetics will increase nearly 16 fold in the coming years. This trend is closely linked to the fact that nearly one-third of the American population is overweight. Weight is a major concern in both the development of and the treatment strategies for Type II diabetes. Exercise is an important, yet often neglected modality in the treatment of diabetes, and has been shown to decrease insulin requirements and improve glucose tolerance[35,36]. Along with diet and medical interventions, exercise needs to be a cornerstone in the treatment and, more importantly, the prevention of diabetes.

A 1991 study used data from the University of Pennsylvania Alumni Health Study to determine the effect of exercise on the subsequent development of Type II diabetes[37]. The authors found that leisure-time physical activity was inversely related to the later development of diabetes. Moreover, the protective effect of exercise was strongest in the highest-risk patients: obese patients, hypertensive patients and those with a family history of Type II diabetes. Overall, the occurrence of Type II diabetes was found to be reduced by 6% for every 500 kcal per week increase in physical activity. Sports activities such as jogging, bicycling and swimming at moderate intensity were effective. This retrospective study of nearly 6000 male patients supports the hypothesis that regular physical activity lowers the risk of developing non-insulin dependent diabetes. It would seem reasonable, then, that targeting high-risk patients by providing guidance and counselling on exercise would be a positive step in curbing the growing epidemic of Type II diabetes.

As with CAD, obesity and overall mortality, no controlled clinical trials have been conducted on Type II diabetes and physical activity. Large epidemiological studies, such as the University of Pennsylvania study, do support the role of exercise in the prevention of diabetes, and the Surgeon General has advocated this as a useful preventive strategy[20]. As with CAD, one of the benefits of exercise in diabetes is probably in producing an improved overall risk factor profile, that is, improving blood pressure, body fat composition and lipoprotein profiles.

Osteoporosis

A mounting concern in women's health over the past few years has been postmenopausal bone loss. This is probably attributable to several factors. First, there are higher percentages of women living to ages where the complications of osteoporosis become apparent. Second, the widespread availability of dual-energy X-ray absorbiometry (DEXA) scanners allows for the accurate quantitation of bone loss. Third, the advent of non-hormonal treatments and preventive strategies for osteoporosis has produced new medical interventions for this disease process. Finally, the social and economic impact of complications of osteoporosis, particularly hip fractures, is enormous. In the early 1980s alone, nearly US4 billion dollars per year were spent on the treatment of osteoporotic fractures. Additionally, hip fractures have a 15–20% 1-year mortality rate[38], making the prevention of such events an important consideration in the care of the postmenopausal woman.

Bone mineral density is dependent on several factors, including hormonal milieu, calcium metabolism and physical activity, among other things. The attention in this discussion is focused on the role that physical activity plays in bone remodelling. Unfortunately, there really are no simple answers regarding what types of exercise may be most beneficial in either maintaining or increasing bone mineral density. The multitude of published studies have differed greatly in the mode, intensity and duration of exercise, making it difficult to provide specific guidelines in prescribing exercise regimens. However, a few generalizations can be made.

Clearly, physical inactivity is a strong risk factor for bone loss. This has been demonstrated in subjects during extended periods of bed rest[39]. In addition, studies comparing the bone density of athletes to that of sedentary subjects support the concept of a higher bone density in the active versus the inactive population[40,41]. The type of exercise that may be most beneficial is unclear, but both resistance and endurance activities (weight lifting and aerobics, for example) seem to have positive effects on bone density[42]. In general, however, weight-bearing exercise is probably more beneficial than non-weight-bearing exercise. A study of female athletes aged 42–50 found that bone mineral density in long-term swimmers did not differ significantly from that of sedentary subjects[41].

A further concern with regard to osteoporosis is the role that estrogen plays in contributing to the preservation of bone mass, both with and without the added stimulating effect of exercise. Some studies suggest that the effects of estrogen and physical activity may be additive; that is, postmenopausal gains in bone density may be greater when hormone replacement therapy is combined with an exercise regimen[43]. Overall, although the optimal regimen for preserving and improving bone density is not known, a moderate-intensity weight-bearing exercise regimen combined with estrogen replacement should be considered in most peri- and postmenopausal women. The role of bisphosphonates and selective estrogen receptor modulators (SERMs) in conjunction with physical activity has been less well explored at this point. The role of these agents combined with exercise, along with further studies of the longitudinal effects of physical activity and the optimal types of activity to maintain bone mass, may be avenues for future research.

Fall prevention

A vital component in the treatment plan for a woman with osteoporosis is the prevention of falls that could lead to osteoporotic fractures. Exercise is not only an important modality in improving bone density, but exercise interventions in the elderly may also decrease fall frequency and thereby decrease the risk of hip fractures. Several studies have shown that physical activity may be useful in preventing falls; other studies have failed to show a significant effect. A meta-analysis of a series of large trials, the FICSIT trials (Frailty and Injuries: Cooperative Studies of Intervention Techniques), found that assignment to an exercise group was associated with a decrease in the risk of falling[44]. The interventions used in these trials, however, were quite varied and included non-

exercise components, so the effect of exercise as a sole modality remains unclear but may well be of benefit. Resistance training to improve overall strength has also been shown to be effective in decreasing fall risk, even in the frail elderly[45].

Exercise probably affects muscle strength and balance, and in that way improves gait stability. The risk of falls in the elderly, however, is a multifactorial problem, and includes factors such as visual acuity, medications, environmental hazards (throw rugs, appliance cords, etc.) and so on. Overall, the ACSM concurs that there is sufficient evidence that strength training and other forms of exercise may reduce fall risk and recommends 'a broad based exercise program that includes balance training, resistive exercise, walking and weight transfer...as part of a multifaceted intervention to reduce the risk of falling'[10].

Cancer prevention

One of the less obvious benefits of exercise, and certainly a concern for most patients, is the correlation between exercise and several types of cancer. The most studied associations have been in the area of colon and breast cancer, but a small number of studies have also looked at the relationship between exercise and endometrial and ovarian cancer. The data on these processes are too few to reach a conclusion, but some of the data indicating an inverse relationship between colon cancer and exercise and the volume of controversial literature with regard to exercise and breast cancer are discussed below. In general, the mechanisms for the positive effects of exercise on neoplastic processes are unclear. However, sharing with patients some of the positive correlations may help to motivate a healthy move towards a more physically active life-style. Along with the standard American Cancer Society guidelines for screening for breast and colon cancer, consideration should be given to emphasizing exercise as part of a healthy life-style, and possibly as a component in preventing certain types of cancer.

Colon cancer and exercise

A recent look at the correlation between colon cancer and exercise using data from the Nurses'

Health Study was published in the July 1997 issue of *Journal of the National Cancer Institute*. This study found a significant inverse association between leisure-time physical activity and the incidence of colon cancer in this large cohort of women. It found that moderate-intensity exercise for 1 h per day decreased the risk of colon cancer by 46%. Significantly, this effect was independent and separate even from an elevated BMI, a previously known risk factor for colon cancer[46]. The mechanism for the positive effect of exercise in colon cancer is unclear; some proposed theories include decreased gastrointestinal transit time, increased immune function and altered prostaglandin levels.

The positive benefit of exercise for prevention of colon cancer in men has been well reported in the past. Previous studies looking at the correlation in women have not shown a significant association between colon cancer and exercise. However, the studies were smaller, used different measures of physical activity and had other methodological differences. Approximately 29 studies have looked at the correlation between colon cancer and physical activity[20]. Unlike the Nurses' Health Study, which examined leisure-time activity, a majority of these studies looked only at occupational physical activity. Despite these differences and some conflicting results, many of these studies also found a protective role for exercise in the development of colon cancer.

It should be mentioned that several studies looked at rectal cancer as a separate entity from colon cancer. The studies that used this as an end-point found no statistically significant association between physical activity and rectal cancer risk.

Breast cancer

The evidence for the role of exercise in decreasing breast cancer risk is inconsistent. Some studies have shown a protective effect and others have shown no significant association. Specific findings are well outlined and reviewed in other sources[20,47]. There are some general deficiencies in many of these studies which should be pointed out. First, many failed to obtain information on hormonal factors (pregnancies, age at menarche, current menstrual status), and this could be a potential confounding factor. In addition, housework and child care-related activity was often not included in assessments of overall physical activity. Furthermore, as with many studies on physical activity, there can certainly be a recall bias, particularly in reporting past participation in exercise regimens. The Surgeon General's report concludes that 'despite numerous studies on the subject, existing data are inconsistent regarding an association between physical activity and breast cancer'[20].

Exercise and mood

Depression is one of the most common presenting problems in the out-patient primary care setting, and women tend to report a higher prevalence of depression and other affective disorders than do men. Exercise may have multiple psychological benefits, including improving self-esteem and body image, providing a sense of well-being and improving mood, as well as decreasing mild stress and anxiety. Multiple studies suggest a positive correlation between physical activity and mood. A 1990 nationwide Canadian survey showed an inverse relationship between symptoms of depression and physical activity in adults over 25 years of age[48]. Another study compared 12 weeks of aerobic exercise to traditional psychotherapy in the treatment of mild to moderate depression, and found that exercise reduced depression symptoms to a greater degree than did therapy[49]. Several other large studies have revealed an inverse relationship between exercise and depression[50,51]. The Iowa 65+ Rural Health Study reported a decrease in depression symptoms in men and women aged 65 and older who walked on a daily basis[52].

Mood swings and mild to moderate depression and anxiety may accompany the menopause. A recent study looked at the effects of exercise both on mood and on reporting of menopausal vasomotor symptoms. The researchers found that exercise had a positive effect on mood, and that immediately after exercise, women had a significant decrease in reported vasomotor symptoms[53].

Exercise may thus be an important adjunct to hormone replacement therapy in treating symptoms of the menopause.

Adverse effects of exercise

As discussed to this point, exercise may have multiple health benefits, but there are potential adverse effects of exercise. The most common are orthopedic injuries, and these tend to be sports-specific. Runners are subject to overuse injuries of the lower extremities. Conversely, swimmers more often suffer shoulder injuries. Compared with males, female athletes demonstrated similar sports-related injury rates overall[54]. Strains and sprains of the ankle and knee are the most commonly reported musculoskeletal injuries[55]. The majority of orthopedic injuries are self-limited and often related to overuse. Most are probably preventable with the use of a moderate-intensity, graded exercise program.

Adverse cardiac events, such as angina, acute myocardial infarction, arrhythmias and sudden death can be a concern with either starting a new exercise regimen or increasing the intensity of an established program. However, as discussed above, the benefits of physical activity in reducing CAD and coronary risk factors probably far outweigh the potential for adverse cardiac events. As recommended by the ACSM, women over the age of 50 who wish to embark on a new exercise regimen or women with risk factors for heart disease or other chronic medical problems should consult a physician prior to starting training[8,9].

Conclusion

A majority of patients lead a sedentary life-style, which has profound implications on the development of multiple disease processes. Exercise counselling should be an integral consideration in preventive health strategies. Women, particularly those over age 65, are at particular risk for an inactive life-style, and many of the physiological changes associated with aging and the menopause can be positively impacted upon by exercise. Public health efforts should be increased towards high-risk groups such as menopausal women, as exercise is an important component in maintaining good health.

References

1. Centers for Disease Control. Sex-, age- and region-specific prevalence for sedentary lifestyle in selected states in 1985. The Behavioral Risk Factor Surveillance System. *Morbid Mortal Weekly Rep* 1987;36: 195
2. Centers for Disease Control. CDC Surveillance Summaries. *Morbid Mortal Weekly Rep* 1990;39:8
3. Hahn RA, Teutsch SM, Rothenberg RB, Marks GS. Excess deaths from nine chronic diseases in the United States. *J Am Med Assoc* 1986;264:2654-9
4. Pate RR, Pratt M, Blair SN, *et al*. Physical activity and public health: a recommendation from the Centers for Disease Control and Prevention and the Americal College of Sports Medicine. *J Am Med Assoc* 1995;273:402-7
5. McTeirnan A, Stanford JL, Daling J, Voigt LF. Prevalence and correlates of recreational physical activity in women aged 50-64 years. *Menopause* 1997;5:95-101
6. Caspersen CJ, Christenson GM, Pollard RA. Status of the 1990 physical fitness and exercise objectives: evidence from the NHIS 1985. *Public Health Rep* 1986;101:587-93
7. Lee C. Factors related to adoption of exercise among older women. *J Behav Med* 1993;16:323-34
8. American College of Sports Medicine. Position stand: the recommended quantity and quality of exercise for developing and maintaining cardio-respiratory and muscular fitness and flexibility in healthy adults. *Med Sci Sports Exercise* 1998;30: 975-89
9. American College of Sports Medicine. Position stand: exercise and physical activity for older adults. *Med Sci Sports Exercise* 1998;30:992-1008
10. Kohrt W, Malley M, Coggan AR, *et al*. Effects of gender, age and fitness level on response of V_{O_2} max to training in 60-71 year olds. *J Appl Physiol* 1991; 71:2004-11

11. Seals D, Hagberg J, Jurley B, Ehsani A, Hollozy J. Endurance training in older men and women: I Cardiovascular responses to exercise. *J Appl Physiol* 1984;57:1024–9

12. Frontera WR, Meredith CN, O'Reilly KP, Knuttzen HG, Evans WJ. Strength conditioning in older men: skeletal muscle hypertrophy and improved function. *J Appl Physiol* 1988;64:1038–44

13. Hubley-Kozey CL, Wall JC, Hogan DB. Effects of a general exercise program on passive hip, knee and ankle range of motion of older women. *Top Geriatr Rehabil* 1995;10:33–44

14. Leslie DK, Frekany GA. Effects of an exercise program on selected flexibility measures of senior citizens. *Gerontologist* 1975;4:182–3

15. American College of Sports Medicine. *ACSM's Guidelines for Exercise Testing and Prescription*, 5th edn. Baltimore: Williams and Wilkins, 1995

16. Lewis BS, Lynch WD. The effect of physician advice on exercise behaviour. *Prev Med* 1993;22:110–21

17. Yusuf HR, Croft JB, Giles WH, *et al.* Leisure-time physical activity among older adults United States, 1990. *Arch Intern Med* 1996;156:1321–6

18. Simoes EJ, Byers T, Coates RJ, *et al.* The association between leisure-time physical activity and dietary fat in American adults. *Am J Public Health* 1995;85:240–4

19. Patterson RE, Haines PS, Popkin BM. Health lifestyle patterns of US adults. *Prev Med* 1194;23:453–60

20. US Department of Health and Human Services. *Physical Activity and Health: A Report of the Surgeon General.* Atlanta, GA: US Department of Health and Human Services, Centers for Disease Control and Prevention, National Center for Chronic Disease Prevention and Health Promotion, International Medical Publishing, 1996

21. Blair SN, Kohl HW, Paffenbarger RS, Clark DG, Cooper KH, Gibbons LW. Physical fitness and all cause mortality: a prospective study of healthy men and women. *J Am Med Assoc* 1989;262:2395–401

22. *Vital Statistics of the United States, 199.* Vol. II, *Mortality Part A*, USDH&HS, PHS, CDC, NCHS, Hyattsville, MD, 1996, DHHS Publ. No. (PHS) 96–101

23. Siegel AJ. Medical conditions arising during sports. In Shangold M, Miran G, eds. *Women and Exercise: Physiology and Sports Medicine*, 2nd edn. F.A. Davis, 1994:261–78

24. Powell KE, Blair SN. The public health burdens of sedentary living habits: theoretical but realistic estimates. *Med Sci Sports Exercise* 1994;26:851–6

25. Gibbons LW, Blair SN, Cooper KH, *et al.* Association between coronary heart disease risk factors and physical fitness in healthy adult women. *Circulation* 1983;67:977–83

26. National Task Force on the prevention and treatment of obesity. Long term pharmacotherapy in the management of obesity. *J Am Med Assoc* 1996;276:1907–15

27. Kuczmarski RJ, Flegal KM, Campbell SM, Johnson CL. Increasing prevalence of overweight among US adults. *J Am Med Assoc* 1994;272:205–11

28. Bray GA. The energetics of obesity. *Med Sci Sports Exercise* 1983;15:32–40

29. Van Itallie T. Health implications of overweight and obesity in the United States. *Ann Intern Med* 1985;103:983–8

30. Jeffery RW. Community programs for obesity prevention: the Minnesota Heart Health Program. *Obesity Res* 1995;Suppl 3:283–8s

31. Gwinup G. Effect of exercise alone on the weight of obese women. *Arch Intern Med* 1975;135:676

32. Brownell KD. Behavioral, psychological and environmental predictors of obesity and success in weight reduction. *Int J Obesity* 1984;8:543

33. Pavlou KN, Krey S, Stefee WP. Exercise as an adjunct to weight loss and maintenance in moderately obese subjects. *Am J Clin Nutr* 1989;49:1115

34. Wing RR. Changing diet and exercise behaviors in individuals at risk for weight gain. *Obesity Res* 1995;Suppl 3:277–82

35. Soman VR, Koivisto VA, Deibert D, Felig P, DeFronzo RA. Increased insulin sensitivity and insulin binding to monocytes after physical training. *N Engl J Med* 1979;301:1200–4

36. Rauramaa R. Relationship of physical activity, glucose tolerance and weight management. *Prev Med* 1984;13:37–46

37. Helmrich SP, Ragland DR, Leung RW, Paffenbarger RS. Physical activity and reduced occurrence of non-insulin dependent diabetes mellitus. *N Engl J Med* 1991;325:147–51

38. National Institutes of Health. *Consensus Development Conference on Osteoporosis*, Vol. 5, No. 3. Washington, DC: Government Printing Office, 1984

39. Donaldson CL, Hulley SB, Vogel JM, Hattner KS, Bayers JH, McMillan DE. Effect of prolonged bed rest on bone mineral. *Metab Clin Exp* 1970;19:1071–84

40. Kirchner EM, Lewis RD, O'Connor PT. Efect of past gymnastics participation on adult bone mass. *J Appl Physiol* 1996;80:225–32

41. Dook JE, James C, Henderson NK, Price RI. Exercise and bone mineral density in mature female athletes. *Med Sci Sports Exercise* 1997;29:291–6

42. Nilsson BE, Westlin NE. Bone density in athletes. *Clin Orthop* 1971;77:179–82

43. Kohrt WM, Sneed DB, Slatopolsky E, Birge SJ. Additive effects of weight-bearing exercise and estrogen on bone mineral density in older women. *J Bone Miner Res* 1995;10:1303–11

44. Province MA, Hadley EC, Hombrook MC, *et al.* The effects of exercise on falls in elderly patients: a preplanned meta-analysis of the FICSIT trials –

Frailty and Injuries: Cooperative Studies of Intervention Techniques. *J Am Med Assoc* 1995;273: 1341–7

45. Fiatarone MA, O'Neill EF, Ryan ND, *et al.* Exercise training and nutritional supplementation for physical frailty in very elderly people. *N Engl J Med* 1994;330:1769–75

46. Martinez ME, Giovannucci E, Spiegelman D, Hunter DJ, Willet WC, Colditz GA. Leisure time physical activity. Body size and colon cancer in women. *J Natl Cancer Inst* 1997;89:948–54

47. Gammon MD, Schoenberg JB, Britton JA, *et al.* Recreational physical activity and breast cancer risk among women under 45 years. *Am J Epidemiol* 1998;147:273–80

48. Stephens J, Craig CL. *The Well Being of Canadians: Highlights of the 1988 Campbell's Survey.* Ottawa: Canadian Fitness and Lifestyle Research Institute, 1990

49. Griest JH, Klein MH, Eicchens RR, *et al.* Running as a treatment for depression. *Comp Psychiatry* 1979; 20:41

50. Camacho JC, Roberts RE, Lazarus NB, Kaplan GA, Cahen RD. Physical activity and depression: evidence from the Alameda County study. *Am J Epidemiol* 1991;134:220–31

51. Paffenbarger RS, Lee IM, Leung R. Physical activity and personal characteristics associated with depression and suicide in American college men. *Acta Psychiatr Scand* 1994;Suppl 377:16–22

52. Mobily KE, Rubenstein JH, Lemke JH, O'Hara MW, Wallace RB. Walking and depression in a cohort of older adults: the Iowa 65+ Rural Health Study. *J Aging Physiol Activ* 1996;4:119–35

53. Slaven L, Lee C. Mood and symptom reporting among middle-aged women: the relationship between menopausal status, hormone replacement therapy and exercise participation. *Health Psychol* 1997;16:203–8

54. Whiteside P. Men's and women's injuries in comparable sports. *Physician Sports Med* 1980;8:130

55. Rettawen K. Athletic injuries: comparison by age, sport and gender. *Am J Sports Med* 1986;14:218

13

Gynecological problems

Hugh R. K. Barber

The word menopause and climacteric are often used interchangeably. This is not correct. Strictly speaking, the word menopause means the final cessation of menstruation. In its broadest sense, it gives a grossly erroneous idea that yesterday all was well, but today everything has changed and this will continue indefinitely. It also implies that a hysterectomy causes a menopause. This is wrong. Menopause occurs if the ovaries are removed or cease to function. Climacteric, meaning a period of change, is a better word because it expresses the all-important concept of a time-scale, but is not in common use. Therefore, it is important to stick to the word menopause and define it as it is used in this chapter.

The menopause is centered on the ovary and its end-built obsolescence. The events of the menopause start when the active ovary begins to fail and ends with the final lapse of the ovary into inactivity. The duration of these events is extremely variable, and can cause as much trouble before menstruation ceases as after the last period. The end of the menopause merges into the postmenopausal period.

The climacteric is that phase in the life of a woman which marks the interval of transition from reproductive age to the age at which reproductive function is lost. This stage is characterized by progressive endocrine changes that lead to the menopause, the final menstrual period that signals the end of cyclic ovarian function. The perimenopause is defined arbitrarily to include the last few years of the climacteric and the first year after the menopause.

It is to be emphasized that menopause is a natural physiological process and only rarely is it a pathological state. The menopause usually occurs at about age 50–52 and may be abrupt, or gradual, over a period of months. It is the events underlying the changes that are responsible for most of the clinical features. These include the loss of estrogen support to the secondary sex organs and, to a lesser extent, to other structures, such as bone, urinary tract, skin and hair. It is the consequent release from feedback inhibition of the hypothalamic-pituitary complex.

There are two types of menopause classified according to cause. One, physiological menopause, occurs at about age 51 and results because the oocytes (follicles) responsive to gonadotropins disappear from the ovary and, second, the few remaining oocytes do not respond to gonadotropins. Spontaneous cessation of menses before age 40 is called premature menopause or premature ovarian failure. Cessation of menstruation and the development of climacteric symptoms and complaints can occur as early as a few years after menarche. The reasons for premature ovarian failure are largely unknown. However, autoimmune disorders and certain viral diseases, as well as genetics, may play a role in ovarian failure.

Artificial menopause is the permanent cessation of ovarian function brought about by surgical removal of the ovaries or by radiation therapy. Irradiation to ablate ovarian function is rarely used today. Artificial menopause is employed as a treatment for endometriosis and estrogen-sensitive neoplasms of the breast and endometrium. More frequently, artificial menopause is a side-effect of treatment of intra-abdominal disease, that is, ovaries are removed in premenopausal women because the gonads have been damaged by infection or neoplasia, or replaced beyond salvage by endometriosis.

Symptoms in geriatric gynecological patients

The most frequent symptoms that occur among in-patient admissions include genital bleeding, and this is present even in the very elderly. A rule of thumb that has been useful in discussing the problem of bleeding in the postmenopausal woman is that, among those with vaginal bleeding, one-third will have a neoplasm, one-third will have a benign process and in one-third the cause will not be able to be determined. It must be emphasized that in this age group vaginal bleeding must be looked upon as a malignancy until it is ruled out. Genital displacement in elderly women is very common. Urinary incontinence is frequently associated with genital displacements and constitutes not only a medical, but also a social, nursing and sociological problem, especially in very old women. Pruritus vulvae is a very frequent symptom. The genital disorders most likely to affect the menopausal patient include those resulting from the cessation of ovarian function with consequent hypoestrogenism, dermatological diseases of the vulva, uncertainties concerning sexual activities, neoplasms that are more common after the menopause, and symptomatic relaxation of the pelvic supporting structures. The genitalia of the menopausal patient are less likely to develop benign neoplasms. Sexually transmitted diseases are less frequently encountered in the older patient, but are being diagnosed with increasing frequency in recent times because of a more liberal attitude in the life-style of the elderly.

History and pelvic examination

The setting for a meeting with the patient must be well structured. The medical evaluation and examination should be conducted in a relaxed and unhurried manner, and the patient given as much privacy and personal attention as possible. Ideally, a team, consisting of a social worker, nurse clinician and nutritionist, together with a physician, should work with the patient to institute the necessary medical care and support services. The confidence of the patient must be gained, a relaxed and friendly atmosphere created, and the practitioner must be prepared to be unhurried as he or she starts to take a history from the menopausal patient. The word menopause has been shrouded in the mystery of silence. Many patients are upset by hearing the word. It is the responsibility of the physician to explain carefully that the menopause is just one part of an overall life process. It must be explained to the patient that the only change is that she will not become pregnant. All other bodily functions will continue as before, and her mind will remain as sharp as before the menopause.

Patients in the early postmenopausal period are able to give a useful history of their obstetric and gynecological experience or the age at which menopause occurred. However, in the late menopausal period, it may be difficult to obtain this information directly from the patient. It is important, therefore, to have a relative or a close friend available, but often this is not possible. Some elderly patients may present or be referred for so-called vaginal bleeding, but on close questioning are uncertain whether the bleeding is coming from the urethra, vagina or the anal area.

It is important to obtain a careful obstetric, menstrual, postmenopausal and gynecological history. The patient should be asked about drug ingestion, particularly whether she has ever taken any type of hormone or is currently taking hormones. The patient must be questioned about the use of over-the-counter drugs or the use of herbal medicines. The eating habits and nutrition of these patients are most important to explore. The elderly woman living alone may live on tea and toast and develop an anemia.

The most recent epidemiological data suggest that anxiety disorders are exceedingly common, occurring more frequently in women than in men across all age groups. It is estimated that approximately 5% of all women, at some time in their lives, will have an anxiety disorder of sufficient severity to interfere with their ability to function in their usual roles. An estimated 10–15% of females over the age of 65 experience anxieties sufficiently severe to warrant medical intervention. The prevalence of anxiety disorders in the elderly demands a basic understanding by the physician of the numerous ways in which these disorders may present: anxiety in the elderly may present as neurological, gastrointestinal, cardiovascular and respiratory symptoms. The most common genitourinary symptoms are pruritus vulvae/vaginae or pruritus ani, or the occurrence of dyspareunia.

The Victorian concept that all sexual activity ends at the time of the menopause has been shown to be totally inaccurate. Many studies have shown that women are able to function sexually very late in their lives. Therefore, it is very important to ask about sexual function. The way in which the inquiry about sexuality is approached confirms and supports the patient's feelings that she is still considered a woman and, if carried out in an open but discerning manner, reinforces the patient's regard for the physician. Sexuality and sexual function in the menopausal and postmenopausal years is now receiving a great deal of attention in the literature.

In 1953, Kinsey reported that the sexual activity of an unmarried woman remains relatively constant until age 55, whereas that of an unmarried man declines progressively from adolescence. Kinsey concluded that, in women, age has no effect on sexual activity until late in life, and he suggested that the subsequent reduction in sexual activity may be due primarily to diminution in the sexuality of the male partner. Since women commonly outlive their partner, it is important to inquire discreetly about masturbation. This provides an opportunity to explain to the patient that masturbation is not harmful to either bodily or mental health.

It seems that women who are sexually active during this period of their lives are approximately 10 kg heavier than those who are not. Thus, in terms of estrogen storage and conversion, as well as in terms of sexual activity, some adiposity is probably rather important. This focuses attention on the importance of diet. It is an important challenge to examine the impact of nutrition on some of the age-related processes.

By this time in the history taking, the patient should relate well to the responsible physician and, having gained the patient's confidence, it is time to ask if there is any sexual dysfunction. Disinterest in intercourse is often a result of dyspareunia secondary to an atrophic vaginal mucosa, introital stricture or decreased vaginal distensibility resulting from estrogen deficiency or inability to lubricate. Although the true significance of sexual dys-

function in the menopause is difficult to measure, it is important for the physician to work with the patient in an attempt to find reasons for the dysfunction. Some patients often ask for a consultation with a sex counsellor and the physician should co-operate by making this referral.

When significance of a complaint is not readily apparent, the physician should listen carefully and question the patient further. The history is all important in establishing a good patient–physician relationship.

Gynecological examination

The findings on physical examination vary greatly, depending on the time elapsed since menopause and the severity of estrogen deficiency. Older women often question the need for periodic gynecological examinations after the menopause. It is important to impress upon the patient that they should continue to protect their health. Age does not prevent the development of cancer of the genitalia or breast. Although the incidence of some genital malignancies may plateau after the menopause, that of some cancers, particularly of the endometrium, vagina, vulva and ovary, actually increases.

Many menopausal patients recognize that they have atrophic vaginal and vulvar tissue and that examination may be painful. Therefore, they are inclined to avoid routine examinations. It is important that the patient receives as little discomfort and pain as possible during the examination. An explanation about the examination often dispels some of the anxiety and may put the patient at ease.

The examining physician should carefully observe the vulva, urethra and Bartholin's and Skene's glands, and it is important to palpate the texture of these structures. Since menopausal women may have atrophic vaginal or vulvar tissue resulting from hypoestrogenism, it is important to use a small speculum or Peterson's speculum. The speculum should be inserted by holding the blades parallel to the introitus, slowly turning the speculum so that the posterior blade rests against the posterior wall of the vagina and, with gentle pressure downwards, opening the vagina without disturbing the sensitive organs that lie anteriorly.

Once the speculum is in place and the cervix is identified, any vaginal secretion should be removed and a careful Pap smear taken, attempting to get into the cervical canal, if possible, also taking a smear of the posterior fornix. Although it is most important to screen the endometrium, it is better not do to it at this particular time, but later in the examination, or schedule it as a separate examination after the patient has established confidence in the physician–patient relationship.

A one-finger vaginal examination should be carried out at the beginning and the finger should be very carefully directed around the entire length and breadth of the vagina, in addition to exploring the fornices and the area under the urethra. Having done this, the uterus should be outlined as to size, shape and mobility, and then the adnexal area is carefully examined. It is important to explain each step of the examination to the patient and to assure the patient that, if there is any pain, the examination will be stopped immediately. Unfortunately, in the elderly, the vagina is often conical and inelastic, limiting a proper adnexal examination.

Rectovaginal bimanual examination is often preferable to vaginal abdominal bimanual examination in the menopausal patient. This allows the rectovaginal septum, cardinal ligaments and uterosacral ligaments to be carefully examined. A rectal examination should be carried out and any blood on the finger identified, and, in those patients in whom blood is not identified, one of the tests for occult blood should be carried out.

Having completed the routine examination, the physician must make a judgement about whether to attempt an endometrial aspiration at this particular examination or to have the patient return at another time for the endometrial aspiration. It is important to be as gentle as possible, otherwise the patient will not return for additional examinations. Using ultrasound, it is possible to measure the thickness of the endometrium and, when significantly over the baseline level, curettage is probably indicated.

In addition to the physical and pelvic examinations, a Pap smear, Schiller test, colposcopy and biopsy must be carried out to establish the diagnosis of any early lesion.

The breasts are considered a part of the upper genital tract and should be carefully examined. The examination must be done in an unhurried manner, and all quadrants should be examined. The patient should be examined while lying down, as well as sitting up. The American Cancer Society has published pamphlets demonstrating the ideal breast examination to be carried out by the physician. During the examination, it is important for the physician to teach the patient breast self-examination. This is the 1–2–3 method: first while taking a shower, then in front of a mirror and, last, while lying down.

Vulva

The vulvar and vaginal tissues of most women who are several years menopausal and who are not on estrogen replacement therapy are more or less atrophic. The vulva presents an atrophic appearance, the skin is thin and flabby, and there is loss of subcutaneous fat and hair. The labia tend to blend into the surrounding skin. The shrinkage, loss of elasticity and dryness of vaginal mucosa are due to estrogen withdrawal. Puckering of the vulvar tissue with atrophy of the introitus, even in multiparous women, may make penile intromission exquisitely painful, and deflection of the penis anteriorly by a rigid perineum may create pressure on the urethral meatus causing urethritis, local inflammation and dysuria. Loss of, or graying of, pubic hair is often psychologically traumatic to these women. An attempt must be made to assure them that it is a normal process and has no pathological significance. It may reassure the patient that her partner is probably in her age group and has decreased eyesight and probably does not notice the change in the pubic hair.

Many vulvar diseases are similar in different age groups. In the postmenopausal patient, there is an increase in the incidence of diabetic vulvitis, hypotrophic dystrophy and lichen sclerosus. Patients with these lesions often present with burning, pruritus or difficulty in coitus. Intertrigo is frequently seen in obese, postmenopausal patients who have difficulty in bathing and cleansing their perineums and vulvae. As a consequence, the skin covering their perineums, genital crura folds, labia majora and thighs is constantly moistened by preparations and soiled by urine. Those with intertrigo usually complain of perineal itching and burning.

Inspection shows the area to be superficially denuded, shiny, hyperemic and moist; a scanty, malodorous discharge may cover the affected areas. Treatment is best effected by good hygiene, clearing up any infection with a bactericidal cream or fungi with an antimycotic cream. After the area has been cleared of any irritation and infection, the patient may protect herself by using cornstarch in the area.

Senile angiomata are small, usually multiple, up to 3 mm in diameter, red, elevated papules that bleed freely when scrubbed or scratched. They are quite innocent, but the bleeding caused when they are traumatized frightens patients. This usually occurs after a hot bath when the area is vigorously rubbed with a bath towel. Angiomata and telangiectasias are not excised unless the patient is unduly alarmed or disturbed by their presence. They can then be treated by laser therapy.

Sebaceous cysts of the vulva form small, rarely 1-cm diameter, yellowish-gray nodules in the skin covering the labia. The foul smelling, purulent material extruded when a sebaceous cyst becomes infected and ruptured, as is often the case, or the discovery of a small lump in the vulva, may be quite disturbing to the patient. Very large sebaceous cysts that become repeatedly infected should be removed.

Clitoral phimosis may cause an inspissated smegma to collect beneath the prepuce, producing discomfort. The area is usually very red and resembles balanitis in men. Persistence of the inflamed area is treated surgically by making an incision over the top of the prepuce and removing the inspissated smegma.

The urethral caruncle is a small, reddened, sensitive, fleshy outgrowth at the urethral meatus. Most represent an ectropion of the urethra or infections at the urethral meatus. Occasionally there are vascular anomalies or benign or malignant neoplasms, which may also cause caruncle formation. The vast majority of caruncles are benign, but any persistent lesion which becomes progressively larger must be biopsied and treated according to the findings. The caruncles may occur at any age, but postmenopausal women are most commonly affected.

The vulvar dystrophies are a group of conditions characterized by disordered growth, sometimes disordered maturation, of the vulvar squamous epithelium. Their etiology is unknown, although recently an association between vulvar dystrophy and achlorhydria has been demonstrated, and a papillomavirus has been identified in some cases. A rationalized and simplified classification and nomenclature of vulvar dystrophies has been established. It includes lichen sclerosus, hypertrophic dystrophy and mixed dystrophy.

Dystrophic lesions appear as white patches in the epithelium known as leukoplakia. In addition, the mucocutaneous tissue becomes dry, shrivelled and brittle, a condition clinically known as kraurosis vulvae. These are clinical terms, similar to dystrophy used to describe the gross appearance of the lesion. They do not indicate specific pathological disease entities. Leukoplakia can be caused by a wide variety of abnormalities other than dystrophy. The diagnosis of specific conditions depends largely on careful histological evaluation.

White lesions of the vulva were once treated as a group. They were considered premalignant. The white appearance of the lesion is due to the keratin, a deep pigmentation and relative avascularity. All three of these mechanisms are present in the vulvar dystrophies. It is now recognized that white lesions of the vulva are not premalignant or malignant. Much of the confusion in the past resulted from the fact that there was no uniform terminology.

The skin of the vulva consists of two parts: dermis and epidermis, which interact and, therefore, modify each other. Each group does not necessarily respond to the same nutritional or other conditioning patterns. Estrogen lack has little effect on vulvar epidermis. However, it has a considerable effect on the dermis, reversing fibrosis and shrinking of the introitus and loss of fat from the labia majora. The vulva is not part of the integument. Embryologically, from the mons pubis to the anus, it is an organ. Its lymphatic drainage and blood supply are its own, and not merged with those of the surrounding skin, although they are related in varying degrees to the connecting vaginal mucosa.

Relief may be obtained by using the following method: place a folded paper tissue in the freezing part of the refrigerator and coat it with plain yogurt; it can be applied to the vulva and will give relief without causing an ice burn. It has no direct therapeutic value.

Based on clinical and histological characteristics, the vulvar dystrophies may be subdivided into three groups: lichen sclerosus, hyperplastic and mixed. In the latter two groups, it may occur with or without atypia.

Lichen sclerosus is the most common of the three groups of white lesions. It usually occurs in postmenopausal patients, but it can affect persons of all ages, including children. Clinical examination reveals the skin of the vulva to be thin, atrophic, parchment-like, dry, and white or yellow. The final diagnosis should be made on histological examination.

Lichen sclerosus is best treated with testosterone applications, which result in some epithelial activation, perhaps by blocking chalone receptor sites or by simply activating the growth potential and increasing the blood supply to the epithelium. Current reports indicate that testosterone is metabolized in much larger quantities in skin from lichen sclerotic patients than in normal vulvar skin. Although not always successful, testosterone ointment can be applied freely for 2–3 weeks, then once or twice a week, or more frequently if the pruritus returns, and finally is needed to promote patient comfort. Testosterone propionate ointment has its greatest benefit when there is burning rather than itching. Judicious use of corticosteroid ointment may help to reduce the disturbing edema of the prepuce and clitoris, but if it is continued for any length of time it may be dangerous because the thin skin is then easily ulcerated. Testosterone propionate 2% is made up in white petrolatum in 60-g units.

Hyperplastic dystrophy is also called hyperplastic vulvitis, neurodermatitis and leukokeratosis. The resulting clinical picture is one of thickening and lightening of the vulva and adjacent skin. Unlike lichen sclerosus, the perineal and perianal areas are seldom affected. Pruritus is always present and, owing to the uncontrollable urge to scratch, changes occur in the primary lesion.

Since these patients present with marked itching, therapy must be directed towards controlling this symptom. It is important to teach the patient proper hygiene. Any soap with detergent should be excluded. For example, Ivory® soap is very alkaline and dries the area and aggravates the itching and burning. The patient should be instructed to use baby soap or Neutrogena®. The tense, nervous patient, particularly one whose focus is on the vulvar itching, should be treated with a mild tranquilizer for a short period of time. Atarax® (hydropyzine hydrochloride) is used widely among dermatologists as an adjuvant treatment for itching. Topical corticosteroids provide the backbone for treatment. They should be applied twice a day. Although the itching is controlled rather rapidly, it takes about 6–8 weeks before any visible change is seen in the gross lesion. Patients who do not respond to the corticosteroids should have cream made up of eurax and corticosteroids, consisting of 30% eurax and 70% corticosteroids, and should be made up in 60-g lots. The cream should be applied twice daily until the itching is controlled. The patient can then resume using topical corticosteroids and switch to the eurax and corticosteroid combination only when the itching is bad. Burning is best treated with testosterone propionate 2% in white petrolatum. Progesterone in oil 400 mg in 4 oz aquaphor has been successfully used in most cases of dystrophy that were unresponsive or unsuited to testosterone.

Approximately 15% of all cases of vulvar dystrophy show a mixed pattern. Both lichen sclerosus and hyperplastic dystrophy can be found on the same vulva, and constitute the condition known as mixed dystrophy. In studying these lesions, some areas show the gross and microscopic features of lichen sclerosus, while others show the features of hyperplastic dystrophy. A wrinkled, parchment-like appearance usually signifies an area of lichen sclerosus, and heaped-up white plaque is usually associated with a hyperplasia. It is important to take multiple biopsy specimens from these lesions. In a differential diagnosis, lichen sclerosus with hyperkeratotic plaques, superimposed fungal infections and carcinoma *in situ* must be considered.

The management is similar to that of other dystrophies. Attention should be given to soap, underclothes and personal hygiene. Pantihose seem to aggravate the problem. The vulva should be treated with corticosteroids and, when the hyperplastic areas disappear, it may be necessary to treat the lichen sclerosus with 2% testosterone propionate in petrolatum base. The corticosteroids and testosterone preparations may have to be alternated. In order to control the itching in some resistant cases, it may be necessary to give alcohol injections, but this is very infrequent. Laser therapy has been employed in some of these patients, but there are not enough data to determine its value accurately.

Vitiligo may occur in the vulva. It is usually associated with a generalized condition of the skin. It may occur early in life and is seen more often in the female than in the male. Hyperkeratosis presents clinically as elevated, thickened patches of white skin or mucosa. Chronic inflammatory lesions may become hypertrophic because of the irritation from scratching. Senile atrophy occurs in elderly women. It is usually accompanied by shrinkage and by very dry, thin tissue, often with multiple telangiectasias present.

Carcinoma *in situ* of the vulva is perhaps the most puzzling dystrophy, and the one which the physician relates to carcinoma of the cervix to which it bears a superficial relationship. The possibility exists that carcinoma *in situ* is a sexually transmitted disease, at least in an associated or triggering role. Carcinoma *in situ* of the vulva may be either unifocal or multifocal, two-thirds being multifocal. Whether this represents exposure to persistent carcinogens on the one hand, or a single stimulus on the other, is unclear. It is important to rule out microinvasion or frank invasion in any vulvar lesion.

The treatment of *in situ* lesions may be observation, removal or destruction. However, it is important to make certain of the diagnosis by using a biopsy technique to document the histology. Although the treatment of carcinoma *in situ* has gone through many phases from simple vulvectomy, skinning procedures or applications of 5-fluorouracil, the use of laser surgery is now playing an increasingly important role in the management of these lesions.

In addition to *in situ* carcinomas, there is at least a 20%, probably greater, association of the vulvae with malignancies in other organs perhaps quite unrelated. The cervix is the most common site, but breast and gut are also common.

Paget's disease is not truly a dystrophy; however, as it is a hyperplastic change within the epithelium and is confined by the basement membrane, it is considered in the *in situ* category. Pruritus is predominant as a symptom, and soreness comes much later. It should not be confused with fungal infestation which causes soreness and redness of the vulva. The typical picture is a velvety red background with white patches scattered throughout the area. It is important that a biopsy be taken that is deep enough to encompass the epidermis and dermis so that a sweat gland or Bartholin's gland cancer is not missed. Having made an accurate diagnosis of carcinoma *in situ*, the patient with Paget's disease can be treated as any other *in situ* patient, with wide local excision. The biopsy must be carried down through the dermis so that the invasive cancer is not missed. The breasts must be carefully evaluated as there may be a concomitant breast lesion.

Primary malignant disease of the vulva represents about 5–10% of female cancers. The most common lesion is epidermoid cancer, which may be invasive or intraepithelial, and is primarily seen in women well over age 60 years. Epithelial dysplasia coexists with about 50% of invasive cancers, and is considered by many oncologists to be a premalignant vulvar disease. A second primary malignancy affecting the cervix, breast or uterus is found in about 50% of patients, often in association with a primary vulvar neoplasm. It is obvious that these patients should have careful evaluation with biopsy. Treatment of invasive cancer of the vulva is primarily surgical with radical or modified radical excisional vulvectomy and superficial inguinal node dissection. The decision about excision of the deep nodes is usually left to the responsible surgeon. Radiotherapy is often given to the nodes deep in the pelvis, and the results are equal to those obtained by surgical excision.

Vagina

The reduction of estrogen support for the vaginal tissues is responsible for most of the common symptoms associated with vaginal disorders. The vaginal epithelium is thin and relatively avascular and inelastic; rugae disappear and the epithelium presents a dry, glazed appearance. These conditions cause no discomfort for many patients, but those who are sexually active may complain of dyspareunia even if they had no coital distress when they were younger.

The most common symptoms suggestive of vaginal disease are leukorrhea, frequency and urgency of urination, dyspareunia, itching and bleeding. In this age group, 80% of the patients studied cytologically are estrogen deficient. Older patients who complain of these symptoms may have no findings other than those associated with atrophic vaginitis. In the absence of a proven pathogen, the most common treatment for atrophic vaginitis is topical estrogen cream. This should be carried out for at least 1 month. The patient should be instructed to insert about one-quarter of an applicator of estrogen cream into the vagina every third or fourth night for approximately 2 months. Inserting a full applicator of cream usually results in some of the cream running out. Having been mixed with vaginal secretion, it may cause a marked irritation around the vulva.

Trichomonas vaginalis and occasionally candida may be superimposed upon some atrophic vaginitis. The diagnosis should be made and, in addition to treating the atrophic vaginitis, trichomonas infestation should be treated with metronidazole for 10 days by mouth, or by metronidazole gel vaginally for 5 days, and the candida infestation treated with topical antifungal agent for approximately the same time. Postmenopausal patients are often helped by douching once a week with a half-cup of vinegar in approximately a quart of lukewarm water. This substitutes for the acidity of the normal vagina.

Women who have been treated for carcinoma *in situ* of the cervix by hysterectomy should have routine Pap smears, because the transformation zone has been found to extend to the vagina in 5% of normal women. Occasionally *in situ* lesions will be identified in the vagina. These lesions should be biopsied and then treated. Treatment with 5-fluorouracil, laser surgery and surgical excision are usually the methods chosen. Having treated the patient, a structured regimen for Pap smears must be instituted.

Primary vaginal carcinoma is uncommon, accounting for less than 1% of cancers of the female reproductive tract. It is usually epidermoid, presenting as an ulcer high in the posterior vaginal fornix. Any persistent lesion of the vagina must be biopsied, and the decision then made about its management. In this age group, radiation therapy is usually the method of treatment chosen.

Cervix

The histology of the cervix is quite different from that of the corpus with regard to its epithelium, glands and stroma. The epithelium is of two varieties, the stratified squamous and the glandular–columnar. The stratified squamous epithelium lines the pars vaginalis or portio, and it has inconspicuous subepithelial papillae and no cornification. This epithelium extends to the external os with some variation of demarcation line. The glandular–columnar epithelium is tall, non-ciliated and picket-fence in appearance and within the endocervical canal. Nuclei are deeply stained and basal, and the cytoplasm, which is rich in mucins, stains faintly basophilic or is neutral and unstained. The transition zone, of vital importance clinically with respect to carcinoma of the cervix, may be gradual or abrupt. In the postmenopausal patient, the squamocolumnar junction is found higher in the endocervical canal than is generally seen in the premenopausal patient.

The cervix presents an atrophic picture similar to the vulva and the vagina in the postmenopausal patient. The cervix shrinks to become flush with the vaginal vault and presents as a relatively avascular fibrous nodule; the cervical canal may become stenosed. Vaginal bleeding is a signal for further evaluation of the patient. Bleeding may occur as a result of atrophic vaginitis, with or without infection, or benign polyps of the cervix, but cervical cancer can and does occur in the elderly population, and cervical smears, colposcopic examination, biopsies and possibly fractional curettage are indicated if the lesion is present on the cervix or cervical smear shows abnormal cytological findings.

Cervical erosion, ulcer and ectropion are three conditions that become increasingly important with aging. In erosion of the acquired type, there is a loss of superficial layers of the epithelium by a local destructive influence which may be unclear etiologically. It may be the result of pH change or bacterial toxicity, or a combination of the two.

The basal cuboidal cells have been exposed. A congenital form of erosion may also be a pathogenetic factor. Cervical ectropion is manifested by an inflamed and edematous endocervical mucosa, which hangs out of the endocervical canal and is easily visible. True cervical ulcers present gross and histological findings as with any ulcer. There is complete loss of epithelium, revealing a base of more or less active granulation tissue with an increasingly fibrous base with time.

Non-specific cervicitis is extremely common and often afflicts almost every multiparous female. A variety of organisms have been implicated. The non-specific cervicitis most commonly results from child-bearing, instrumentation, pH change, contaminating coitus, estrogen depletion, cervical eversion and others. Chlamydia is starting to be found in the menopausal and postmenopausal patient, as well as in the young patient. This is also true of the human papillomavirus. Occasionally, herpes simplex type 2 may cause a lesion on the cervix. The increasing incidence of chlamydia, human papillomavirus and herpes simplex virus 2 being found in the vagina and on the cervix of the menopausal and postmenopausal woman may represent a change in life-style today.

Whereas carcinoma *in situ* of the cervix occurs premenopausally, the average age being 38 years, the invasive phase of this disease affects white women with a peak occurrence in the 40–49 year range, after which the rate remains constant with advancing age. However, in the past few years, it has been found that the incidence of carcinoma *in situ* of the cervix appears to be increasing in the postmenopausal period. Again, this may be the result of a change in life-style.

Invasive cancer of the cervix is encountered less often in the postmenopausal patient than in the younger patient. This difference between the age groups is due in no small part to the widespread use of Pap smears. Even so, elderly patients should be examined for cervical carcinoma just as they were premenopausally. In patients under 70 with a stage IB or IIA carcinoma, radical hysterectomy and pelvic node dissection is usually chosen unless there is a medical contraindication. However, in stages IIB, III and IV, radiation therapy is the treatment of choice.

Uterus

The uterus undergoes retrogressive changes and becomes small and atrophic. Leiomyomas tend to atrophy, although they may still present problems. There are many causes for postmenopausal genital bleeding, but endometrial carcinoma must be ruled out when it occurs in this age group. Bleeding may be a result of estrogen therapy, a collection of bloody fluid in the endometrial cavity bursting through an occluded cervix, an estrogen-producing ovarian tumor, a lesion of the vagina or vulva, or coital, instrumental or digital trauma. Whatever its presumed cause, it is mandatory that such procedures as are necessary be performed to exclude endometrial cancer or other genital cancer. Endometrial biopsies and lavages are often ill-suited for study in the endometrium of the postmenopausal patient. The use of ultrasound to measure the thickness of the endometrium may help in making the diagnosis. If there is any question, the patient should be hospitalized in an ambulatory setting and, under anesthesia, have a careful pelvic examination and a fractional curettage. Carcinoma of the endometrium ranks as the fifth most common cause of death in women in whom cancer develops and who are 75 years of age or older. Diabetes mellitus, obesity, certain ovarian tumors and hypertension are among the risk factors for uterine cancer. Any treatment with estrogens, anticoagulants or a number of other medications, as well as the possibility of blood dyscrasias, should always be included in the differential diagnosis. In patients who are unable to distinguish bleeding from the urethra, vagina or anal canal, it may be necessary to perform cystoscopy and sigmoidoscopy, in addition to investigating the reproductive tract.

The management of endometrial cancer has evolved from using preoperative radiation followed by hysterectomy to doing surgery as an initial procedure, and then making a decision about the type and extent of external radiation. All patients with carcinoma of the endometrium are given a radiation implant into the vagina. This has reduced the number of vaginal vault recurrences. Patients with a normal-sized uterus and well-differentiated adenocarcinoma confined to stage

IA G1 can be treated with surgery alone, without additional radiation therapy.

Ovary

Ovarian cancer is the leading cause of death from gynecological cancer. It is the most frustrating problem that the physician faces in gynecology. It is not possible to make an early diagnosis, as evidenced by the fact that 60–70% are already in stages III and IV when they present for initial examination and treatment. The overall survival rate for the truly invasive epithelial ovarian cancers is seldom better than 25% 5-year survival.

Ovarian tumors have a complex classification, but may be considered under the headings of gonadal–stromal, germ cell, mixed, common epithelial ovarian cancer and metastatic tumors. The greatest number of cases of common epithelial ovarian cancer occur between ages 50 and 70, with a peak incidence of occurrence at about age 77. It is obvious that the ovary becomes too old to function, but never becomes too old to form a cancer. Although it has been stated that there are no early symptoms of ovarian cancer, reports in the literature contradict this statement. A great number of women with ovarian cancer have vague abdominal complaints for a long time before the diagnosis is made. Many of these women have had a thorough work-up, including barium enema and gastrointestinal series, but a serious attempt at a pelvic or rectal examination has not been carried out. It is important, therefore, to rule out ovarian cancer in any woman over age 40, particularly one who is nulliparous or had a history of involuntary sterility or multiple spontaneous abortions, and who presents with vague abdominal symptoms that are not identified by careful work-up. These patients must be watched very carefully, including the use of tumor markers and vaginal color Doppler ultrasound, and, if indeed the suspicion is great enough, the patient should have surgical exploration. It is important to examine patients over age 35 years every 6 months. They should be instructed to take an enema or to insert two Dulcolax® (bisacodyl) rectal suppositories before coming in for a pelvic examination. Any woman who is more than 2 years postmenopausal and presents with a palpable ovary that is normal in size and consistency for the premenopausal years must have a careful work-up, and, if on repeat examination findings are confirmed, surgical exploration should be carried out without delay. This ovarian finding has been designated the postmenopausal palpable ovary syndrome. This syndrome does not refer to the small cysts that are found on ultrasound examination and may be a normal finding in women as old as 80 years of age. The cyst probably represents the last follicle left in the ovary, followed by connective tissue surrounding the cavity giving a small coin-like lesion.

Of the gonadal–stromal tumors, the granulosa theca cell tumor is the most important. These tumors occur at any age, but may become manifest during the climacteric with the average age at 52. About 65% occur in the postmenopausal period. Probably as a result of their frequent hormone production, numerous associated conditions are found along with these tumors, and include such entities as endometrial carcinoma, leiomyomas, breast carcinoma and mammary dysplasia. Approximately 25% of these tumors are functioning and about 25% are malignant. The bilaterality rate is about 5%. The Sertoli–Leydig cell tumor is associated with masculinization when it functions, but only about 25% do so. They have a malignancy rate of about 25% and about 5% are bilateral. When the gonadal–stromal tumors appear in the menopausal and postmenopausal years, the treatment is total hysterectomy, bilateral salpingo-oophorectomy, cytological washing and omentectomy as deemed in the best interest of the patients.

The germ cell tumors usually occur in the child-bearing years, and most commonly occur from birth to age 20. They are seldom seen in the postmenopausal period, but, when they are diagnosed at this time, the treatment is total hysterectomy, bilateral salpingo-oophorectomy, omentectomy and triple anti-cancer chemotherapy.

The ovary is unique in that not only does it give rise to a great number of primary tumors and malignancies, but is itself a recipient of metastases from a variety of organs. Since breast and colon cancers are among the leading killers of women from cancer and have a propensity for metastasizing to the ovary, it is important to do a very thorough evaluation in any patient suspected of having ovarian cancer. Although all metastatic tumors to the ovary are referred to as Krükenberg, this is not strictly correct. The Krükenberg tumor is usually a metastatic tumor that involves both ovaries, giving them a kidney-shaped appearance, and, on microscopic examination, has a characteristic signet ring cell dispersed with an inactively responsive connective tissue. The usual primary is somewhere along the gastrointestinal tract, most often the stomach, particularly the pyloric end.

The treatment for common epithelial ovarian cancer is surgical removal of uterus, tubes, ovary, omentum and appendix, and possible lymph node sampling. The surgery should be aggressive without creating inordinate morbidity and mortality. External X-ray therapy is reserved for special findings as far as treatment of the common epithelial ovarian cancer is concerned. It should be used to treat supraclavicular and inguinal nodes and, if there is an area that is against the pelvic wall, it should be outlined by metal clips and radiation directed to that area. Also, radiation therapy has value in the management of germ cell tumors and gonadal–stromal tumors. For the common epithelial ovarian cancer, the adjuvant treatment of choice is a combination of anti-cancer chemotherapy, and the drugs most often employed are Platinol® (cisplatin) and Taxol® (paclitaxel). Since these patients are elderly, it is important to make sure that renal function is within normal limits before *cis*- platinum is administered. Taxol is now used for both first- and second-line therapy.

Fallopian tube

Primary adenocarcinoma of the Fallopian tube accounts for less than 1% of the malignant neoplasms of the female genital tract. However, the true incidence is difficult to assess as, in many cases, the primary site of origin of the neoplasm cannot be determined. Some cases of ovarian and endometrial carcinoma spread to the Fallopian tube. Although the reverse is also true, lesions of ambiguous origin are not usually assigned to the tube, in view of the greater frequency of ovarian and uterine carcinoma.

Fallopian tube adenocarcinoma usually occurs in postmenopausal patients between the ages of 45 and 55 years. Approximately 60% of patients are infertile, which may be the result of the pre-existing inflammation. The tumors are usually asymptomatic until they infiltrate locally or metastasize. The patient may then present with a triad of pain, serosanguinous or watery vaginal discharge, or frank bleeding. Any adnexal mass in postmenopausal patients should suggest the possibility of ovarian or tubal carcinoma. The spread is similar to that found with the common epithelial ovarian cancer, and the same treatment is employed for carcinoma of the tube as is employed for carcinoma of the ovary.

Breast

Carcinoma of the breast is the second leading cause of death from cancer among women. There are approximately 175 000 new cases and 43 300 women are anticipated to die of the disease in 1999. One woman in eight will develop a carcinoma of the breast by age 70.

Although breast cancer is covered in another chapter in this book, it is important that attention be directed towards reducing breast cancer mortality. The principles that should be followed are:

(1) Breast examinations are an integral part of the routine gynecological examination for all patients.

(2) Patients must receive instructions in the proper technique of life-long periodic breast self-examination.

(3) Proper ambulatory surgical facilities for performing breast biopsies must be developed.

(4) The final diagnosis of pathology rests on careful histological examination of a biopsy specimen (biopsy is recommended for all true, solid, three-dimensional masses).

(5) Research, both basic and clinical, and etiology, diagnosis and treatment of breast lesions are to be encouraged. Innovative screening programs for high-risk patients must be included in this effort. Residency training programs in obstetrics and gynecology must include specific instructions in early detection techniques of breast carcinoma, including biopsy examination. The American Cancer Society has monographs on the step-like

fashion for breast examination by the physician, as well as monographs for the patient to learn breast self-examination.

(6) Research should be directed to evaluate designer estrogens (selective estrogen receptor modulators or SERMs) and their role in the prevention and treatment for the patient who has survived breast cancer.

(7) Tamoxifen, the first known SERM has extended millions of lives by acting as an antiestrogen in breast cancer. It is suggested, but not conclusive, that it may prevent breast cancer.

Cystourethrocele and uterine descensus

It is generally agreed that the support of pelvic structures depends on the endopelvic fascia, the uterosacral and cardinal ligaments, and levator muscles. This intact fascial system with its attachments to the vaginal fornices and upper two-thirds of the lateral vagina provides a well-supported vaginal tube, which in turn is the most important supporting structure for the uterus and vaginal vault. Traumatic (obstetric) stretching, wear and tear of living, occupational and unusual athletic endeavors, heredity and postmenopausal attenuation of pelvic and perianal muscles all contribute in varying degrees to the development of pelvic relaxation. Additional contributing factors that promote uterine descensus are chronic obstructive pulmonary disease (COPD), and asthma and other chronic lung diseases. These are commonly associated with cystocele and in women who have urinary stress incontinence. However, urethrocele is not a cause of urinary incontinence. It is interesting that in women with large cystoceles there is seldom any stress incontinence. However, these patients often have repeated bouts of cystitis. Patients with large cystoceles often have to put their finger in their vagina and push the bladder upward in order to empty their bladder. The patient with a large cystocele may pull on the trigone of the bladder and, as a result, has a constant urge to pass urine. Nothing short of surgery will correct this condition.

The essentials of diagnosis include:

(1) Sensation of vaginal fullness, pressure of falling out;

(2) Feeling of incomplete emptying of the bladder, urinary frequency and perhaps the need to push the bladder up in order to empty the bladder completely;

(3) Presence of soft, reducible mass bulging into the anterior vagina and distending the vaginal introitus;

(4) With straining or coughing, increased bulging and descent of the anterior vaginal wall as well as the urethra.

Although a degree of cystocele is demonstrable in virtually all parous women during the childbearing years, their condition may not progress and may not cause symptoms.

The importance of physiological and anatomical factors in the problems of prolapse and incontinence has led to the adoption of the term 'pelvic floor dysfunction'. When examining living persons, the pelvic floor is a convex, dynamic structure that must continually expand and contract in response to different stimuli and conditions. It must contract to help maintain urinary and fecal continence, yet it must relax to allow the expulsion of urine and feces. It has a role in normal sexual responsiveness in females and may play a role in the generation of an orgasm at the peak of sexual excitement.

Treatment in such cases is not usually required until after the menopause, when the pelvic fascial and muscular supports become attenuated by slowly progressive involutional changes. The cystocele requires surgical repair if there are repeated bouts of cystitis or trigonitis, or if the cystocele becomes so large that the patient cannot adequately empty her bladder, with repeated bouts of cystitis, or the cystocele protrudes outside the vaginal introitus and causes an ulceration of the vaginal wall. A large cystocele may result in pulling on the trigone, giving rise to a constant urgency. The various types of pessaries do not usually help cystoceles and very often create stress incontinence. Many older women tolerate large cystourethroceles and some degree of descensus without complaint, but massive procidentia (complete prolapse) is always disabling, and is occasionally associated with trophic ulceration of the exposed vaginal mucosa or with kidney dysfunction caused by kinking from displacement of both ureters. The uterus gradually descends from the axis of the vagina taking the vaginal wall with it. It may present clinically at any level, but is usually classified as one of three degrees: first, cervix still inside the vagina; second, cervix appears outside the vulva, cervical lips become congested and ulcerated; and third, complete prolapse. This is sometimes called complete procidentia. (Procidentia means 'parts of the body falling out of place'.) The uterovaginal prolapse represents the herniation of the genital tract through the pelvic diaphragm. The uterus and vagina are held in the pelvis by the cardinal and uterosacral ligaments and by the pelvic floor musculature, mainly the levator ani. When these ligaments and muscles become ineffective, the uterus and vagina descend (prolapse) through the gap between the muscles. The causes of prolapse are:

(1) Stretching of muscle and fibrous tissue which occurs with repeated childbirth;

(2) Increased intra-abdominal pressure which occurs in women with a chronic cough or asthma and in women who undertake heavy industrial work;

(3) A constitutional predisposition to stretching of the ligaments as a response presumably to years in the erect position.

Thus, nulliparous women can develop prolapse. However, in those that do, a thorough neurological examination should be carried out, as well as careful metabolic and endocrine studies as indicated.

It is often reported that obesity might increase the load on the pelvic floor; however, this is probably not the case, because the abdominal viscera presents essentially a fluid-like mass, and the pressure at the bottom of a column of fluid is related only to the height of the column and not to its overall diameter.

Management

These conditions are probably best treated surgically, and even the most elderly can tolerate the surgery fairly well. However, there are some women for whom it is well advised not to perform surgery, and a vaginal pessary of the Gellhorn, disc type or Smith–Hodge type may support the uterus and bladder. Although the patient will require scheduled visits for removal and cleansing of the pessary, it decreases the need for an operation. The pessary is usually considered as the last resort measure. However, when indicated, it can be a great comfort to a very sick old woman with severe heart disease, emphysema and the presence of a procidentia.

Rectocele

Bulging of the posterior vaginal wall and underlying rectum through the rectovaginal fascia results in a rectocele. If the prolapse is at the level of the middle third of the vagina, the rectovaginal septum is often involved and the rectum prolapses with the vaginal wall. This is called a classic rectocele. If the lowest part of the vagina is prolapsed, the perianal body is involved rather than the rectum.

A mild degree of rectocele (rarely causing symptoms) is usually present in all multiparous patients. A large rectocele may cause a sense of pelvic pressure, rectal fullness or incomplete evacuation of stool. Occasionally a patient may find it necessary to reduce the posterior vaginal wall manually in a backward direction to evacuate stool effectively from the lower rectum. Distinguishing a high rectocele (involving the entire rectovaginal septum) from an enterocele may sometimes be difficult. Generally, with the patient straining, a rectovaginal examination will confirm the presence of abdominal contents sliding into the enterocele sac so that an enterocele, as opposed to rectocele, presents as a true hernia. Since pessaries are not helpful for either a rectocele or an enterocele, surgical repair is indicated when symptoms interfere with the quality of life.

Enterocele

An enterocele results when the small bowel pushes the peritoneum between the rectum and the vagina. Large enteroceles occasionally give upper abdominal distress because of the pull on the mesentery of the bowel. If the upper part of the posterior vaginal wall prolapses, the pouch of Douglas is elongated and small bowel or omentum may descend, pushing the peritoneum in front of it. This has been called the classic enterocele. Enterocele is usually associated with uterine prolapse and is sometimes called vault prolapse or hernia of the pouch of Douglas. The diagnosis is made from the following:

(1) An uncomfortable pressure and a falling out sensation of the vagina;

(2) Association with uterine prolapse or subsequent to hysterectomy in any age group, most commonly in postmenopausal women;

(3) Demonstration of a mass bulging into the posterior fornix and upper posterior vaginal wall;

(4) Occasionally the enterocele will put traction on the mesentery of the small bowel, causing upper abdominal discomfort.

The diagnosis is made by having the patient stand and by inserting the index finger into the rectum and the thumb into the vagina, and asking the patient to strain or cough. An impulse of the small bowel against the examining fingers is almost certain to be an enterocele. If the enterocele is large and bulges through the introitus, or if there is a great deal of abdominal discomfort, the enterocele should be repaired surgically. It is important in repairing an enterocele to have a high ligation of the peritoneal sac and closure of the transversalis fascia, and an additional insurance against recurrence is to bring the uterosacrals together and close off the cul-de-sac.

Stress incontinence

Urinary incontinence and lower genital tract disorders become more frequent after the menopause. The lower urinary tract and the lower genital tract are of the same embryonic origin and influence each other in physiological and pathophysiological conditions.

Stress incontinence is defined as involuntary loss of urine due to a sudden increase in intra-abdominal pressure such as occurs with laughing, coughing or sneezing. About 50% of parous women occasionally experience stress incontinence. It must be distinguished from overflow incontinence, urgency incontinence, enuresis and incontinence resulting from a neurological disorder.

The causes of genuine stress incontinence are urethral sphincter incompetence or anatomical scarred urethra (iatrogenic or traumatic), or urethral denervation. During the stress of coughing, the proximal portion of the urethra drops below the pelvic floor. An increase in intra-abdominal pressure induced by coughing transmits to the bladder, but not to the urethra. Since the urethral resistance is overcome by the increased bladder pressure, leakage of urine results. On urodynamic evaluation, there is a decrease in the functional length of the urethra, decreased urethral closure pressure and abnormal response of the sphincteric mechanism in reaction to stress, assumption of the upright position and bladder filling. Stress incontinence occurs when the urethra sags away from its attachments to the symphysis. It may appear before the menopause, but for many women it becomes increasingly distressing after the age of 60. Loosening of the pelvic supporting tissue, damaged years earlier by vaginal delivery and aggravated by years of standing and straining, becomes more marked after estrogen secretion decreases following the menopause.

The function of the levator ani muscles can be compromised in two ways: first, there can be direct injury to the muscle, resulting in mechanical disruption of the entire muscle; second, damage to nerves supplying the muscles could lead to their inability to contract, even though they themselves remain intact. Damage to the nerve supply of the muscle probably explains why the Kegel exercises fail to control stress incontinence in some women.

Urodynamic studies are important for correct diagnosis. These include X-ray findings such as cystourethrograms, the Bonney or Marchetti test in which there is support given to the posterior urethrovesicle angle and observing whether any urine is lost on straining, and direct electronic cystometry. This procedure is favored over others for differentiating bladder instability due to cystitis and nerve or muscle dysfunction. Urodynamics means the determination of bladder tone and its response to gradual distention with normal saline. This will provide a measurement of capacity (the normal bladder can hold about 700 ml) and of any residual urine after voiding (as with cystocele). About 50 ml are instilled at a time, and the bladder wall given time to accommodate. The manometer indicates detrusor contractions and, if they are frequent and occur early on, an irritable bladder is diagnosed. Cystometry cannot determine the cause.

Half the women with stress incontinence can avoid surgery if they have good pubococcygeal tone and faithfully practice pubococcygeal exercises (puckering the vagina and urethral supporting tissue in a manner comparable to stopping a stream of urine). This is called a Kegel perineal exercise. The patient is advised to carry out this exercise for 2 min at least four times a day. It takes approximately 2 months before any positive results are seen in a great number of cases. Incontinence will recur if the exercises are not continued. If the Kegel exercises are done properly, and there is absolutely no response, it probably represents damage to the nerve supply of the muscles which leads to their inability to contract, even though they themselves remain intact.

Three-quarters of women with stress incontinence are asymptomatic after surgery that is carried out to repair a cystourethrocele and return the urethra to its normal position above and behind the symphysis. The most commonly employed operation to restore the urethrovesicle angle is the Marshall–Marchetti–Krantz operation or the Burch operation. These procedures are not effective if loss of urine is due to another cause.

Exogenous estrogens and endometrial cancer

It has been estimated that approximately 25% of women of menopausal age have symptoms of such severity as to warrant estrogen therapy. Although the evidence is not conclusive, it is suggested that estrogen replacement therapy has long-term metabolic benefits by reducing the incidence of stroke, heart disease, osteoporosis and fractures, and by slowing aging of the brain. Those that have been receiving estrogen replacement for 5 or more years have a decrease of Alzheimer's disease by 60%. A

number of case–control studies, however, have indicated that this form of treatment is associated with an increased incidence of endometrial cancer, with a risk ratio ranging between 5 and 15. These studies were based on case–control studies that are cheap, quick and easy to perform because they are retrospective. The problem involves an accurate and rigid selection of the case controls and, without this, the study has very little value. Using an alternative analytical method, Horwitz and Feinstein showed that the risk ratio was close to one. Although there is still slight concern about the relationship of exogenous estrogens to carcinoma of the endometrium, the physician should not be discouraged from using estrogen therapy when indicated. The judicial use of progesterone when giving estrogen replacement therapy will cut the incidence of carcinoma of the endometrium almost to zero.

The common symptoms that can be helped by estrogen replacement therapy include flushes, flashes, sweats, insomnia and dry vagina. As the patient gets older, the flushes and sweats disappear, but the dry, atrophic vagina becomes worse. Since osteoporosis is usually seen in the postmenopausal period, the issue of estrogen replacement therapy as a preventive treatment or a method of preventing the progress of osteoporosis is raised. Therefore, although the risk of endometrial cancer is increased, the physician must treat the symptomatic patient. The protection provided to the cardiovascular system by estrogen therapy is an indication to continue estrogen therapy for the duration of the patient's lifetime. The use of low-dose progesterone when giving estrogen replacement therapy does not seem to affect the lipid profile, but does protect the endometrium.

Occasionally this will cause vaginal bleeding, but, if the patient is monitored and has endometrial screening, it should not be a deterrent to keeping these women comfortable. Some women who have atrophic vulvitis and vaginitis, which do not always respond to estrogen by mouth, must have a supplemental estrogen vaginal cream. It is important to teach the patient to rub the estrogen cream on the outside, particularly around the posterior fourchette and just into the introitus. It is important to instruct the patient to start the estrogen vaginal cream just above the anus and rub it carefully into the perineum, particularly the posterior fourchette. This increases the amount of vulvar and vaginal tissues and usually stops the itching and discomfort that occurs with intercourse.

In the past couple of years, alendronate therapy has been shown to restore bone mass, but, when discontinued, the loss of bone mass continues. In the elderly, alendronate therapy is often associated with gastrointestinal symptoms, particularly esophagitis. Ideally, the alendronate must be taken first thing in the morning on an empty stomach with a glass of tap water. Carbonated water and fruit juices must be avoided at this time. Following the ingestion of alendronate and one glass of tap water, the patient is instructed not to eat or drink anything for half an hour, and the patient must not lie down during this time.

Recently, designer estrogens (SERMs) have been introduced. These agents behave like estrogen in some tissues, but block its action in others. The drug raloxifene has demonstrated ability for maintaining bone density in postmenopausal women. Reports indicate that it provides protection against endometrial cancer and breast cancer. Like estrogen replacement therapy, it increases the incidence of blood clots in veins. The media publicity has been great for the recent designer estrogens, but more data must be accumulated before they are prescribed for every patient.

Osteoporosis

Although the subject is covered in detail in another part of this book, it is important to review it briefly in this chapter. Many women visiting their family practitioner or the obstetrician/gynecologist, especially those in the postmenopausal years, inquire about osteoporosis. Osteoporosis has been called the silent disease. Technically this is because it usually produces absolutely no symptoms until a fracture occurs. In reality, osteoporosis is not a disease *per se*, but rather the end result of severe or prolonged bone loss. Osteoporosis is a painful, disfiguring and debilitating process. It is a women's issue. Osteoporosis cannot be cured, but with alendronate bone mass can be restored. However, it can be prevented and the symptomatology relieved. A great number of women visiting their

gynecologist for backache after they have been thoroughly evaluated by an orthopedic doctor may be found to have osteoporosis. Usual X-ray studies cannot identify osteoporosis until it is far advanced. When it shows up on the usual radiographs, there is about a 30% bone mass loss. However, by use of single photon absorptiometry or dual photon absorptiometry, a diagnosis can be made at an early stage and the patient treated for symptoms, and hopefully the progress of the osteoporosis stopped. In an overall evaluation, osteoporosis is really a pediatric disease. Therefore, prevention should start in early childhood, including a well-balanced diet, structured exercise and, above all, prohibition of smoking and drinking.

The patient who is predisposed to developing osteoporosis is a postmenopausal woman who is slender in weight, with very fair skin and small bone structure. There are other contributing factors that may predispose the patient to osteoporosis, namely a family history of the disease, Asian background, nulligravida, lack of physical activity, poor diet, calcium deficiency, vitamin D deficiency, smoking, alcohol, change in estrogen balance and change in calcium metabolism. Therapy for established disease includes calcium supplements, at least 1500 mg, vitamin D 400 IU, estrogens, androgens, fluoride and calcitonin. Alendronate has recently been introduced and has the ability, when calcium supplements and vitamin D are given, to restore bone mass. Treatment should be carried out under strict control conditions. It can be stated that osteoporosis cannot be cured, but, with alendronate, bone mass can be restored, but can only be maintained if alendronate is given continuously. However, the patient can be made more comfortable by treatment, and it may be possible to prevent osteoporosis from progressing. Structured exercise and a well-balanced diet are particularly important in dealing with osteoporosis. The new designer estrogens have been effective in preventing and treating osteoporosis and, although the reports are suggestive, they are not conclusive.

Cardiovascular disease

There is a relationship between the loss of ovarian function and the development of heart disease.

Approximately 450 000 American women die of heart attacks each year. Studies have shown the relationship between ovarian function, coronary atherosclerosis and mortality. Up until the menopause, women have less coronary heart disease problems than men, but, within the first 10 years after the menopause, women who have not been given estrogen replacement have a rate as high or higher than that for men, whereas women who have been taking estrogen have a much lower rate of coronary heart disease. Therefore, it is obvious that the use of appropriate doses of estrogen may offer postmenopausal women protection against coronary heart disease. The protective effect of low doses of estrogen is mediated through a decrease in the low-density lipoproteins (LDLs) and an increase in the high-density lipoproteins (HDLs). If the dosage of estrogen is too high, hypertension may be produced, but this is very seldom seen in women taking appropriate doses of estrogen. In addition, it should be added that estrogen replacement therapy has not been associated with an increased incidence of stroke, embolism or thrombophlebitis. Women receiving estrogen replacement therapy must be warned about the danger of smoking while taking estrogens.

Probably the most important indication for long-term hormonal therapy is the prevention of cardiovascular disease. This causes ten times more death than breast cancer in the postmenopausal population. Estrogen therapy reverses the negative lipoprotein changes that usually occur after the menopause. However, there is some evidence that estrogen may not benefit women with established coronary artery disease (CAD). Among women who have an intact uterus, a progestational agent should be added to the estrogen as part of the hormone replacement therapy. By the use of medroxyprogesterone acetate in small doses, such as 5 or 2.5 mg, the beneficial effect of estrogen on the lipid profile is not adversely affected. The role of the designer estrogen remains to be determined as far as the value in preventing cardiovascular disease is concerned.

There is increasing evidence in the literature that estrogen replacement therapy returns sex hormones to the premenopausal level, and it has been proposed as one method for reducing cardiovascular disease. In postmenopausal women treated with estrogen replacement therapy, it is anticipated that there will be a 50% decrease in all-cause mortality, compared to women who did not receive estrogen replacement therapy. On further examining the analysis of the data, it is evident that the largest effect on mortality was in decreasing ischemic heart disease. Although not every woman is a candidate for estrogen replacement therapy, if this treatment is prescribed judiciously and with full knowledge of its clinical effects, it can both offer patients lower mortality for cardiovascular disease and enhance quality of life. Recently it has been shown that estrogen therapy can slow aging of the brain and, if the patient has been taking estrogen replacement therapy for 5 or more years, it decreases the incidence of Alzheimer's by 60%. The effect of designer estrogens on the brain is to be determined.

Sexuality

With better nutrition, more cholesterol in the diet, more rest and better health, women are maintaining an interest in sexual function well into their postmenopausal years. Continued sexual outlets and functioning are the most important factors in maintaining sexual interest and capacity in the menopausal woman. If for any reason a woman is sexually inactive for some years in the postmenopausal period, there may be difficulty with re-institution of sexual function.

Women generally experience little serious loss of sexual capacity because of age alone. Those changes that do occur are mainly in the shape, flexibility and lubrication of the vagina. These can be traced directly to lowered levels of the hormone estrogen during and after the menopause. Women who have severe problems can be treated successfully with estrogen replacement therapy and are then able to carry on an active sex life.

In 1953 Kinsey reported that the sexual activity of unmarried women remains relatively constant until age 55, whereas that of unmarried men declines progressively from adolescence. Among married couples also, the frequency of sexual intercourse appears to decline in a similar fashion with aging. Kinsey concluded from these observations that, in women, age has no effect on sexual activity until very late in life, and suggested that subsequent reduction in sexual activity may be due primarily to diminution in the sexuality of the male partner.

Alterations in sexual response associated with aging are a result of generalized decrease in tone, strength and elasticity of tissues and lengthening of response time. In older women it may take 3-5 min for vaginal lubrication to occur, whereas in the young woman it takes only 15-20 s. At the same level of arousal, the older woman will have a smaller volume of lubrication. Again, provided that she is in good health and especially if there has been continuing of sexual function, lubrication for intercourse will be adequate. Use of commonly available lubricants may be helpful. Currently, Upsher-Smith Laboratories, Inc. has introduced Lubrin®, a vaginal lubricating insert which is unscented, colorless and convenient, as well as Replens®, which provides long-lasting lubrication for sexual intercourse. Some women find that Astro-Glide® serves as an adequate lubrication.

Sexual dysfunction may be life-long, in the sense that the woman has brought the condition into her marriage or other relationships, or it may have been acquired after a period of successful functioning. The dysfunction may affect both partners, or it may be situational in the sense that it is present in only one partner, usually the male. Many instances of sexual incompatibility are based on insufficient foreplay or preparation by the partner. Although the blame may be assigned to the partner, the failure is that of the woman herself, for she should assume responsibility for her own sexual pleasure and be able to communicate effectively her needs to her partner. If her partner rejects the explicit request, the problem is of general marital dysfunction and not strictly sexual.

The menopausal woman complaining of sexual inadequacy is often told by her physician that loss of sexual function is to be expected with the change of life and there is nothing to be done about it. Although sexual behavior is the sum total of the individual make-up, including chromosomal sex, gender identification, gonadal adequacy, childhood rearing, environmental influences, a possible hypothalamic sensitization and hormone factors, there is a definite role for hormone therapy in modifying sexual responsiveness. A combination of estrogen and androgen is often beneficial. Con-jugated estrogen or its equivalent in a dose of 0.625 mg, or 5 mg of methyltestosterone, is recommended. In some women, methyltestosterone, 10 mg three times a day for 2 weeks, will often increase the libido and fantasy level, and, if the patient indulges in intercourse, the desires will continue without needing any further stimulation from hormonal therapy. Androgens are not important for the physiological sexual response, but they are critical for the cognitive aspects of a woman's sexual functioning, such as desire. In women for whom intercourse is difficult because of shrinkage secondary to estrogen withdrawal, hormonal cream is often beneficial. This should be applied locally on the outside, around the inside lip of the small labia, up around the clitoris, and particularly around the posterior fourchette. It is important not only to apply the estrogen cream, but also to rub it into the tissue. The treatment should be carried out two to three times a week until the tissue has undergone a period of rejuvenation. The treatment should then be continued at less frequent intervals. A quarter of an applicator of estrogenic cream inserted into the vagina every 2-3 weeks usually keeps the upper part of the vagina pink and moist.

Some women seek advice about masturbation. Since they are elderly, they feel that it is a sign of some abnormal psychological condition. The patient must be instructed that it has no harmful physical or psychological effects. However, if the patient raises a moral issue about masturbation, it is best to refer her to her clergyman.

Masters and Johnson have shown that all four stages of the response cycle (excitement, plateau, orgasm and resolution) are somewhat diminished with increased age. In the excitement phase, breasts are less engorged and the sexual flush may be absent. The clitoris enlarges normally, but there is no noticeable change in the labia majora. Vaginal lubrication is reduced. Vaginal ballooning occurs later in the plateau phase and is often less marked. Orgasms continue to occur, but their duration is shorter, and muscular contraction may also be less intense. Uterine spasms may render some orgasms painful. The resolution phase is rapid in elderly women and occasionally, because of urethral trauma, is accompanied by a desire to void. Decrease in the strength of vaginal contractions occurring with orgasm is another change that occurs in elderly women. This effect is recordable and documented. However, older women may report no diminution in the experience of pleasure or release gratification.

Viagra® (sildenafil citrate) is receiving a great deal of media attention at present. However, it needs to be investigated in more detail and is not recommended at this time.

Major gynecological surgical procedures in the aged

Advances in preoperative, operative and postoperative management have considerably reduced the hazards of surgery for the postmenopausal patient. Older women are increasingly requesting surgery for gynecological problems in order to improve the quality of their lives.

A number of published studies have demonstrated that there is very little increase in the morbidity or mortality or length of stay in hospitals for patients undergoing major and minor gynecological surgery when compared with the younger age group, provided that due respect is paid to the patient's general condition. Most procedures can be performed with regional or local anesthesia with minimal discomfort to the patient, if general anesthesia is contraindicated. The majority of operative procedures are for the definitive treatment of genital prolapse and the diagnosis of the cause of postmenopausal bleeding, followed by surgery for uterine and vulvar lesions. Patients who are 90 years and older can undergo successful major surgery. The problem is that, in the postanesthesia stage, the patient may appear to be confused, and stroke and emboli must be ruled out.

As the postmenopausal population increases and women no longer accept age alone as a barrier to active life, more elective surgery will be demanded by patients and performed by gynecological surgeons.

Disorders of the female genital organs are certainly not among the major causes of death. Yet they give rise to important illnesses producing discomfort and disability and, therefore, warrant treatment. Most of the gynecological complaints of elderly women are related to genital prolapse. These conditions cause daily discomfort and anxiety. Contrary to the practice in younger patients, most of the operations in the elderly are carried out by the vaginal route. Vaginal hysterectomy is the procedure most often chosen to correct uterine prolapse. However, in rare situations, either the Manchester or LeFort operations may be employed.

Medical advancements in diagnosis and treatment and the better understanding of physiological and pathophysiological processes in the elderly now justify the performance of major operations in this group. Reports from numerous authors have shown that age alone does not contraindicate surgical intervention if due regard is paid to the patient's general condition. Better anesthesia and antibiotic therapy have resulted in greater security in the postoperative course. It is important for the physician to bear in mind that sexual activity in some women continues into very old age. Therefore, vaginal surgery should be performed with this in mind.

The duration of operation should be kept as short as possible, because the prolonged lithotomy position invites more complications than does prolonged anesthesia. Many postmenopausal patients develop hallucinations and disorientation following the anesthesia. This gives rise to the question of whether the patient has thrown an embolism or has had a cerebral accident. Unfortunately, these patients must be subjected to the usual evaluation for these conditions.

Mini-heparinization should be carried out in these patients starting the evening before surgery, continuing through surgery and for the first few days postoperatively. Contraindications to surgical intervention should not include chronological age.

Summary

Aging is a process that is continuous from conception to death. Aged is a term used to identify persons generally according to some established arbitrary chronological decision. In this conceptual system of the unitary man, aging is a developmental process. Moreover, aging is a continuously creative process directed towards a growing diversity of field pattern and organization. It is not a running down. The aged need less sleep and the pattern frequency of sleep/wakefulness is more diverse. Aging is not a disease. New life-styles are being promulgated by the postmenopausal patient. It is obvious that the postmenopausal patients represent a significant part of the population and that they add stability through their maturity and wisdom.

Strictly speaking, the word menopause means a final cessation of menstruation. This gives the grossly erroneous idea that yesterday all was well, tomorrow has changed; it also implies that a hysterectomy causes the menopause. This is incorrect. Menopause occurs if the ovaries are removed or cease to function. Climacteric, meaning the period of change, is a better word because it expresses the all-important concept of a time-scale, but is not in common use.

The quality of life for the postmenopausal woman can be significantly improved by active investigation and treatment of gynecological disorders, such as postmenopausal osteoporosis, and consideration of the best method of administering hormones and rehabilitation plans when illness strikes. Whereas patients were considered elderly at age 60, this has now been advanced to a retirement age of 70. With the improvements in technology, food, rest, leisure-time and a variety of methods of physiotherapy, patients are staying younger much longer than previously. Surgical intervention should never be excluded simply on the basis of chronological age.

Loss of urine control or urinary incontinence is especially common in postmenopausal women, but occurs in men as well. At least one in ten patients aged 65 or older has a problem with this. Incontinence can range from the discomfort of slight losses of urine to the disability and shame of severe frequent wetting. Persons who are incontinent often withdraw from social life and try to hide their problem from their family, friends and even their doctors. Relatives of an incontinent person often do not know about the choices of treatment, and are made to believe that nursing-home care is the only option. These reactions are unfortunate because in many cases incontinence can be treated and controlled, if not cured. Incontinence is not an inevitable result of aging. It is caused by specific changes in bodily function which often result from disease or use of medication. If untreated,

incontinence can increase the risk of skin irritation and might raise the risk of developing bed-sores. Some patients are put in a nursing home for incontinence and not incompetence.

Incontinence may be brought on by illness that is accompanied by fatigue, confusion and hospital admission. Incontinence is sometimes the first and only symptom of urinary tract infection. Curing the infection will usually relieve or clear up the incontinence. It is important to differentiate stress incontinence, urgency incontinence and overflow incontinence. They all have different etiologies and treatment. There are methods of diagnosis, and the treatment ranges from medication to behavioral management techniques, exercises, a variety of surgery and often prosthetic devices. In the rare instance in which the incontinence cannot be totally cured, specially designed absorbent underclothing is available. Many of these garments are no more bulky than normal underwear, can be worn under everyday clothing, and free a person from the discomfort and embarrassment of incontinence. It is important to remember that incontinence can be treated and often cured. Even incurable problems can be managed to reduce complications, anxiety and family stresses.

Sexuality in postmenopausal life is a healthy sign, and free discussion should be had with the patient so that she understands that it is all part of her life and is not to be stopped because society in the past has frowned upon this. The Victorian age is over. Many menopausal and postmenopausal patients have adopted a new life-style which parallels the freedom of younger patients.

Most women want and are able to lead an active, satisfying sex life. With age, women do not ordinarily lose their physical capacity for orgasm nor men their capacity for erection and ejaculation. There is, however, a gradual slowing of response, especially in men, which is a process currently considered a part of normal aging, but perhaps eventually treatable or even reversible. In the postmenopausal patient, sex often improves because of several factors. One is that her husband has reached a stable level in business and the children have grown up, so a couple have more time together. In addition, ovarian androgen secretion increases for a period of time after the menopause. In patients who have been studied, it has been found that a relatively higher testosterone/estrogen ratio in women after the ovaries have undergone follicular depletion may contribute to increased libido and fantasy.

A pattern of regular sexual activity, which may include masturbation, helps to preserve sexual ability. When problems occur, they should not be viewed as inevitable, but rather as a result of disease, disability, drug reaction or emotional upset that may require medical care.

Women generally experience little serious loss of sexual capacity because of age alone. Those changes that do occur affect mainly the shape, flexibility and lubrication of the vagina. These can be traced directly to lowered levels of the hormone estrogen during and after the menopause. Women who have severe dryness can be treated successfully with estrogen.

The incidence of illness and disability increases with age. Although they can affect sexuality in later life, even the most serious diseases rarely warrant stopping sexual activity. Public acceptance of sexuality in later life is gradually increasing. Physicians can expect that the day will come when special aspects of sexuality in the postmenopausal patient are generally understood and when diagnosis and treatment of sexual problems is refined to a greater degree. It is obvious that the postmenopausal patient has developed a new life-style that is much more liberal than previously.

Osteoporosis is not a disease *per se*, but rather is the end result of severe or prolonged bone loss. Osteoporosis cannot be cured, but it can be prevented. Recently, alendronate has been approved by the Food and Drug Administration (FDA) and can restore bone loss, but must be continued otherwise the bone mass will decrease. Estrogen replacement therapy is a vital factor in osteoporosis therapy, as well as an important factor in treating other symptoms of the menopause. Articles have appeared which indicate that the relative risk in using estrogen therapy far outweighs the benefits, but recently this concept has been challenged, and most physicians believe that the benefits far outweigh any risk. One risk factor relates to stimulating the development of endometrial carcinoma. It has never been shown that estrogen is a cell transformer, but merely a stimulator and a promoter. It has been shown that, combined with progesterone

therapy, the endometrium is protected against development of a malignant process. It is the height of professional responsibility to provide estrogen when it is needed, and to withhold it when it is contraindicated or not needed.

The problem of the menopause and the management of gynecological problems during this period has taken on added significance in the past three decades. Women are living longer and can anticipate spending approximately one-third of their lives in the postmenopausal period. It is important, therefore, for physicians to be prepared to handle the problems that arise during this time.

Acknowledgements

The author wishes to express his thanks to Ruzena Danek, Julia Chai, Bridget McGuire and Elizabeth Armour for their assistance in the preparation and editing of this manuscript.

Bibliography

Andrews W. What's new in preventing and treating osteoporosis? *Postgrad Med* 1998;104:89

Avioli L, ed. *The Osteoporosis Syndrome.* New York: Grune and Straton, 1983

Barber HRK. *Ovarian Carcinoma. Etiology, Diagnosis and Treatment.* New York: Masson Publishing, 1981

Barber HRK, Sommers SC, eds. *Carcinoma of the Endometrium. Etiology, Diagnosis and Treatment.* New York: Masson Publishing, 1981

Brown ADG. Postmenopausal urinary problems. *Clin Obstet Gynecol* 1977;4:181

Cancer Facts and Figures - 1999. American Cancer Society.

Coutifaris B, Chryssicopoulos A, Botsis D. Primary carcinoma of the fallopian tube. *Int Surg* 1980;65:83

DeLancy JO. Anatomy and biomechanics of genital prolapse. *Clin Obstet Gynecol* 1993;36:897

Frederick EJ Jr. *Vulvar Disease.* Philadelphia: WB Saunders, 1976

Gruis MG, Wagner NN. Sexuality during the climacteric. *Postgrad Med* 1979;65:197

Hoffman RH, Gardner HL. Vulvar dystrophies. *Clin Obstet Gynecol* 1978;21:1801

Huffman JW. Gynecologic disorders in the geriatric patient. *Geriatr Gynecol Postgrad Med* 1982; 71:38

Huffman JW. The diagnosis and treatment of gynecologic disorders in elderly patients. *Compr Ther* 1983;9:54

Jordan VC. Designer estrogen. *Sci Am* 1998;279:60-7

Judd HL. Hormonal dynamics associated with the menopause. *Clin Obstet Gynecol* 1976;19:775

Kaplan HS. *The Illustrated Manual of Sex Therapy*. New York: Quadrangle/New York Times, 1975

Marshall VF, Marchetti KE. The correction of stress incontinence by simple vesicourethral suspension. *Surg Gynecol Obstet* 1949;88:509

Masters WH. The sexual response cycle of the human female: vaginal lubrication. *Ann NY Acad Sci* 1959;83: 301

McKeithen WS. Major gynecologic surgery in the elderly female. *Am J Obstet Gynecol* 1975;59:63

Romoff A (with Yalof I). *Estrogen, How and Why It Can Save Your Life*. New York: Golden Books, 1999

Sagar PM, Pemberton JH. Dysfunction of the posterior pelvic floor and disorders of defecation. *J Pelvic Surg* 1993;1:92

Te Linde RW. Prolapse of the uterus and allied conditions. *Am J Obstet Gynecol* 1966;94:444

Wall LL. The muscles of the pelvic floor. *Clin Obstet Gynecol* 1993;36:910

Yancik R, Ries LD, Yates JW. Ovarian cancer in the elderly: an analysis of surveillance, epidemiology and end results program data. *Am J Obstet Gynecol* 1980;154: 639-47

14

Urological problems

Nina S. Davis

Introduction

The majority of urological problems in the post-menopausal woman involve the bladder and urethra. The cumulative effects of childbirth, lifestyle, systemic disease, pelvic surgery, endocrinological change, tissue aging and gravity can alter both the constitutional integrity of the urethrovesical unit and its relations with the pelvic floor. The consequences of these structural and anatomical changes are far-reaching and can cause disorders ranging from bladder instability to recurrent urinary tract infection. In the female geriatric population, symptoms most commonly include frequency, dysuria, nocturia, urgency, a sensation of incomplete emptying, and stress and urge incontinence[1]. In many instances, patients present with a complex of these symptoms, indicating that a combination of factors may be operative. This complicates diagnosis and treatment. It is therefore necessary to obtain a thorough history, a detailed abdominal and pelvic examination, and judicious testing to identify the relevant problems. Specific therapy, intervention that has a greater likelihood of being effective, can then be instituted.

This chapter focuses on those disorders which most commonly prompt referral of the postmenopausal woman for urological evaluation: urinary incontinence, hematuria and urinary tract infection. Whereas in the earlier part of the 20th century lower urinary tract dysfunction was poorly understood and therapy was largely based on empirical experience, more recent basic science and clinical investigation has produced new knowledge regarding the pathophysiology and treatment of these conditions. Additionally, panels of experts have critically reviewed the literature and established standards of practice, thereby providing a more rational approach toward patient assessment and care[2]. The material presented is based on such diagnostic and therapeutic principles.

Normal anatomy and physiology of the bladder and urethra

The bladder is a muscular organ that lies in the true pelvis. It functions as a urinary reservoir. The body of the bladder comprises interdigitating smooth muscle fascicles (detrusor) arranged in a random fashion. The bladder base at the level of the trigone demonstrates a more complex architecture with a longitudinal muscle layer overlying the detrusor, the latter taking on a circular configuration. The bladder is lined by transitional epithelium (urothelium) which is covered by a glycocalyx. This mucopolysaccharide coating is a barrier to infection and affects mucosal permeability[3].

The urethra, which is approximately 4 cm in length, begins at the bladder neck and courses along the distal third of the anterior vaginal wall to the external meatus. It is lined by transitional epithelium that gradually changes to non-keratinized stratified squamous epithelium distally. Passive coaptation of the urethral wall is maintained by a subepithelial layer of spongy vascular tissue, an important component of the female continence mechanism[4]. The mucosal and submucosal layers are both estrogen-sensitive. In men there are distinct sphincteric entities that effect continence; however, maintenance of female continence is more complex and dependent upon both intrinsic urethral musculature and pelvic floor support. The entire length of the wall of the female urethra consists of a thick, longitudinal smooth muscle layer surrounded by a thinner circular layer. The distal two-thirds of the urethra is enveloped by striated muscle which forms the external sphincter. Its fibers become attenuated posteriorly, inserting into the vaginal wall to form the compressor urethrae which, on contraction, closes the urethra against the anterior vaginal wall. Just proximal to the vaginal vestibule, the urethrovaginal sphincter is formed as the striated muscle encompasses the urethra and vagina. Contraction of this sphincter in conjunction with the bulbospongiosis muscle produces tightening of the urogenital hiatus. Continence, as well as prevention of prolapse, is also dependent on the integrity of the pelvic floor musculature and fasciae and the ligamentous attachments of the pelvic viscera[5-7].

It is important to understand the innervation of the bladder and proximal urethra, as it is the basis for all pharmacological manipulation of vesicourethral function. Both autonomic and somatic nerves supply the bladder and urethra. Parasympathetic fibers from S2–S4 travel via the pelvic nerve to the pelvic plexus and stimulate cholinergic receptors in the bladder wall, producing contraction of the detrusor muscle. Sympathetic fibers from T10–L2 course through the hypogastric plexus and reach the bladder neck via the hypogastric nerve, increasing α-adrenergic tone and outlet resistance. In addition to the α receptors in the bladder neck and proximal urethra, there are scattered β-adrenergic receptors in the bladder body that facilitate relaxation of the detrusor during filling. Somatic nerves derived from the S2–S4 cord segments supply the striated sphincter via the pudendal nerve. Voluntary contraction of the sphincter is mediated by acetylcholine.

The normal micturition cycle consists of a filling/storage phase and an emptying phase, which are modulated by the pontine motor nucleus of the central nervous system (CNS) as well as the peripheral autonomic and somatic nerves. During the filling phase, the bladder accommodates increasing volumes of urine, while the detrusor pressure remains lower than urethral pressure. This distensibility or compliance is facilitated by the viscoelastic properties of the bladder wall, by central suppression of reflex contractions and by sympathetic detrusor relaxation. Intraurethral pressure remains high owing to increased α-adrenergic tone at the bladder outlet and contraction of the external sphincter. Normal voiding is initiated by voluntary relaxation of the striated sphincter followed by reflex relaxation of the bladder neck and proximal urethra. Finally, parasympathetically mediated contraction of the detrusor results in expulsion of vesical contents. Normal voiding is therefore a coordinated event, and the disruption of any step in the process can result in significant dysfunction.

Pathophysiology of the aging bladder

Age-associated disorders of the bladder and urethra result from intrinsic and extrinsic changes that alter the composition, relations and function of the urogenital organs. Alterations in estrogen levels are the *sine qua non* of the menopause, producing a number of effects on the pelvic organs. There is decreased cellularity and thinning of the vaginal and urethral epithelia, as well as a decrease in tissue elasticity and increase in friability. The vagina atrophies and shortens, causing the urethral meatus to recede along the anterior vaginal wall[8,9]. Atrophy also contributes to pelvic floor prolapse. Vaginal secretions are reduced in volume and lose their protective acidity. This change in vaginal pH is thought to promote urethritis and cystitis in menopausal women.

Estrogen receptors have been identified in the urethra and bladder, particularly the trigone, so hypoestrogenism in the menopause negatively impacts urethral closure mechanisms and predisposes to incontinence. There is also indirect evidence that lack of estrogen diminishes bladder stability, as one study found that estrogen supplementation in a group of postmenopausal women reduced nocturia[10]. A number of animal studies have suggested that hormone withdrawal can affect receptor density and sensitivity in the bladder and urethra. Restoration of normal estrogen levels reverses these effects, increasing the number and response of muscarinic and adrenergic receptors. Furthermore, reduced estrogen levels may provoke a global decrease in responsiveness to nerve stimulation[9]. Indeed, a generalized decline in smooth muscle tone has been associated with aging.

On a structural level, anatomical and ultrastructural studies have identified distinct degenerative changes in aging smooth and striated muscle that may predispose to dysfunctional states, even though these abnormalities may be present in individuals without evident genitourinary pathology. One of the best established characteristics of the aging bladder is fibrosis. Although initially thought to be indicative of outlet obstruction, it has been demonstrated in the bladder walls of normal elderly women[11]. Both collagen and elastin are increased in the geriatric bladder, but the functional significance of this finding is not altogether clear[12,13]. In order to understand better the functional correlates of such structural changes, a number of investigators have performed histological analyses on tissues obtained from normal and symptomatic patients. Levy and Wight[14] focused on the submucosa, as it constitutes 25% of the thickness of the bladder wall. Bladder biopsies were studied with both optical and electron microscopy. The authors found progressive separation and disorganization of the collagen fascicles, which was most pronounced in the face of obstruction. In urgency alone, the collagen could barely be detected. In an elegant and detailed series of papers correlating urodynamic findings with ultrastructural data from detrusor biopsies, Elbadawi and colleagues[15-18] identified histological patterns that consistently accompanied given clinical entities. They described a 'dense band' pattern of degeneration in the normal aging bladder. Associated degeneration of muscle cells and axons produced impaired contractility. A 'dysjunction pattern' correlated with detrusor instability, and 'myohypertrophy' was characteristic of obstruction. Combinations of these patterns correlated with complexes of the related symptoms. More recently, changes in the striated sphincter with aging have been examined[19]. Accelerated apoptosis, programmed cell death, appears to be responsible for muscle cell loss. This is postulated to induce stress incontinence in the elderly.

Functionally, mechanical factors contribute in large part to the loss of pelvic floor support provided by the pelvic and perineal muscles. Injury to the perineal body during parturition disrupts the urogenital sphincter, enlarges the urogenital hiatus and attenuates the urogenital plate. The processes of childbirth and aging partially denervate and weaken the levator ani. This loss of muscular support means that there is greater transmission of intra-abdominal forces to the pelvic fasciae, causing them to become lax or to tear[20]. In this way, cystoceles, enteroceles and rectoceles form, and may present singly or in combination as pelvic floor prolapse.

Problems of the aging bladder and urethra: urinary incontinence

Urinary incontinence is one of the most prevalent and costly problems afflicting the elderly, and it affects predominantly postmenopausal women. In the geriatric population, the incidence of female incontinence is twice that of men[21]. Although lower urinary tract dysfunction and incontinence are commonly associated with the climacteric, they are not direct sequelae of ovarian failure[22]. They are, rather, entities that derive from complex age-related anatomical and physiological changes, which may be modulated by constitutional and situational factors. This often results in patients presenting with confusing constellations of symptoms. It is therefore imperative that a comprehensive evaluation be conducted to determine the exact nature of a patient's problems. The importance of accurate diagnosis and appropriate therapy cannot be overstated, as incontinence in all of its forms can profoundly restrict life-style, making an invalid of an otherwise healthy individual.

Classification of incontinence

Over the years, a number of classification systems for incontinence disorders have been proposed in an effort to standardize diagnostic categories, and to guide therapeutic decision-making. Most have proved cumbersome and complicated, and have been abandoned. In general, descriptive nomenclature is used to classify subtypes of incontinence regardless of the etiology. The following terminology is in general use.

Genuine stress incontinence (SUI) refers to urinary leakage that results from provocative maneuvers such as coughing, sneezing, laughing or lifting. It is produced by anatomical abnormalities including urethral hypermobility, pelvic floor prolapse and intrinsic sphincter deficiency (ISD) or loss of natural urethral coaptation.

Urge incontinence (DI), popularly known as 'over-active bladder', describes the spontaneous expulsion of urine which is variably associated with a sudden strong desire to void. It usually results from an uninhibited detrusor contraction. Synonyms for this type of incontinence include detrusor instability and detrusor hyperreflexia; however, the latter term is reserved exclusively for dysfunction related to a neurological defect. Age-related changes in the bladder wall, disorders of innervation, inflammation, neoplasia, loss of normal anatomical relations of the bladder and urethra, urethral obstruction or incontinence surgery may all cause bladder instability. Often patients present with symptoms of both SUI and DI, which is referred to as mixed incontinence. One must then determine which is the predominant disorder and focus therapy accordingly.

A unique subset of geriatric patients present with DI in conjunction with impaired bladder contractility (acronym DHIC), such that the usual symptoms of bladder instability are accompanied by valsalva voiding to augment emptying and increased post-void residuals because emptying is not complete[23]. DHIC may mimic many other pathological voiding states, so urodynamics are particularly beneficial in making the diagnosis. The implications for treatment are also significant, since anticholinergics may produce retention in patients with DHIC, and surgical interventions for presumed SUI may result in postoperative exacerbation of irritative voiding symptoms or persistent incontinence.

Overflow incontinence describes the spontaneous loss of urine that occurs when the bladder has exceeded its capacity. This entity is seen infrequently in postmenopausal women and is usually associated with an areflexic (flaccid) bladder owing to diabetes or to a stroke. Anticholinergic medications are a common iatrogenic etiology.

Total incontinence denotes constant urinary leakage. This is a rare type of incontinence in women and usually signifies the presence of a vesicovaginal fistula. Severe intrinsic sphincter deficiency may occasionally masquerade as total incontinence.

Although not a generally accepted diagnostic category, the term functional incontinence has been used to refer to incontinence that results from physical limitations that prevent prompt toileting or from other environmental impediments to controlled urination[2].

Evaluation of the incontinent patient

It is critical to the accurate diagnosis and treatment of incontinence disorders to obtain an in-depth history and complete physical examination. In taking the history, determining basic information such as onset, course, nature and duration of symptoms is a good departure point. Often a patient will trace the onset of her symptoms to a particular event such as childbirth or pelvic surgery. The obstetric history, including number of pregnancies, as well as types of deliveries and their complications, should be elicited. Details related to the menopause are also relevant; the physician should explore specific symptomatology and the administration of hormone replacement therapy (HRT) and its efficacy. The patient should be asked whether she has sought consultation for the same problems previously, what treatments, if any, were instituted, and how successful the treatments were. The review of symptoms should focus on the presence or absence of diabetes, neurological disease, defecation problems, and back or pelvic pain. In asking about medications, the examiner must be vigilant for agents with anticholinergic effects that may impede urination.

Further questioning should then be directed towards differentiating the type of incontinence a patient may have. Special care should be taken to distinguish stress from urge incontinence, as activity that increases intra-abdominal pressure may stimulate uninhibited detrusor contractions as well as spontaneous leakage. Sometimes patients will complain of unprovoked leakage which may be intermittent or constant. Such 'unconscious incontinence' may be due to involuntary bladder contractions without cortical awareness, vaginal voiding (common in obese individuals), severe stress incontinence such that gravity alone produces urinary loss, drainage from a urethral diverticulum, or a vesicovaginal or ureterovaginal fistula[24]. Past surgeries, especially pelvic operations and prior incontinence procedures, must be detailed, as they can produce urethral scarring leading to ISD, fistulae or urethral obstruction such as may be seen after suspension procedures for incontinence. Finally, the patient's voiding habits must be determined, including daytime frequency and nocturia, number and type of pads used, and effects on life-style. Contributory factors to incontinence in the elderly have been described extensively by Resnick[25], who has also systematized them into a mnemonic, DIAPPERS (delirium, infection, atrophic vaginitis, pharmaceuticals, psychological, excessive urine output, restricted mobility and stool impaction).

Although it is important to evaluate the patient as a whole, the key components in the assessment of the incontinent patient are the abdominal and pelvic examinations. The abdomen should be inspected for scars and distention. Palpation will reveal focal areas of tenderness, masses and hernias. The region of the bladder should be percussed. If there is any question of incomplete emptying, a bladder scan can be done to establish an elevated residual.

As the patient moves down the table into the lithotomy position, observe for leakage, a clue to SUI related to ISD. On initial inspection of the perineum, the presence of vulvar lesions should be noted, the degree of atrophy should be assessed and the length of the perineal body should be evaluated. Often a caruncle, an erythematous polypoid mass, is visible at the urethral meatus. Its only clinical significance is that it may sometimes, especially when large, produce bleeding. Significant degrees of pelvic floor prolapse are often marked by protrusion beyond the introitus. The examiner must determine the nature of the prolapse, whether it represents cystocele, rectocele or enterocele, or a combination of these. This is abetted by the 'half-speculum examination', which allows separate manipulation of the anterior and posterior vaginal walls. Prior to this, however, palpation of the pelvic floor musculature is used to assess its strength, and palpation of the urethra permits the detection of urethral cysts or diverticulae or the gritty firmness of urethral carcinoma. When compression of the urethra produces a purulent meatal discharge, the diagnosis of a urethral diverticulum is established. However, it should be noted that this entity is seen infrequently in the postmenopausal population. A cough test should be performed to reproduce stress incontinence and to

assess the degree of prolapse engendered by this maneuver. Furthermore, it is important to note the extent of urethral mobility produced by the cough. A fixed urethra can be a clue to ISD. The presence of a vaginal discharge should prompt a wet-prep examination and/or culture as appropriate. The integrity and support of the vaginal wall, uterus and cervix should be evaluated. Bimanual examination will allow further assessment of the bladder and pelvic organs, if present, and will detect pelvic masses or tenderness. The bulbocavernosus and anocutaneous reflexes should be elicited to test the integrity of spinal segments S2–S4.

A urinalysis should always be included as part of the initial examination. Often an occult infection is detected, and treatment of this alone can significantly improve or eradicate incontinence. The presence of microscopic blood in the urine should alert the examiner to the possibility of a genitourinary neoplasm. Hematuria and urinary tract infection are discussed in more detail later in this chapter.

Urodynamic testing in the evaluation of incontinence

Objective assessment of vesicourethral function using urodynamic studies is indicated for the evaluation of patients with mixed incontinence and those who have failed empirical medical therapy. In the case of chronic neurological disorders, urodynamics is used to establish the baseline functional status of the lower genitourinary tract, to detect abnormalities that may compromise upper tract function (high storage and voiding pressures), and to re-evaluate bladder and urethral function when a change in symptoms is noted. Additionally, urodynamic studies are integral to the diagnosis of ISD and to the evaluation of postsurgical voiding dysfunctions. The range of testing should be tailored to the individual patient. For instance, if one wishes to establish the presence of ISD, one need only to perform leak-point pressure testing. Alternatively, if a patient complains of stress and urge incontinence as well as problems passing her urine, a full complement of tests should be performed. A complete urodynamic evaluation consists of the following tests.

Uroflowmetry measures the pattern and rate of urinary flow. In normal micturition, there is no hesitancy in initiating voiding. To have a valid study, it is desirable that the patient void at least 150 ml. It should take no longer than 23 s to discharge a bladder volume of 400 ml[26]. In women, maximal flow is not affected by age and ranges between 15 and 36 ml/s. A common uroflow abnormality is the 'stutter-step' intermittency characteristic of abdominal straining. Diminished voiding velocities usually indicate obstruction. Following voiding, a catheter is usually placed to check the post-void residual volume and to begin cystometric testing.

Cystometry is a test of bladder storage which assesses capacity and compliance. It also offers an indirect means of determining bladder sensation. A normal bladder should maintain low pressures during filling. In this study, the bladder is filled at a steady rate with fluid or gas and several parameters are evaluated including filling pressure, sensation, capacity, compliance, the presence of uninhibited (involuntary) detrusor contractions and the ability to suppress voiding. In general, the filling pressure should not exceed 5–10 cmH$_2$O, and the capacity ranges from 300 to 400 ml. Sustained storage pressures $\geq$40 cmH$_2$O produce renal damage via transmission of pressure to the upper tracts[27].

Voiding pressure-flow study is used to evaluate the emptying phase of the micturition cycle by providing information related to voiding pressures and bladder contractility. It is useful for detecting bladder outlet obstruction or abnormal voiding patterns. After her bladder is filled to capacity, the patient is asked to void to completion. The flow rate and pattern, as well as voiding pressures, are noted. A post-void residual volume can also be measured. Voiding pressures in women are generally low because of the diminished outlet resistance conferred by their short urethras. Failure to relax the external sphincter during voiding, however, results in the characteristic pattern of a reduced flow rate with an elevated voiding pressure. In elderly women, it is much more common to see a reduced flow rate and a low voiding pressure with or without an elevated post-void residual, consistent with a decompensated or flaccid bladder. Generally, voiding pressures should be less than 60 cmH$_2$O. This study complements the uroflow nicely as it provides corroborative data.

Electromyography (EMG), in most cases, is not performed as an isolated study. It is an adjunct to cystometry and pressure–flow testing, and allows simultaneous assessment of striated (external) sphincter function. It is a critical component of the neurophysiological evaluation. Normally, the sphincter exhibits increasing tone as the bladder fills or when attempting to suppress an uninhibited contraction or stress leakage. Conversely, EMG activity should be negligible during voiding. When detrusor–sphincter dyssynergia is present, there is an inappropriate increase in EMG activity during voiding, creating elevated voiding pressures and reduced urinary velocity. This may occur in association with neurological disease or functional disorders.

Leak-point pressure testing (LPP) as used in this context refers to abdominal LPP, otherwise known as 'valsalva' or 'stress' LPP. It is a test of urethral competence. The patient is asked to perform straining maneuvers, and the pressures at which urethral resistance is overcome and leakage occurs are measured. This study is used to distinguish stress incontinence due to ISD from that due to urethral hypermobility. Classically, LPPs less than 60 cmH$_2$O are indicative of ISD, and those over 90 cmH$_2$O are characteristic of hypermobility-related urinary loss[28]. A mixed situation exists for pressures between 60 and 90 cmH$_2$O, and clinical correlation usually allows identification of the predominant cause of the patient's leakage. The distinction is important, as treatment of SUI is based on the mechanism of leakage. Patients with ISD do not usually do well after standard bladder neck suspension procedures. Rather, these patients fare better with pubovaginal slings or intraurethral collagen injections.

Videourodynamics is a specialized form of urodynamic testing involving measurement of urodynamic parameters with simultaneous fluoroscopic visualization of the bladder and its outlet. Basically, dynamic cystography results when contrast is used for bladder filling instead of the usual irrigant. The advantages of this method include being able more precisely to correlate the measurements with actual function, to identify artifacts and to define better the patient's anatomy.

Videourodynamics are therefore particularly valuable in evaluating patients with complicated voiding complaints. Recently, Nitti and colleagues found that the diagnosis and etiology of subtle outlet obstruction in women could be most accurately established using videourodynamic pressure–flow studies[29].

Urodynamics in the postmenopausal woman A number of studies have been performed using urodynamics to characterize detrusor dysfunction in the aging bladder. There is a consensus that bladder capacity and flow rates are universally diminished and that post-void residuals are higher[30,31]. Detrusor sensory function is thought to be impaired as well[32]. Changes in urethral function with aging are much more difficult to measure, and findings are contradictory in many instances; however, one large study demonstrated lower urethral pressure and decreased sphincteric function with age[33]. It is not clear to what extent age-related changes in vesicourethral function contribute to the pathogenesis of incontinence and other disorders.

Supplemental testing in the evaluation of incontinence

When significant pelvic floor prolapse is present or when the exact nature of a patient's incontinence is not clear, it is often beneficial to perform a resting and straining cystogram. This simple radiographic examination can provide anatomical information that is invaluable in planning surgical intervention. The study consists of placing a urethral catheter, and instilling contrast into the bladder. The catheter is plugged so that the contrast cannot escape. Lateral films are taken with the patient at rest, then bearing down. The degree of bladder descensus and changes in the urethrovesical angle with straining can be assessed. In cases of anterior vaginal wall prolapse of uncertain etiology, a cystogram allows the practitioner to distinguish a cystocele from an enterocele. If there is little or no change in the urethrovesical angle with straining, the diagnosis of ISD is suggested; however, in classic SUI, there is rotatory descent of the bladder and urethra, producing a funnel-like appearance of the bladder neck. Whereas cysto-graphy is a static study, videourodynamics provides real-time fluoroscopic imaging that is correlated with measurements of lower genitourinary tract function. Therefore, videourodynamics is superior to cystography and is the preferred imaging modality for the evaluation of incontinence.

Cystoscopy is another means of assessing vesicourethral anatomy, but is rarely indicated in the evaluation of incontinence. It should be considered only in cases of sterile hematuria or pyuria, bladder pain, recent onset of irritative voiding symptoms or suspected genitourinary pathology.

Treatment of urinary incontinence

When counselling patients regarding treatment options for incontinence, it is useful to present the choices in terms of three broad categories: pharmacological agents, physiotherapy/behavioral therapy and surgical interventions. With the prevalence of direct-to-consumer advertising by the pharmaceutical companies, patients will often come to the office requesting a specific medication. Alternatively, patients may have spoken with friends who have had a successful outcome from a particular treatment, and they want similar therapy. In either case it is important to determine the exact nature of the patient's disorder and to recommend the most appropriate treatment, whether or not it is what the patient has asked for. All options should be reviewed briefly with each patient and explanations given as to why a particular intervention is or is not applicable to her situation.

Pharmacological therapy In general, medical therapy works best for urge incontinence and for mild stress incontinence without significant associated pelvic floor prolapse. A summary of the most common medications, their mechanisms of action, dosages and notes regarding usage are provided in Table 1. Two caveats apply: anticholinergic agents should not be used in patients with narrow-angle glaucoma nor in those with a tendency to retain urine. Indeed, if a patient is prescribed an anticholinergic and she subsequently reports worsening of her symptoms, especially increased frequency, one must suspect urinary

Table 1 Pharmacological agents used in treatment of incontinence

Classification/name	Dosage	Comments
Antihistamine/decongestant		
Phenylpropanolamine/chlorpheniramine	one capsule bid	first-line drug for SUI
Smooth muscle relaxant		
Flavoxate 100 mg	1–2 tablets tid or qid	rarely used; better for inflammatory conditions
Anticholinergic		
Propantheline 15 mg	1–2 tablets tid or qid	adult use uncommon
Anticholinergic/smooth muscle relaxant		
Dicyclomine 10 mg	1–3 tablets tid	used infrequently
Hyoscyamine 0.125/0.375 mg	one tablet q4 h/bid	both are excellent for urge incontinence
Oxybutynin 5 mg	one tablet tid or qid	
Tolterodine 1/2 mg	one tablet bid	best tolerated; costly
Tricyclic antidepressant		
Imipramine 10/25/50 mg	one tablet qd or bid	both used for SUI and voiding dysfunction
Amitriptyline 10/25/50 mg	one tablet qd or bid	

bid, twice a day; tid, three times a day; qid, four times a day; q4 h, every 4 h; qd, once a day; SUI, genuine stress incontinence

retention. If a particular medication is initially effective, but becomes less so acutely, urinary tract infection should be ruled out. All bladder relaxant medications can cause severe dry mouth, constipation, palpitations and asthenia, which often prompt discontinuation of the drugs. Tolterodine, a new antimuscarinic agent, produces the fewest adverse effects and is best tolerated, especially by the elderly.

Physiotherapy and behavioral interventions Although Kegel exercises have long been advocated for the enhancement of pelvic floor muscular support, they are often performed incorrectly, and there is no evidence that they have any prophylactic benefit in the prevention of pelvic floor prolapse or urinary incontinence[34]. While such self-directed methods of pelvic floor exercise are usually ineffective in the treatment of urinary incontinence, a properly designed and supervised regimen combining behavior modification, pelvic muscle rehabilitation and, when necessary, biofeedback or electrical stimulation of muscles or nerves can dramatically improve or cure incontinence[2,34,35]. These techniques are also quite effective in the treatment of functional voiding disorders and pelvic pain syndromes. Because rehabilitative pro-

grams are non-invasive and involve little risk to the patient, they have been promoted as first-line therapy for incontinence[2], however, patients should only be referred for behavioral/physical therapy if they are motivated and willing to make the time commitment required to achieve success. In general, it takes 6–12 weeks to realize significant improvement and up to 6 months to attain maximal benefit[35].

Many patients choose behavioral/physical therapy because the 'holistic' nature of the treatment is more appealing than medication or surgery. Such services are usually provided by nursing personnel in continence centers or by specially trained physical therapists in rehabilitation facilities. It has been shown that frequent monitoring of patients' progress and offering positive reinforcement reduce attrition and enhance performance[36]. With pelvic floor exercise alone, 70–80% of patients improve, 40–50% are completely satisfied with the results of therapy and 20% are completely dry[35].

A voiding diary is a useful tool in tailoring a therapeutic plan for the incontinent patient. It details the patient's fluid intake, voiding schedule, and number and timing of leakage episodes. Suggested behavioral interventions might then include timed or prompted voiding, adjustment of fluid intake, a bowel regimen or dietary restriction of bladder irritants such as caffeine or artificial sweeteners. Behavioral therapies are primarily indicated for detrusor instability and urge incontinence, although developing more healthful bladder habits is applicable to any rehabilitative regimen.

For SUI, exercise instruction with various adjuncts such as biofeedback or weighted vaginal cones is indicated. Often, insurers will cover temporary home use of biofeedback devices. More sophisticated techniques such as electrical stimulation can also be used to identify and to strengthen the pelvic floor musculature, particularly in those patients who have difficulty localizing their muscles.

In cases of refractory urge incontinence, neuromodulation via low-level stimulation of the sacral nerve roots can provide significant relief. Stimulation of a wire placed percutaneously in the S3 sacral foramen produces detrusor inhibition. This is a relatively new technique whose role in the treatment of incontinence and other pelvic floor disorders is currently limited.

In summary, behavioral interventions and physiotherapy are very effective in properly selected, motivated patients with mild to moderate SUI without significant pelvic floor prolapse, urge incontinence, functional voiding disorders and neurogenic vesicourethral dysfunction.

Surgical treatment of stress urinary incontinence Surgical modalities may be employed in the treatment of both stress and urge incontinence, but operative interventions are most frequently used to treat SUI, particularly in conjunction with repair of pelvic floor prolapse. When a patient is found to have a cystocele, rectocele, and/or enterocele in addition to urethral hypermobility or ISD, all must be corrected in order to restore normal pelvic support and continence. Often a hysterectomy will be required, either because of associated uterovaginal laxity or vault prolapse or because of a concomitant gynecological disorder[37]. If a significant cystocele occurs in the absence of incontinence, a suspension procedure should nevertheless be done to maintain urethrovesical support.

In incontinent patients with urethral hypermobility as the sole defect of pelvic support, or who require restoration of normal urethrovesical relations as well as repair of pelvic floor prolapse, a number of suspension procedures are available. These can be performed using either an abdominal or a vaginal approach. Since repair of various types of prolapse is most commonly done via the vagina, the additional morbidity of a large abdominal incision can be obviated by a vaginal suspension procedure. With the recent advent of bone anchors that can be placed transvaginally, even the usual small suprapubic (mons) incision can be avoided. These purely transvaginal approaches are particularly advantageous in the obese patient.

The principle of all suspension procedures is to correct SUI due to urethral hypermobility by restoring the bladder neck and urethra to their normal retropubic position. An additional benefit of these procedures is that they will correct modest cystoceles. Suspension procedures alone are contraindicated in the presence of moderate to severe cystoceles, as they accentuate the prolapse and may create obstruction. The transabdominal or retropubic approaches include the Marshall–Marchetti–Krantz procedure and the Burch colposuspension. The methods of transvaginal urethropexy include anterior colporrhaphy and the needle suspensions: the Pereyra and Raz procedures with their numerous modifications. Sling procedures utilize a number of different tissues to suspend and create a buttress for the bladder base and urethra. The simplest of these is a vaginal wall sling. As originally conceived, a segment of rectus fascia was excised and used to fashion the sling. This continues to be a popular method. More recently, synthetics such as Dacron® have been used, and cadaveric tissue such as fascia lata is becoming increasingly prevalent.

Laparoscopic variations on the retropubic techniques have also been advocated for effecting resuspension of the bladder neck and urethra. Unfortunately, a recent report suggests that such procedures do not hold up over time[38]. Indeed, there is significant controversy as to which suspension procedure is most effective in the long term and is therefore 'the best'. Patient selection is certainly a critical factor as is technique. A recent review[2] reported cure rates of 62% for anterior repair, 78% for retropubic suspensions, 84% for needle suspension procedures and 89% for pubovaginal slings. Because of such data, some urologists have begun performing only pubovaginal slings to treat all forms of SUI.

As with all surgery, suspension operations may be associated with significant morbidity. In addition to the usual risks of bleeding, infection, deep vein thrombosis/pulmonary embolism, injury to bladder, ureters and urethra, and failure of the procedures, they may produce bladder instability and outlet obstruction with urinary retention. Overcorrection or overly high suspension of the bladder neck is a common mechanism of obstruction. Obstruction may also result from placement of suspension sutures too medially or from sling migration. As one might surmise, the more involved the surgery, the greater the risk of a serious complication. Therefore, the various sling procedures have the highest complication rates[2]. Use of synthetic sling material is associated with a higher infection rate and with urethral erosion. Pubovaginal slings may cause permanent retention in 5–10% of cases; hence, patients must be prepared to perform clean intermittent catheterization postoperatively.

Pubovaginal slings are also indicated in cases of SUI due to ISD, as they produce urethral coaptation as well as support. Other choices for the treatment of ISD include the artificial urinary sphincter and periurethral collagen injection. The artificial sphincter can be quite difficult to place in female patients and has a significant rate of urethral erosion, infection and mechanical malfunction. It is therefore used infrequently. A popular alternative to either the pubovaginal sling or the artificial urinary sphincter for the treatment of sphincteric incontinence is injection of a periurethral bulking agent to enhance urethral thickness, to restore urethral coaptation and to increase outlet resistance. Although autologous fat and Teflon® paste have been used for this purpose, glutaraldehyde cross-linked bovine collagen enjoys the greatest usage. It is injected either transurethrally via a special needle passed through the working channel of a cystoscope or periurethrally using a spinal needle inserted adjacent to the urethra, with collagen placement being guided by simultaneous cystoscopy. Both methods have been found to be equally efficacious[39]. One of the major advantages of collagen injection is that it is usually performed in the office using local anesthesia, so it is particularly suited to the older patient who does not want surgery or cannot tolerate it. Patients must be told that it often takes at least two sessions to achieve complete continence and that additional treatments may be required in the future to maintain dryness.

Proper patient selection is critical to the success of collagen injection. The patient with low abdominal leak point pressures, preferably less than 65 cmH$_2$O, normal vesical function and adequate pelvic support is an ideal candidate. In one series with up to 46 months of follow-up, treatment with collagen resulted in 83% of patients being either cured or improved[40]. Morbidity is low and complications consist of temporary retention, irritative voiding symptoms and bleeding.

Surgery for urge incontinence Although urge incontinence is most commonly treated with medical therapy, surgery may be used in refractory cases, particularly those resulting from a neurological injury or disorder. Bladder augmentation involves interposition of a portion of bowel into the bladder wall to interrupt detrusor contractions. In most cases, subsequent bladder emptying is incomplete and clean intermittent catheterization is required. A special form of augmentation, autoaugmentation, involves splitting the bladder muscle at the dome leaving the mucosal layer to expand, increasing bladder capacity and compliance. Finally, as described above, permanent implantation of an S3 nerve root stimulator can significantly diminish detrusor overactivity in selected patients.

Problems of the aging bladder and urethra: hematuria

Hematuria, either gross or microscopic, is one of the most common reasons for referral to a urologist as it is the sign most frequently associated with genitourinary pathology. Even a single episode of gross hematuria is reason for concern and demands investigation; however, what constitutes significant microscopic hematuria is controversial. Many consider only one red blood cell per high-power field to be significant, while others feel that three or more are necessary to prompt further study. If a patient is a smoker or is otherwise at risk for genitourinary disease, any degree of hematuria should be pursued. The conventional work-up consists of intravenous pyelography (IVP) followed by cystoscopy. However, for patients with painful hematuria, a history of urolithiasis or other indicator of a renal or ureteral stone, unenhanced helical computed tomography (CT urography or CTU) has supplanted IVP as the radiographic study of choice in many centers. CTU consists of a CT scan of the abdomen and pelvis without intravenous contrast. Often, a plain radiograph of the abdomen is included in the study for correlation in the sagittal plane. The advantage of CT urography is that it is faster than IVP and it will demonstrate non-opaque stones. Because bladder lesions may be small and are not well seen on radiographic studies, cystoscopy must always be performed, even if the preceding imaging study shows a genitourinary lesion that might be responsible for the hematuria. Cystoscopy is particularly beneficial when it is performed at the time that the patient is actually bleeding, as it often allows localization and identification of the source.

In women aged 40–60, the most common causes of hematuria are acute urinary tract infection, stones and bladder tumors, primarily transitional cell carcinoma. Those 60 years of age or older present most commonly with bladder cancer and urinary tract infection. Among patients over the age of 50, genitourinary malignancies are associated with microscopic hematuria in 7.5% of cases, but the incidence increases to 34.5% in those with gross hematuria[41]. Although rare, urethral carcinoma is the only urinary cancer that is more prevalent in women than men. It does produce hematuria, but patients usually present with a urethral mass and symptoms of urethral obstruction. Renal cell carcinoma, although less common than bladder cancer, must also be ruled out in the patient with hematuria.

A number of non-malignant lesions may cause hematuria in the postmenopausal woman and should be considered in the differential diagnosis. Caruncles are polypoid lesions of the urethra that may bleed or, less frequently, produce discomfort. They are inflammatory in nature and do not appear to undergo malignant transformation. Intervention is rarely indicated, but if they are bothersome to the patient or if they are actively bleeding, they are easily removed under local anesthesia in the office. Other inflammatory disorders may affect the bladder and mimic cancer. Chronic cystitis, which resembles carcinoma *in situ* (CIS) of the bladder and produces identical irritative symptoms, may not have an apparent microbial etiology at the time of diagnosis. It can only be distinguished from CIS by biopsy. Tuberculosis may affect any portion of the genitourinary tract and can cause asymptomatic hematuria and pyuria.

In diabetic patients or those who abuse non-steroidal anti-inflammatory drugs, IVP may demonstrate calyceal blunting characteristic of papillary necrosis, and, during the acute phase, sloughed papillae may appear as polypoid intra-renal or ureteral masses. At such times, patients will not only report gross hematuria, but they will often note passage of tissue fragments in the urine.

Painful hematuria, gross or microscopic, is most commonly produced by renal or ureteral calculi. Associated irritative symptoms occur when a stone lies in the distal ureter near the bladder. Such symptoms often indicate that passage is imminent.

Finally, conditions unique to the postmenopausal woman may produce microscopic hematuria. Those women taking HRT, particularly the estrogen–progesterone combinations, can experience overt or occult vaginal bleeding. Contamination of the urine with vaginal secretions then results in small quantities of blood in the urine. Conversely, in women who are not being treated with hormone replacement, atrophy alone, because of the associated tissue fragility, may give rise to microscopic hematuria.

Problems of the aging bladder and urethra: urinary tract infection

The prevalence of urinary tract infection (UTI) increases with age, and the incidence of bacteriuria in community-based populations of women 65 years of age and older ranges from 9 to 33%[42]. Rates are higher in institutionalized patients, and they are at greater risk of complicated UTIs and sepsis. This group presents special problems not directly related to the menopause and is not included in further discussion.

Bacteria gain access to the urinary tract in an ascending fashion from the perineum and vagina, which are chronically colonized with microorganisms. Factors that facilitate development of infection in the menopausal woman include atrophic changes in the mucosa of the urethra and vagina, age-related changes in local or systemic immune responses, increased residual urine due to neurogenic dysfunction or a cystocele, and perineal soiling owing to urinary or fecal incontinence[43].

Urinary tract infections may be asymptomatic or they may present with dysuria, frequency, urgency, urge incontinence, suprapubic pressure or pain, back pain and fever. On office evaluation, the infected patient may exhibit suprapubic tenderness and fullness. Costovertebral angle tenderness is infrequently seen. The urethra and bladder base may also be tender to palpation. The degree of estrogenization of the vulva should be assessed. A midstream clean-catch urinary specimen should be obtained and sent for culture as appropriate. Catheterization to obtain an uncontaminated specimen for culture is rarely needed; however, if vaginal contamination is a concern, catheterization is indicated. All urine specimens should first be centrifuged and examined in the office under a microscope. Dipsticks alone are inaccurate in the diagnosis of infection. Variable degrees of hematuria, pyuria and bacteriuria may be noted. When the urinary specific gravity is extremely low, bacteria may be missed because of a dilution effect. In such cases, culturing of the urine is dictated by patient symptoms, the presence of significant pyuria or the presence of nitrites on dipstick. Conversely, if large quantities of bacteria are seen in conjunction with epithelial cells, vaginal contamination must be suspected. Often, large quantities of bacteria without associated epithelial cells are found in cases of asymptomatic bacteriuria.

Often, physicians will empirically treat the uncomplicated, sporadic UTI. Cultures should be obtained, however, in patients with recurrent or persistent symptoms, and therapy should be directed towards the responsible organism. If a patient remains symptomatic, but cultures are negative, stone disease or tumor must be ruled out. Work-up consisting of IVP or renal ultrasound with cystoscopy, as indicated, should be performed in any patient who does not respond to appropriate antibiotic therapy. Localization studies may also be necessary when the source of a persistent infection is not clear.

The treatment of UTI is governed by several general principles. Reduction of known risk factors to prevent infection is most optimal. It has been shown that estrogen supplementation after the menopause can help prevent recurrent UTI[44]. Holistic remedies such as drinking cranberry juice, and maintaining healthy vaginal acidophilus colonization via eating yogurt with live cultures or taking acidophilus tablets, remain quite popular and are supported by scientific data. A recently published report found that a group of tannins known as proanthocyanidins, which are found in both cranberries and blueberries, impair bacterial adherence to mucosal surfaces[45]. When patients do develop an uncomplicated UTI, treatment with a 3- or a 7-day regimen of antibiotics is appropriate. In the absence of culture data, the choice of antibiotic should be based on the suspected organism, a history of antibiotic hypersensitivity, potential side-effects, unfavorable effects on the vaginal and fecal flora, and cost.

Complicated UTIs occur in diabetics as well as in patients who are immunocompromised, who have genitourinary tract abnormalities or who have undergone recent surgery. These individuals should always be cultured and should be treated with a 10- to 21-day course of an antimicrobial that is specific to their organism. Six-month prophylaxis with a single daily dose of a low-level antibiotic may be considered in patients who have recurrent UTIs without underlying pathology. This allows restoration of the patient's natural defense mechanisms. Prolonged prophylaxis is rarely indicated, but may be instituted in patients who have a high risk of morbidity from UTI. In general, asymptomatic bacteriuria is not treated.

References

1. Bent AE, Richardson DA, Ostergard DR. Diagnosis of lower urinary tract disorders in postmenopausal patients. *Am J Obstet Gynecol* 1983;145: 218-22

2. Fantl JA, Newman DK, Colling J, *et al*. *Urinary Incontinence in Adults: Acute and Chronic Management*. Clinical Practice Guideline, No. 2, 1996 Update. Rockville, MD: US Department of Health and Human Services. Public Health Service, Agency for Health Care Policy and Research, March 1996. AHCPR Publication No. 96-0682

3. Steers WD. Physiology and pharmacology of the bladder and urethra. In Walsh PC, Retik AB, Vaughan ED, Wein AJ, eds. *Campbell's Urology*, 7th edn. Philadelphia: WB Saunders, 1998:870-915

4. Raz S, Caine M, Zeigler M. The vascular component in the production of intraurethral pressure. *J Urol* 1972;108:93-6

5. Delancey JOL. Structural aspects of urethrovesical function in the female. *Neurourol Urodyn* 1988;7: 509-20

6. Delancey JOL. Pubovesical ligament: a separate structure from urethral supports ('pubourethral ligaments'). *Neurourol Urodyn* 1989;8:53-62

7. Mostwin JL. Current concepts of female pelvic anatomy and physiology. *Urol Clin North Am* 1991; 18:175-95

8. Brown ADG. Postmenopausal urinary problems. *Clin Obstet Gynecol* 1977;4:181-206

9. Longhurst PA, Kauer J, Leggett RE, *et al*. The influence of ovariectomy and estradiol replacement on urinary bladder function in rats. *J Urol* 1992;148: 915-19

10. Fantl JA, Wyman JF, Anderson RL, *et al*. Postmenopausal urinary incontinence: comparison between non-estrogen-supplemented and estrogen-supplemented women. *Obstet Gynecol* 1988;71:823-8

11. Holm NR, Horn T, Hald T. Detrusor in ageing and obstruction. *Scand J Urol Nephrol* 1995;29:45-9

12. Susset JG, Servot-Viguier D, Lamy F, *et al*. Collagen in 155 human bladders. *Invest Urol* 1978;16:204-6

13. Cortivo R, Pagano F, Passerini G, *et al*. Elastin and collagen in the normal and obstructed urinary bladder. *Br J Urol* 1981;53:134-7

14. Levy BJ, Wight TN. Structural changes in the aging submucosa: new morphologic criteria for the evaluation of the unstable human bladder. *J Urol* 1990; 144:1044-55

15. Elbadawi A, Yalla SV, Resnick NM. Structural basis of geriatric voiding dysfunction. I. Methods of a prospective ultrastructural/urodynamic study and an overview of the findings. *J Urol* 1993;150: 1650-6

16. Elbadawi A, Yalla SV, Resnick NM. Structural basis of geriatric voiding dysfunction. II. Aging detrusor: normal versus impaired contractility. *J Urol* 1993; 150:1657-67

17. Elbadawi A, Yalla SV, Resnick NM. Structural basis of geriatric voiding dysfunction. III. Detrusor overactivity. *J Urol* 1993;150:1668-80

18. Elbadawi A, Yalla SV, Resnick NM. Structural basis of geriatric voiding dysfunction. IV. Bladder outlet obstruction. *J Urol* 1993;150:1681-95

19. Strasser H, Tiefenthaler M, Steinlechner M, *et al*. Apoptosis of rhabdosphincter cells: the main cause of urinary incontinence with advancing age? *J Urol* 1999;161(Suppl):254

20. Brooks JD. Anatomy of the lower urinary tract and male genitalia. In Walsh PC, Retik AB, Vaughan ED, Wein AJ, eds. *Campbell's Urology*, 7th edn. Philadelphia: WB Saunders, 1998:89-128

21. Payne CK. Epidemiology, pathophysiology, and evaluation of urinary incontinence and overactive bladder. *Urology* 1998;51(Suppl 2A):3-10

22. Versi E. Incontinence in the climacteric. *Clin Obstet Gynecol* 1990;33:392-8

23. Resnick NM, Yalla SV. Detrusor hyperactivity with impaired contractile function: an unrecognized but common cause of incontinence in elderly patients. *J Am Med Assoc* 1987;257:3076-81

24. Erickson DR, Davies MF. Office urogynecology. *AUA Update Series* 1999;18:81-8

25. Resnick NM. Geriatric incontinence. *Urol Clin North Am* 1996;23:55-74

26. Boone TR, Kim YH. Uroflowmetry. In Nitti VW, ed. *Practical Urodynamics*. Philadelphia: WB Saunders, 1998:28-34

27. McGuire EJ, Woodside JR, Borden TA. Prognostic value of urodynamic testing in myelodysplastic children. *J Urol* 1981;126:205-9

28. McGuire EJ, Fitzpatrick CC, Wan J, *et al*. Clinical assessment of urethral sphincter function. *J Urol* 1993;150:1452-4

29. Nitti VW, Tu LM, Gitlin J. Diagnosing bladder outlet obstruction in women. *J Urol* 1999;161: 1535-40

30. Brocklehurst JC, Dillane JB. Studies of the female bladder in old age. I. Cystometrograms in non-incontinent women. *Gerontol Clin* 1966;8:285-305

31. Madersbacher S, Pycha A, Schatzl G, *et al*. The aging lower urinary tract: a comparative urodynamic study of men and women. *Urology* 1998;51:206-12

32. Wagg AS, Lieu PIC, Ding YY, *et al*. A urodynamic analysis of age associated changes in urethral function in women with lower urinary tract symptoms. *J Urol* 1984;156:1984-90

33. Collas DM, Malone-Lee JG. Age-associated changes in detrusor sensory function in women with lower urinary tract symptoms. *Int Urogynecol J* 1996;7: 24-9

34. Lightner DJ. Conservative management for urinary incontinence. *AUA Update Series* 1999;18:113–20

35. Payne CK. Conservative therapy for female urinary incontinence. *AUA Update Series* 1996;15:269–80

36. Bo K, Hagen RR, Kvarstein B, *et al*. Pelvic floor muscle exercises for the treatment of female stress urinary incontinence. III. Effect of two different degrees of pelvic floor muscle exercises. *Neurourol Urodyn* 1990;9:489–502

37. Timmons M, Addison WA. Vaginal vault prolapse. In Brubaker LT, Saclarides TJ, eds. *The Female Pelvic Floor: Disorders of Function and Support.* Philadelphia: FA Davis, 1996:262–8

38. McDougall EM, Portis A. The laparoscopic bladder neck suspension fails the test of time. *J Urol* 1999; 161(Suppl):105

39. Faerber GJ, Belville WD, Ohl DA, *et al*. Comparison of transurethral versus periurethral collagen in women with intrinsic sphincter deficiency. *Tech Urol* 1998;4:124–7

40. Kennelly MJ, McGuire EJ. Intrinsic sphincter deficiency. In O'Donnell PD, ed. *Urinary Incontinence.* St Louis: Mosby, 1997:207–13

41. Sultana SR, Goodman CM, Byrne DJ, *et al*. Microscopic hematuria: urological investigation using a standard protocol. *Br J Urol* 1996;78:691–6

42. Nicolle LE. Urinary tract infection. In O'Donnell PD, ed. *Geriatric Urology.* Boston: Little, Brown and Co., 1994:399–409

43. Karafin LJ, Coll ME. Lower urinary tract disorders in the postmenopausal woman. *Med Clin North Am* 1987;71:111–21

44. Parsons CL, Schmidt JD. Control of recurrent lower urinary tract infection in the postmenopausal woman. *J Urol* 1982;128:1224–6

45. Howell AB, Vorsa N, Der Marderosian A, *et al*. Inhibition of adherence of p-fimbriated *Escherichia coli* to uroepithelial-cell surfaces by proanthocyanidin extracts from cranberries [Letter]. *N Engl J Med* 1998;339:1085–6

15

The breast in the menopause

Bernard A. Eskin

Earlier chapters have described the significant intracellular changes associated with estrogen and progesterone in the female reproductive organs. With the onset of the menopause, almost all of the tissues of the breast show the marked effects of estrogen and/or progesterone deprivation. It is apparent that these hormones have an important effect on the growth and metabolism of the breast. The changes caused by these reduced reproductive steroids can be readily separated from those due to aging. The breast may serve well to distinguish these two prime factors of the mature years.

The overall major function of the human breast is supposedly the preparation and delivery of milk, which results in the ability to feed the young. The breast has the capacity through biochemical intracellular units to synthesize milk, a highly nutritious substance for the newborn. Despite the decrease in nursing in some cultures, the breast continues to command attraction for the emotional and sexual responses.

Ducts run separately throughout the tissues of the breast, beginning internally with the terminal duct or acinar which contains the major synthetic plant (Figure 1). The milk is then delivered to the baby through a series of ducts running through the breast and terminating into larger ducts, externally through the nipple. These independent ductal activities require internal and external stimuli. The active tissues, which constitute 20% of the breast, are essentially elastic, pliable and relatively soft. The remainder of the breast consists of layers of adipose and connective tissue, which have responsibilities for protection and support. All or any of the components may age, atrophy or become diseased or abnormal. This characteristic brings about benign and malignant changes which may lead to pain, illness and death.

Because of the anatomical location, breast tissues are exposed and easily examined (Figure 2). Characterization of breasts in reproduction, appearance and sexuality has led to many conflicts and myths. Mammary gland tissues are extremely active in the reproductive years because of the hormone cycles, and for that reason have an increased tendency for dysfunction. When reproduction wanes, the diseases that occur become more serious and the rate of malignancy increases.

In this chapter, a brief review of the anatomy and physiology of the breast is presented for both the reproductive and the postreproductive woman for comparison. In addition, a short medical overview of benign and malignant breast disease is described. Finally, the breast modifications which result from estrogen-progesterone replacement therapy in the menopausal woman are discussed.

Anatomy

Human mammary glands lie bilaterally on the pectoralis muscles, with the skin overlying. This occurs on the chest from the second rib to the sixth or seventh intercostal space (Figure 1). Laterally they extend into the apical area and medially towards the lateral aspect of the sternum.

In the cross-section of the breast it is noted that the skin superficially has two layers with a thinned areola in the tissue center. The areolar region contains an elevated nipple, which has in its center apices through which the primary ducts open (Figure 2). Smooth muscle is arranged circularly and longitudinally below the areolar area with potential for erection and contraction of the apices. There are usually 15–20 openings into the nipple, each representing a duct–lobule system. The nipple contains nerves, elastic tissue and

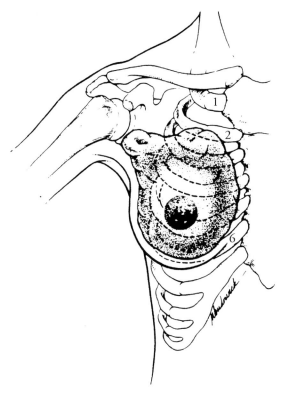

Figure 1 On the chest wall the breast extends from the second to sixth ribs and from the lateral border of the sternum to the midaxillary line. The long axis is towards the axilla, the tail of Spence. From reference 1, with permission

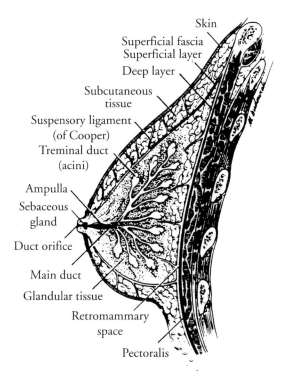

Figure 2 Glandular and supporting framework of the breast. The drawing is of 1-cm breast tissue sections, fixed in metholsalicylate and studied by trans-illumination. From reference 1, with permission

muscle which participate in the erectile patterns. The nipples hypertrophy with nursing and sexual arousal. On the circumference of the nipple-areolar complex, small glands secrete a thick lipid substance which protects the nursing mother from injury.

Below the skin, there is a thicker, fascial sheath which completely surrounds the underlying breast tissues from the skin to the pectoralis muscle fascia. The first layer below the fascia contains a good deal of fat irregularly arranged as a protective coat through which the lactiferous (milk) ducts travel.

Within the breast, the smallest units are the internally located terminal ducts or acini, which effectively produce the secretions. Acini are multicellular (2–4 cell thicknesses) and have myoepithelial structures on the basement membranes. The myoepithelial cells appear similar to smooth

muscle and are endocrine activated (Figure 3). Tertiary and secondary ducts (two-cell layered) extend from these terminal bud-like structures and eventuate into the primary ducts which enter the areolar–nipple area. The combination of these terminal, secondary and primary ducts with connective tissues and blood vessels forms larger units called lobules. Each lobule has a primary duct termination.

The subdermal or superficial fat externally and the layer noted anterior to the pectoral muscle (secondary fat) essentially buffer the breast. There appears to be a genetic variability in size and conformity, which may be expressed by fat content and metabolism. The superficial fat is based on hormonal and nutritional intake, while the secondary fat appears to be affected by heredity.

During the ages of reproduction, ducts are firm, regular and easily distinguished. Surrounding the ducts are layers of elastic and fibrous tissue which result in the positioning of the ducts, but provide a mobile cushion.

Endocrinology of the breast

In the prepubertal girl, the primordial cyst begins to develop into immature breast ducts. The cyst is developed by the 4th to 6th year and, by the 8th year, as ovarian estrogen first begins to be secreted (thelarche), differentiation of primary and secondary ducts becomes visible.

Growth and development of the breast is affected by many substances. The most important include thyroid hormones, iodine, insulin, cortisol and eventually functional steroids, estrogen and progesterone (Table 1). At menarche, breast tissues reach maturity and are assessed according to size, appearance and nipple growth (Tanner system). A tertiary duct system, though rudimentary at first, should be present which has the capability of milk synthesis and delivery through the nipple.

Throughout the reproductive years when estrogen and progesterone cyclicity occurs, the breast tissues react to the hormones providing changes by both hypertrophy and hyperplasia of the lining cells. Estrogen increases duct size by hypertrophy of the lining cells, while progesterone causes hyperplasia of these cells with increased chemical activity of prelactation compounds within the terminal ducts.

A third hormone, prolactin, secreted from the pituitary, increases as estrogen reaches its apex near mid-cycle and remains elevated until estrogen

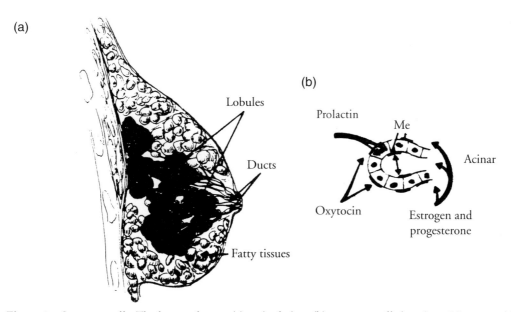

Figure 3 Secretory cells. The human breast: (a) sagittal view; (b) secretory cells in acinar. Me, myoepithelial cells. From reference 2, with permission

Table 1 Breast physiology

Hormone	Development	Alveolar growth	Pubertal changes	Lactation
T_3/T_4	+	+	+	+
Iodine	+	+	+	+
Estrogen	−	−	+	+
Progesterone	−	−	+	+
Prolactin	−	+/−	+	+
Insulin	−	−	−	+
Cortisone	−	−	−	+

T_3/T_4, tri-iodothyronine/thyroxine; +, increase; −, decrease

decreases. Prolactin has the ability to bind lactalbumin to the protein casein in the terminal ducts and, hence, synthesize milk.

During a non-pregnant cycle, when estrogen is available, the amount of secretion generated is minimal and is usually absorbed within the duct system. Periodic evidence of dry inspissated milk on the nipple may represent a breakdown of this physiological action. On the other hand, if stasis of the secretion occurs, it may be impeded within the duct. This results in a fluid-filled segment of the duct which, on expansion, causes inflammatory ductal damage. When a fibrous protective layer forms, the outcome is fibrocystic nodules. The breasts may become uncomfortable for the patient (mastodynia), and this discomfort may continue until there is a decrease in estrogen. Since progesterone increases the duct size, the two hormones together may intensify the pain.

In the reproductive woman, prolactin increases markedly during pregnancy and early postpartum, resulting in synthesis of milk. The flow of milk is maintained by the newborn sucking via sensory pathways from the nipple to the brain, while prolactin levels fall after birth. Posterior pituitary secretions of oxytocin and possibly vasopressin result. These act on the myoepithelial cells of the terminal ducts and cause continuity of milk flow (Figure 3). In the menopausal woman, abnormal prolactin secretion may occur, which results in nipple secretions through the same physiological mechanisms. Such secretions require immediate investigation for an anatomical or endocrinological pathology. Often prolactin surges occur in women with epilepsy or miscellaneous seizures[3].

Breast anatomy remains only partially intact during the premenopause, which results in a number of unpredictable tissue changes particularly if replacement hormones are used. While benign histologically, they take on the characteristics of reproductive breast abnormalities and often become difficult to diagnose by the usual non-invasive techniques.

Menopause

Estrogen and progesterone secretions and related cellular responses decrease slowly from the age of approximately 28, and rapidly after the age of 42 years. The availability of estrogen and progesterone receptors is reduced as estrogen receptor stimulation is lagging. Prolactin, on the other hand, is difficult to assess, as the prolactin receptor cannot be accurately measured[4]. The effect of prolactin on breast tumorigenesis is, thus, not well understood. Modification of the breast tissues begins with an initial loss of subcutaneous fat and connective tissues followed by degeneration of the duct systems. This constitutes thinning of the cellular linings, particularly the secondary and tertiary ducts. The fibrous tissue and elastic tissues begin to disintegrate, and may do so in a manner which appears dysfunctional (Figure 4). Since the skin is involved in the aging process, it becomes thinner with wrinkling and dryness. These latter changes are non-hormonal, but are brought about primarily by cellular degeneration with the

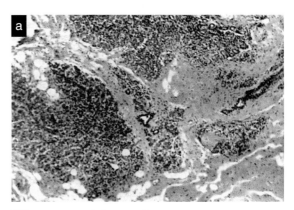
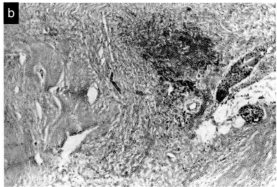

Figure 4 Photomicrographs of female breast tissues (× 7.75). (a) Perimenopausal breast section showing active duct and stromal areas (age 32 years); (b) menopausal breast section with atrophic and inactive tissues (age 69 years). Courtesy of C. Grotkowski and W. Battisti

inability for restoration. The nipple loses some of its vascularity and changes from a red appearance to a light pink.

Elastic tissues and minimal muscular tissue are responsible for the support of the breasts. When a reduction of these elements occurs at menopause, firmness of the breast is lost. Superficial fat dissipates with the loss of estrogen, resulting in a caved-in and elongated appearance. In obese patients where there is an increase in estrone from extraovarian androgen metabolism, the breast tissues sometimes retain a semiactive state for a long period of time with continued support after the menopause has occurred. The prepectoral fat tissues remain at this time and for at least 10 years following the menopause. Initial findings of estrogen receptor β were located in the breast adipose tissues, and this may have a role in estrone responses[5].

During the postmenopause, with further loss of estrogen, glands and ducts atrophy, resulting in a change in all the breast tissues to fat cells as the prominent component. Postmenopausal breasts appear translucent on mammograms, and reverse only when replacement hormones are given.

Diseases of the breast

Benign breast disease

Breast diseases are often considered as age-dependent, peaking during the deceleration period of reproduction. Unfortunately, while benign breast disease morbidity appears to diminish after the menopause, malignancy incidence increases proportionately. An increasing occurrence of breast cancer has been shown with each 5-year increment in age, which becomes convincingly evident in the menopause[6].

Benign breast disease is less likely to occur in postmenopausal women as the menstrual cycles that cause these changes in the breast discontinue. Duct and gland prominence decrease with consequent diminished nodularities. Severe degenerative histological changes occur and are shown in Figure 4.

The most common benign diseases seen in the premenopausal woman fall into a category that has been defined as *fibrocystic disease*. The major patho-

gnomonic findings are benign fluid retention that occurs in the ducts and the accompanying periductal fibrosis. This is often secondary to inflammatory or traumatic responses, notably in the connective tissues. Many pathologists refer to these changes as gross cystic breast disease, which occurs clinically in 60% of all women[7]. Symptoms consist of bumpy and enlarged breasts often accompanied by breast tenderness.

There have been several recent references to the need for reclassification of fibrocystic disease[8]. A suggested classification for benign breast disease is presented in Table 2[9]. Considerations that the pathologists advise are to provide descriptions of 'specific component elements' of the tissues obtained at biopsy, so that experience can be gained in determining which fibrocystic diseases may be precancerous. These features would include cystic morphology, stromal cellular variations and glandular hypertrophy and hyperplasia.

Similarly, radiologists are confounded constantly by the distortions seen on mammography when fibrocystic disease is marked[10]. Needle aspiration of the cysts often helps to improve the acumen of the radiological diagnosis. Needle biopsy is needed when the cited lesion continues to remain uncertain between benign and malignant.

In the menopause, the loss of estrogen–progesterone stimuli is a major factor in the reduction in fibrocystic disease. The breasts are easier to examine both physically and radiographically. The response of the breast tissue to the use of estrogen replacement therapy (ERT) is discussed later in this chapter as it includes women who had

Table 2 Fibrocystic diseases of the breast[9]

Non-proliferative lesions
Breast cysts
Papillary apocrine
Epithelial-related calcifications
Mild hyperplasia
Fibroadenoma

Proliferative lesions without atypia
Moderate or florid hyperplasia
Intraductal papillomas
Sclerosing adenosis

Atypical hyperplasia
Ductal
Lobular

premenopausal fibrocystic disease. The recurrence of these symptoms has been variable with the use of ERT[11].

Breast cancer

Risk factors

Breast cancer is thought to occur as a result of a mutagenic transformation in DNA during mitosis[12]. There have been descriptions of various mutagens (viral, chemical, radiation-induced) which may show responsibility for carcinogenic change, the spontaneous or unknown mutations being most common. Inherited mitotic changes are only responsible for less than 10% of cancers.

Family history is essential in establishing risk levels for breast cancer. First-degree relatives of breast cancer patients carry a two- to three-fold increased risk of developing breast cancer. If the cancer relative was premenopausal and had bilateral disease, the risk increases. Risk for the other breast increases when one breast is cancerous, while cancers of the ovary and endometrium also increase the risk[13,14].

Aging is probably one of the most important factors involved in breast cancer etiology. During the aging process, fragmentation and mutation of DNA increases. As previously stated, breast cancer incidence is greater after age 70 than before 40. Conditions which appear also to increase breast cancer risk are: early menarche (before 11), late menopause (after 50), first-term pregnancy after 30. Reduction in risk has been attributed to: nursing, full-term pregnancies, oophorectomy before age 30[15].

Obesity is a risk for menopausal women, while it appears to be unrelated in the premenopause. This may correlate with the socioeconomic risk which increases in the higher strata. In postmenopausal women, increased mammary gland size may be a risk for breast cancer[16]. Basic concepts become somewhat clouded when these groups are compared, considering diet and medical care. High-fat diets are involved in peripheral estrone metabolism, which may be considered precancerous in the postmenopausal woman while it has no effect on premenopausal women. Intake of coffee, tea, methylxanthine foods and beverages, and alcohol (greater than 3 oz per week) seems to increase the risk. Arguments for and against have been levelled, and all of these proposals seem difficult to assess clinically.

Whether benign disease is a precursor to breast cancer remains a controversial topic, despite numerous studies. Women with fibrocystic disease were considered originally to have a risk factor four times greater than those without[8]. A study from a committee of the American Pathology Association noted that the risk factor level could only be calculated when histopathology was used in the diagnosis[17]. Twenty-six per cent (26%) of women who have proliferative breast nodules can be given a risk rating. This increases if any of the above-described risk factors are also present. About 30% of this risk category have atypical hyperplasia (adenomatous tissue type), which places these individuals at high risk[18]. Atypical hyperplasia, seen on biopsy, in both pre- and postmenopausal women showed a significant increase in breast cancer[19]. From these results, it becomes apparent that a classification is needed that will provide the clinician with a better normal baseline from which to consider when excision should be done in borderline cases. A classification for these benign but premalignant conditions has been suggested. This serves some pathology laboratories and is useful, particularly when discussing the follow-up of benign biopsies as indicated in Table 2[9].

Estrogen therapies

Menopausal women are concerned with the effect of replacement estrogen on the breast. This entire issue is clouded by the oral contraceptive controversy as well as the relationship of estrogen to breast cancer etiology[20]. The level of estrogen (usually ethinylestradiol) given in birth-control hormones has estrogen receptor effectiveness approximately seven times that of the dose used for replacement therapy. When breast cancers are estrogen dependent as shown by positive estrogen and/or progesterone receptor laboratory tissue evaluations, replacement medication is contraindicated, especially in the postmenopause[21]. Except for specific cancer patients, there appears to be no medical or scientific reason against giving estrogen to women in the menopause for their symptomatology[22-24].

No significant increase in risk was shown in a series of relatively acute studies (1–5 years) as well as several chronic therapy series over 12 years in menopausal women. Latency (15–20 years) similarly did not result in breast changes that can significantly change the longevity or comfort of the patient[25]. A recent update by the Cancer Committee of the College of American Pathologists used more specific diagnostic data, with a refining of the degree of risk associated with individual lesions[26]. Long-term studies are continuing in women who are over 70 and taking estrogen replacement, as responses in the geriphase (late menopause) have not yet been fully evaluated. Early data show a mild rise in risk in this group (over age 65). In light of the cardiovascular and bone protection afforded by the estrogen, the protective values must be measured against the risks.

The Cancer and Steroid Hormone Study (CASH) and Centers for Disease Control have evaluated almost 5000 cases of breast cancer (ages 20–54), seeking confirmation of whether there is an increased risk with birth-control pills[22]. Most recent studies from these groups and others have shown no significant differences using age-of-first-utilization data. The research continues, considering several other related reproductive factors as well[27]. In a recent study, for all types of breast cancer considered, hormone replacement therapy (HRT) use was not associated with significantly increased risk (relative risk, RR for use 5 years or less, 1.07; RR for use greater than 5 years, 1.11). 'Exposure was associated most strongly with an increased risk of invasive cancer with a favorable prognosis'[28].

Biochemically, estrogen metabolism can be restricted at certain cell levels mutagenically and receptor-wise. The resulting growth may deviate and become neoplastic in older tissues, where severe atypical pathways of development have been described[29]. Progesterone therapy is a parallel medication taken with estrogen replacement when the patient has a uterus[6]. The endometrium is activated and may become atypical where unopposed estrogen is given to menopausal women. This can lead to endometrial neoplasia. Progesterone may be essential with unopposed estrogen to protect breast tissues in a similar manner. Nevertheless,

the American Association for Reproductive Medicine has stated that it is unnecessary, based on the evidence available, to add progesterone cyclically for breast protection[30].

Some forms of progesterone, such as medroxyprogesterone acetate or megestrol acetate, have been shown to lower the risk when given simultaneously. This breast controversy continues as there are no convincing statistics against the estrogen therapy. In individuals with high risk for breast cancer, the use of progesterone does not appear to change the increasing risk seen after 15 years of estrogen therapy, compared to those women without risk[31].

Incidence of breast cancer in the menopause
Breast cancer remains a serious threat to women of all ages. In the reproductive ages, the breasts are essential for nursing, and are distinctly affected by hormones from the central nervous system, both anterior and posterior pituitary, and the ovary. This sensitive endocrine target organ is affected additionally by the thyroid (and iodine), insulin and cortisone as well as the characteristic changes brought on by estrogens, progesterone and prolactin (see Table 1). During nursing, oxytocin and perhaps vasopressin have an influence on the breasts. The female breast is extremely well vascularized as any surgeon recognizes, and typically is affected by fat metabolism as evidenced by the changes in size and shape. Besides these endocrine activities, the human mammary glands are persistently manipulated by brassières, plastic surgeons and exercising mechanisms. Because of these multiple intrusions, it is not surprising that breast atypia and neoplasia are potential consequences throughout the woman's life.

The estimated cancer incidences have shown most recently that, as the millenium begins, breast cancer dominates all other cancer sites for all women by a large margin. Although lung cancers are increasing, the American Cancer Society statistics for breast cancer during the past 5 years continue to be about 30% of the total cancer rates. About 10% of all women will be subject to neoplasia of the breast in the United States, a high-risk region for the disease. While breast cancer morbidity has increased, the death rate from breast cancer shows a minimal rate decrease. The 5-year relative survival rate now stands at 76%.

Breast cancer increases in women in their forties to seventies, and is evidently a serious disease for the perimenopausal woman. However, mortality is relatively lower, and a less provocative disease pattern is seen in the menopause. Several studies indicate that all women, whether taking estrogen replacement or not, are equally protected[32].

Diagnosis of breast diseases

The general aim of the various breast diagnostic techniques is to differentiate benign from malignant disease. The breast tissues change with the menstrual cycle because of sex hormonal variability during each reproductive month. These functional variations begin tentatively at menarche (onset of bleeding) but plateau during the premenopausal period. Examination of the breasts should be done immediately after menses when steroid hormone levels are lowest. During the premenopause when cycles continue, examinations provide inaccurate and often alarming results even if this rule is followed. Following the menopause, estrogen is often available intrinsically in variable amounts, but less than that required to cause menstruation or estrogen withdrawal bleeding, or provide significant changes in the breast[33].

Techniques commonly used for breast diagnoses are palpation, mammography, ultrasound and histopathological evaluation by fine-needle biopsy or tissue biopsy. Ancillary evaluations by aspiration of cystic structures and nipple excretion testing with cytology are useful. Other methods which have been described are: diaphanography, thermography and chemical determinations by computer densitometry.

Early detection of small breast cancer lesions seems to provide a longer survival for the women. Thus, a commitment to systematic evaluation is advised. In premenopausal women, self-breast examination is taught by the physician or nurse so that a recognizable lesion may be reported immediately to the physician for follow-up. In older women, postmenopausal self-examination becomes more difficult and less accurate because of the increase in fibrous firm tissue. Routine breast examinations by a physician should be a routine every 6 months, or at least yearly. Suggested techniques are described and demonstrated in diagnostic textbooks, as a unified agreement on the method for breast examination has not been achieved[33].

The American Cancer Society and the American Medical Association in 1999 made recommendations that mammography be done routinely:

(1) As a baseline before 40;

(2) Yearly in the forties and fifties;

(3) Thereafter as indicated.

Individuals who are at risk may require mammography more often. The Radiologic Society of America feels that the dangers from the radiation received during low-dose mammography present a much lower risk than the potential of breast cancer[34]. While other suggestions have been proposed as cost-efficient, this routine prevails.

Fibrocystic disease hampers diagnosis since it may distort the physical examination and mammography so that small lesions may be missed. When the cysts are large enough to permit needle aspiration with ultrasound localization the techniques are more reliable. The fibrocystic disease seen in menopausal women tends to be reduced but firmer when the cysts are drained. Several benign lesions can be differentiated by a trained mammographer. When the lesions are suspicious, tissue biopsy is the surest diagnostic technique. Some surgeons feel that needle biopsy is sufficiently accurate and less invasive when the lesion is easily attained.

Both physician palpation and self-breast examination can feel a separate mass at 1 cm. However, growth pattern studies show that a palpable 1-cm lesion has been growing for 8 years. A mammogram can detect the lesion approximately 3 years before palpation using the newest radiographic techniques. For this reason, mammography screening in large community programs reduces mortality as much as 30%. The problems connected with mammography for the patients are cost, discomfort, radiation exposure and inconvenience. There appears to be less radiation hazard to women over 35, when the average dose to the sternum is 50 mrad.

Diagnostic techniques

Several office techniques have become available during the past few years. The improved accuracy of these methods for obtaining an early diagnosis has made it possible for qualified physicians to follow up the presence of a palpable or mammographic lesion. Masses are considered dominant when they can be palpated in two dimensions from the background nodulation. Dominant lesions are not felt until they are 2–3 cm in diameter. Testing methods such as ultrasound and diaphanography have been devised to help differentiate the consistency of these and provide some indication of the content. When a lesion appears to be fluid-filled, aspiration is recommended.

Cytological examination of the aspirate from these cysts is useful primarily when it is thickened, bloody or discolored. Otherwise the aspirate is discarded, particularly if the mass has been eliminated[35]. Should the lesion remain after this procedure, localization with ultrasound or X-ray and biopsy must be done. During the premenopause, abundant cystic changes occur in sensitized breasts; however, in the postmenopause, there are fewer cystic masses unless estrogen replacement is given[36].

Descriptive literature regarding the value of fine-needle aspiration of the breast has become less controversial, while the standard biopsy techniques still seem more reliable, particularly in borderline cases. The false-negative rate for needle aspiration remains variable (3–15%). Pathologists report that, often, cancer cells do not adhere well to the aspirating needle, so that the major flaw in the procedure is that the neoplastic cells, if present, are not always obtainable. Most major centers continue to use this technique because a positive result is usually correct (3.2% false–positive), and this immediate positive report reduces the delay in therapy. Methods for this test are amply described in the literature[37,38].

Again at this time, the age-old question dominates: who should do the diagnostic biopsies? It has been generally acknowledged that invasive diagnostic techniques should be done only by the breast surgeons, since they will have final responsibility for excision and therapeutic support, should cancer be present.

When a mass is seen by mammography, ultrasound or diaphanography which cannot be palpated, the level of suspicion is left to the interpreter. If the lesion is questionable, needle localization of the lesion with a formal biopsy is required. This may increase survival time by reducing metastatic potential[39].

Treatment of breast diseases in the menopause

Benign disease

Benign breast nodules accompanied by pain, often described as mastalgia, are present in 60–75% of all reproductive-aged women and 30% of those in the perimenopausal period. While fibrocystic disease has been considered to be a misnomer for all mastalgias, this diagnostic eponym is generally used by physicians on the basis of the nodularity and discomfort. Periodic breast pain occurs in 95% of all women with ovulatory cycles in the premenopause. The discomfort begins generally after ovulation and continues for variable lengths of time until menses occurs, with the average duration cited as 5 ± 1.3 days.

The menopause does not result in a total loss of estrogen secretion, particularly in the early postmenopause. Perturbations in estrogen are responsible for mastalgias and persistence of fibrous and occasional cystic nodules. The use of ERT may initially cause these characteristics to occur, but the persistence of therapy without modulations eventually results in recovery.

The discomfort described varies from specific localized areas laterally and medially to the total breast area. Mammography may show large multicystic clumps of tissue that often obscure major lesions, particularly small carcinomas which may lie behind them. Large tender cysts may be aspirated directly, localizing with palpation or ultrasound, which results in reducing discomfort. If diagnostic testing has indicated that the mastalgia is the result of non-neoplastic disease, various therapies have been suggested.

Prophylactically, daily vitamins C and E, small doses of antiprostaglandins and dietary avoidance of caffeine have been considered effective in many patients. None of these methods has been shown to have scientific validity. Many plants including sunflower, canola and evening primrose have been sold and used. It has been indicated that the oils of these plants contain some essential fatty acids, such as linoleic and gamma linoleic, which provide prostaglandins. The use of evening primrose oil in mastalgia has depended on uncontrolled studies, but maintains a high therapeutic use[40].

Many treatments that are recommended suppress estrogen activity specifically in the breast tissues. Many of the benign fibrocystic changes have pathognomonic findings of ductile/lobular hyperplasia, periductal fibrosis, increased ductal secretions with expanded cystic structures and adenosis of the cells and hypertrophy of the ducts. Experimentally, these may be produced by estrogen excess, with an increased prolactin stimulation. This has led to the use of drugs which are antiestrogenic with a prolactin-lowering response.

Treatment with danazol (Danocrine®), tamoxifen citrate (Nolvadex®), raloxifene (Evista®) and gestrinone has resulted in improvement of benign fibrocystic changes diagnosed by tissue biopsy and mammograms. Pain has been relieved moderately by these antiestrogenic substances[41]. However, dosage levels are kept relatively low because of the marked side-effects described with the use of these products. Hormone treatment with progesterone shows variable success. Thyroid and cortisone hormone therapy has not been reliably effective.

Use of elemental iodine has produced a high level of improvement with reduced fibrosis[42,43]. Fibrocystic changes due to iodine deficiency were seen to increase with aging, and were more responsive to replacement[44]. Both clinical and basic breast studies have shown that iodine may also be involved in preventing malignant transition where iodine deficiency exists[45,46]. The side-effects appear to be minimal, and a more accurate mammography may be obtainable since the iodine therapy eliminates much of the nodularity and most of the fibrosis.

Malignant disease

Breast cancer has evolved with an eclectic system of therapeutics ranging through surgery, radiation and chemotherapy. Menopausal women present with breast cancer that is more widespread but slower growing than in reproductive women. As with younger patients, the predominant tissue type of breast cancer is the infiltrating duct carcinoma (65–75%). These are better differentiated in older women. Hormonally, the incidence of estrogen receptor-positive tumors increases with age from 30% below 40, to 75% at 75. As expected, progesterone receptors increase in a similar manner[47].

Studies of randomized groups of women with either tamoxifen citrate or cytotoxic therapies showed that the latter reduced the morbidity rate by 25% during the first 5 years, under the age of 50. The antiestrogen tamoxifen citrate reduced the rate by 50% in 5 years in the women who were over 50[48]. A significant increase, however, was observed in the mean percentage of estrogen receptor positivity in ductal tissue[49]. The effectiveness of tamoxifen use can be predicted and monitored by analyses of tumor cell characteristics such as hormone receptor content and proliferation function[49].

When the diagnosis of breast cancer has been made in the menopausal woman, the major factors are: stage, histopathology and receptor status of the tumor. Receptor status is now considered a useful diagnostic step whenever biopsy or excision is done. Both estrogen and progesterone receptors are measured and reported to the oncological or radiation therapist. The estrogen receptor has been further defined as ER-α and ER-β; the former is the common evaluation on which therapy is decided, while the latter receptor has been found in breast and abdominal subcutaneous adipose tissue[50].

Additional important variables are the overall health and age of the patient. The classification used for tumors is presented in Table 3.

The present options for therapy offered to patients of all ages are:

A, biopsy with hormonal therapy;

B, segmental resection (local excision, 'lumpectomy');

C, wide excision of tumor;

D, simple mastectomy;

E, modified radical mastectomy.

Table 3 Staging for breast carcinoma. This staging system provides a strategy for grouping patients with respect to prognosis. Therapeutic decisions are formulated in part according to staging categories but primarily according to lymph node status, estrogen and progesterone receptor levels in the tumor tissue, menopausal status and general health of the patient. The American Joint Committee on Cancer (AJCC) has designated staging by TNM classification. Reproduced from reference 51

TNM definitions

Primary tumor (T):

  TX: primary tumor cannot be assessed

  TO: no evidence of primary tumor

  Tis: carcinoma *in situ*; intraductal carcinoma, lobular carcinoma *in situ*, or Paget's disease of the nipple with no associated tumor. Note: Paget's disease associated with a tumor is classified according to the size of the tumor

  T1: tumor 2.0 cm or less in greatest dimension

    T1mic: microinvasion 0.1 cm or less in greatest dimension

    T1a: tumor more than 0.1 cm but not more than 0.5 cm in greatest dimension

    T1b: tumor more than 0.5 cm but not more than 1.0 cm in greatest dimension

    T1c: tumor more than 1.0 cm but not more than 2.0 cm in greatest dimension

  T2: tumor more than 2.0 cm but not more than 5.0 cm in greatest dimension

  T3: tumor more than 5.0 cm in greatest dimension

  T4: tumor of any size with direct extension to (a) chest wall or (b) skin, only as described below. Note: chest wall includes ribs, intercostal muscles, and serratus anterior muscle but not pectoral muscle

    T4a: extension to chest wall

    T4b: edema (including peau d'orange) or ulceration of the skin of the breast or satellite skin nodules confined to the same breast

    T4c: both of the above (T4a and T4b)

    T4d: inflammatory carcinoma

Regional lymph nodes (N):

  NX: regional lymph nodes cannot be assessed (e.g. previously removed)

  N0: no regional lymph node metastasis

  N1: metastasis to movable ipsilateral axillary lymph node(s)

  N2: metastasis to ipsilateral axillary lymph node(s) fixed to each other or to other structures

  N3: metastasis to ipsilateral internal mammary lymph node(s)

Pathological classification (pN):

  pNX: regional lymph nodes cannot be assessed (not removed for pathological study or previously removed)

  pN0: no regional lymph node metastasis

  pN1: metastasis to movable ipsilateral axillary lymph node(s)

    pN1a: only micrometastasis (none larger than 0.2 cm)

    pN1b: metastasis to lymph node(s), any larger than 0.2 cm

      pN1bi: metastasis in 1–3 lymph nodes, any more than 0.2 cm and all less than 2.0 cm in greatest dimension

      pN1bii: metastasis to 4 or more lymph nodes, any more than 0.2 cm and all less than 2.0 cm in greatest dimension

      pN1biii: extension of tumor beyond the capsule of a lymph node metastasis less than 2.0 cm in greatest dimension

      pN1biv: metastasis to a lymph node 2.0 cm or more in greatest dimension

  pN2: metastasis to ipsilateral axillary lymph node(s) fixed to each other or to other structures

  pN3: metastasis to ipsilateral internal mammary lymph node(s)

Distant metastasis (M):

  MX: presence of distant metastasis cannot be assessed

  M0: no distant metastasis

  M1: distant metastasis present (includes metastasis to ipsilateral supraclavicular lymph nodes)

AJCC stage groupings

Stage 0

  Tis, N0, M0

Continued

Table 3 *Continued*

Stage I
  T1*, N0, M0

Stage IIA
  T0, N1, M0
  T1*, N1**, M0
  T2, N0, M0

Stage IIB
  T2, N1, M0
  T3, N0, M0

Stage IIIA
  T0, N2, M0
  T1*, N2, M0
  T2, N2, M0
  T3, N1, M0
  T3, N2, M0

Stage IIIB
  T4, any N, M0
  any T, N3, M0

Stage IV
  any T, any N, M1

Inflammatory breast cancer
Inflammatory carcinoma is a clinicopathological entity characterized by diffuse brawny induration of the skin
  of the breast with an erysipeloid edge, usually without an underlying palpable mass. Radiologically there may
  be a detectable mass and characteristic thickening of the skin over the breast. The clinical presentation is due
  to tumor embolization of dermal lymphatics or to capillary congestion. Inflammatory carcinoma is classified
  T4d

*T1 includes T1mic; **the prognosis of patients with pN1a disease is similar to that of patients with pN0 disease

C, D and E are done with or without axillary lymph node dissection; B and C are done with axillary node biopsy; D and E are done with axillary dissection.

Adjuvant breast cancer therapy is chemotherapy and/or radiotherapy and/or hormonal therapy given in addition to tumor removal, to decrease the chance of recurrence or distant spread. It may be used before, during or after radiation and similarly before or after mastectomy under the individualized conditions[52]. It is usually started after surgery. Adjuvant radiation therapy begins within 10 days of conservative surgery in postmenopausal women with early lesions. Chemotherapy, once considered inadvisable for postmenopausal women because of apparent poor response and toxicity[36], has now also been added as a therapeutic measure.

Altering the hormonal milieu seems to be somewhat effective in some patients. The idea of providing an undesirable environment for the malignancy while safeguarding the normal cells is the basis for most chemotherapies. However, estrogen and progesterone have minimal effectiveness and are used only if the tumor receptor response is not favorable for growth. Aminoglutethiamide was used to inhibit adrenal steroidogenesis in the postmenopausal patient when estrogen receptors were increased and peripheral steroid pathways to estrogen were to be avoided[48].

Tamoxifen citrate is probably the best antiestrogen therapy available at present. Since breast cancer is slower-growing postmenopausally, the tumor is better differentiated, with a higher estrogen and progesterone receptor-positive index. For this reason, menopausal patients with breast cancer have a greater affinity for tamoxifen therapy. The response rates are 55–80% effective in estrogen and progesterone receptor-positive breast cancer aspirates (cytological sampling) or biopsies (monoclonal or chemical testing). When tamoxifen is used as an adjuvant, 5-year survival increases with or without positive axillary nodes. Side-effects of this medication seem relatively mild. An increased incidence of endometrial carcinoma after prolonged use has been cited, but may be reduced by concomitant progesterone therapy. Endometrial biopsies on an annual basis are indicated when uterine bleeding is present.

Prognosis

Metastasis remains the dread of all concerned. In breast carcinoma the first evidences of this are found in the axillary lymph nodes. The prognoses in general are ascertained first from lymph node biopsies and are usually evaluated as the ratio of nodes that are positive to the number removed (for example, 2 : 10). Other important indicators are: receptor status, primary lesion size and age. An indication of receptor status helps because of the treatments available, such as antiestrogens. Lesion size represents the critical time of neglect before discovery during which metastases may occur[10,48,53].

Since survival rates are higher for menopausal women with early disease, accurate diagnosis during this period is important. Aging results in slower growth and metastases, which is an asset to the survival of the menopausal woman[39].

Estrogen replacement therapy and breast cancer

Women with moderate to severe menopausal symptoms who have breast neoplasia or are at high risk for breast cancer are in a therapeutic dilemma[44]. This problem is dealt with in detail elsewhere in this book (Chapter 21). However, progestational agents, clonidine and tranquilizers have been suggested as a substitute for estrogen replacement therapy. Most often these medications do not provide successful results. When estrogen has been considered as absolutely contraindicated, recent studies have suggested that replacement is permissible if progestational therapy is used concurrently and receptor-positive tumors are not involved. Such therapy requires the consent and understanding of the patient after personal evaluation of risks and benefits.

Women who use estrogen–progestin replacement therapy as a continuous daily regimen may develop larger breasts than those with a shorter period of progestin monthly. As the combined therapy uses an opposed estrogen level, the overall result does not cause any further breast cancer risk[44].

Summary

While the incidence of benign breast disease decreases with aging, the incidence of breast cancer peaks premenopausally and remains high in the postmenopause. It is the most common cancer of the mature woman. Early diagnosis appears to assist in combating the disease and providing quality survival[54].

The available diagnostic techniques consist of breast self-examination, physician palpation, mammography, ultrasound, needle aspiration, needle biopsy and tissue biopsy. It is important to communicate to women the need for availing themselves to this hierarchical process. Several programs are available, but the most logical sequence that remains is characteristic self-examination and reliable physician follow-up. Time frames for mammography suggested by the radiological groups with the American Cancer Society should be followed. These must be modified according to risk factors.

Breast cancer therapeutics for the 21st century are promising because they are relatively effective and provide a holistic approach for the mature woman. Results that have been obtained by surgery/adjuvant therapies will be further improved and simplified. Breast reconstruction has become a commonly available ancillary feature during or after severe surgical procedures. Fascial or prosthetic implants are being used for cosmetic correction. Knowledgeable support groups have become available for breast cancer patients, which increase acceptance by the patient of the therapeutic choices offered. Improved quality of life is an important factor in the selection of the treatment modality chosen by the woman.

Breast changes should be evaluated stringently in the menopausal woman in light of the effective outcome. All physicians who serve the menopausal population should learn and understand the basic factors for current diagnostic techniques and therapies.

References

1. Egan RL. *Breast Imaging - Diagnosis and Morphology of Breast Diseases*. Philadelphia: WB Saunders, 1988
2. Eskin BA. Disorders of prolaction secretion. In Eskin BA, ed. *Issues in Reproductive Technology*. New York: Medical Arts, 1984;171:1–4
3. Malkowicz DE, Legido A, Jackel RA, Sussman NM, Eskin BA, Harner RN. Prolactin secretion following repetitive seizures. *Neurology* 1995;45:448–52
4. Touraine P, Martini JF, Zafrini B, *et al*. Increased expression of prolactin receptor gene assessed by quantitative polymerase chain reaction in human breast tumors versus normal breast tissues. *J Clin Endocrinol Metab* 1998;83:667–74
5. Crandall DL, Busler DR, Novak TJ, Weber RV, Kral JG. Breast and abdominal subcutaneous adipose tissue. *Biochem Biophys Res Commun* 1998;248:523–6
6. Gambrell RD Jr. Hormone replacement therapy and breast cancer. *Maturitas* 1987;9:123–33
7. Schairer C, Brinton LA, Hoover RN. Methylxanthine and benign breast diseases. *Am J Epidemiol* 1986;124:603–11
8. Dupont WD, Page DL. Risk factors for breast cancer in women with proliferative breast disease. *N Engl J Med* 1985;312:146–51
9. Eskin BA. Fibrocystic disease of the breast. In Eskin BA, Asbell SO, Jardines L, eds. *Breast Diseases for the Primary Care Physician*. New York: Parthenon Publishing, 1999:65–73
10. Seidman H, Gelb SK, Silverberg E, *et al*. Survival experience in the Breast Cancer Detection Demonstration Project. *CA* 1987;37:258–90
11. Bergkvist L, Adami H-O, Persson I, *et al*. The risk of breast cancer after estrogen and estrogen–progestin replacement. *N Engl J Med* 1989;321:293–7
12. Wren BG, Eden JA. Do progestogens reduce the risk of breast cancer? A review of the evidence. *Menopause* 1996;3:4–12
13. Kvale G, Heuch I, Eide G-E. A prospective study of reproductive factors and breast cancer. I. Parity. *Am J Epidemiol* 1987;126:831–41
14. Rohan TE, McMichael AJ. Methylxanthines and breast cancer. *Int J Cancer* 1988;41:390–3
15. Willett WC, Stempfer MJ, Colditz GA, *et al*. Moderate alcohol consumption and the risk of breast cancer. *N Engl J Med* 1987;316:1174–80
16. Hsieh CC, Trichopoulos D. Breast size handedness and breast cancer risks. *Eur J Cancer* 1991;27:131–5
17. Cancer Committee of the College of American Pathologists. Is fibrocystic disease of the breast precancerous? *Arch Pathol Lab Med* 1986;110:171–3
18. Bauwens SF. Safety of estrogen therapy for women with fibrocystic breast disease. *Clin Pharm* 1987;6:683
19. London SJ, Connolly JL, Schmitt SJ, Colditz GA. A prospective study of benign breast disease and the risk of breast cancer. *J Am Med Assoc* 1991;267:941–4
20. Soderqvist G, Olsson H, Wilking N, von Schoultz B, Carlstrom K. Metabolism of estrone sulfate by normal breast tissue: influence of menopausal status and oral contraceptives. *J Steroid Biochem Mol Biol* 1994;48:221–4
21. Thorpe SM, Cristensen IJ, Rasmussen BB, Rose C. Estrogens, progestogens, normal breast cell proliferation, and breast cancer risk. *Eur J Cancer* 1993;29A:971–7
22. CASH Study: Centers for Disease Control and NICH, Human Development; Cancer and Steroid Hormone Study. Oral-contraceptive use and the risk of breast cancer. *N Engl J Med* 1986;315:405–11
23. Eskin BA. Malignant potential of benign breast lesions: indications for estrogen therapy. *J Am Med Assoc* 1991;266:1146
24. Hulka BS. Hormone-replacement therapy and the risk of breast cancer. *CA* 1990;40:289–96
25. Wingo PA, Layde PM, Lee NC, *et al*. The risk of breast cancer in postmenopausal women who have used estrogen replacement therapy. *J Am Med Assoc* 1987;257:209–15
26. Fitzgibbons PL, Hensen DE, Hutter RV. Benign breast changes and the risk for subsequent breast cancer: an update of the 1985 consensus statement. Cancer Committee of the College of American Pathologists. *Arch Pathol Lab Med* 1998;122:1053–5
27. Merrill JM. Estrogen replacement therapy after breast cancer. *J Am Med Assoc* 1992;267:568
28. Gapstur SM, Morrow M, Sellers TA. Hormone replacement therapy and risk of breast cancer with a favorable histology. *J Am Med Assoc* 1999;281:2091–7

29. Roth GS, Adelman RC. Hormone receptor changes during childhood and senescence: significance for aging research. *Exp Gerontol* 1975;10:1

30. American Fertility Society. Opinion on Estrogen Replacement. *Fertil Steril* 1987;47(Suppl 1):1-75

31. Steinberg KK, Thacker SB, Smith JS, *et al*. Review: a meta-analysis of the effect of estrogen replacement therapy and the risk of breast cancer. *J Am Med Assoc* 1991;265:1985-90

32. Thomas DB. Do hormones cause breast cancer? *Cancer Res* 1984;52:595

33. Jardines L. Clinical breast evaluation and management of a palpable breast mass. In Eskin BA, Asbell SO, Jardines L, eds. *Breast Diseases for the Primary Care Physician*. New York: Parthenon Publishing, 1999:25-36

34. Gordillo C. Breast cancer screening guidelines agreed on by AMA and other medically related organizations. *J Am Med Assoc* 1989;262:1155

35. Ciatto S, Cariaggi P, Bulgaresi P, *et al*. The value of routine cytologic examination of breast cyst fluids. *Acta Cytologica* 1987;31:301-4

36. Marchant DJ. The surgical treatment of breast cancer. *Maturitas* 1987;9:183-92

37. Watson DPH, McGuire M, Nicholson F, *et al*. Aspiration cytology and its relevance to the diagnosis of solid tumors of the breast. *Surg Gynecol Obstet* 1987; 165:435-41

38. Hindle WH, Nevin J. Breast aspiration cytology: a neglected gynecologic procedure. *Am J Obstet Gynecol* 1983;146:482

39. Sadowsky NL, Semine A, Harris JR. Breast imaging: a critical aspect of breast conserving treatment. *Cancer Res* 1990;65:2113

40. Pye JK, Mansell RE, Hughes LE. Clinical experience for drug treatment of mastalgia. *Lancet* 1985; 2:373-7

41. Peters F. Multicentre study of gestrinone in cyclical breast pain. *Lancet* 1992;339:205-8

42. Ghent WR, Eskin BA, Low DA, Hill LP. Iodine replacement in fibrocystic disease of the breast. *Can J Surg* 1993;36:453

43. Eskin BA, Ghent WR. Determination of iodine pathways in breast diseases by using replacement therapy. *Breast Cancer Res Treat* 1989;14:171

44. Krouse T, Eskin BA, Mobini J. Age related changes resembling fibrocystic disease in iodine-blocked rat breasts. *Arch Pathol Lab Med* 1979;103:631

45. Eskin BA, Funahashi H. Iodine deficiency and breast cancer: Japanese Symposium. *Int Council Cont Iodine Deficiency Disorders (WHO)* 1998;14:48

46. Eskin BA, Grotkowski CE, Connolly CP, Ghent WR. Different tissue responses for iodine and iodide in rat thyroid and mammary glands. *Biol Trace Element Res* 1995;49:9-19

47. Early Breast Cancer Trialists' Collaborative Group. Effects of adjuvant tamoxifen and of cytotoxic therapy on mortality in early breast cancer: an overview of 61 randomized trials among 28 896 women. *N Engl J Med* 1988;319:1681-92

48. Fisher B, Mauer M, Margolese R, *et al*. Five-year results of a randomized clinical trial comparing total mastectomy and segmental mastectomy with or without radiation in the treatment of breast cancer. *N Engl J Med* 1985;312:673

49. Walker KJ, Price-Thomas JM, Candlish W, *et al*. Influences of antioestrogen tamoxifen on normal breast tissue. *Br J Cancer* 1991;64:764-8

50. Crandall DL, Busler DE, Novak TJ, *et al*. Identification of estrogen receptor RNA in human breast and abdominal subcutaneous adipose tissue. *Biochem Biophys Res Commun* 1998;248:523-6

51. American Joint Committee on Cancer. Breast. In *AJCC Cancer Staging Manual*, 5th edn. Philadelphia: Lippincott-Raven, 1997:171-8

52. Asbell SO. Adjuvant therapy. In Eskin BA, Asbell SO, Jardines L, eds. *Breast Diseases for the Primary Care Physician*. New York: Parthenon Publishing, 1999:125-30

53. Winchester DP, Murphy GP, Bowman HE, *et al*. Surgical management of Stages 0, I, IIA breast cancer. *Cancer Res* 1990;65:2105

54. Scanlon EF. Progress in the treatment of early breast cancer. *Cancer Res* 1990;65:2110

16

Cognitive changes in the menopause

Karen L. Dahlman, Jennifer Hoblyn and Richard C. Mohs

Introduction

As the proportion of the population over age 50 increases, the field of geropsychology in general has expanded rapidly. Issues related to the menopause have also become the focus of much attention, with a large amount of this work centered on hormone replacement therapy and its effects on cognition, mood, vasomotor symptoms and sexuality of peri- and postmenopausal women. The intent of this chapter is to present a context in which to understand the effects of aging and of the menopause in particular on cognition. The first part of the chapter defines what constitutes normal aging, in terms of psychological issues and cognitive changes faced in the menopause and afterwards. This is contrasted with profiles of abnormal conditions in peri- and postmenopausal women, including discussions of both dementia and depression. The second part focuses on the effects of hormone treatment on cognitive functioning in peri- and postmenopausal women with and without dementia, as well as in depressed and non-depressed women. The final section evaluates the evidence regarding the impact of hormone replacement therapy on the risk of Alzheimer's disease.

Normal aging and cognition

A key issue in the assessment of aging patients is the need to discriminate between normal age-related intellectual changes and those changes that are clinically significant. Although many cognitive functions decline as part of the normal aging process[1,2], the extent and pattern of the decline varies according to both the individual and the type of function being examined. Aspects of cognitive functioning that deal with well-rehearsed, over-learned activities change very little across the life span. Other cognitive functions, including speeding tasks, processing of unfamiliar information, complex problem-solving, delayed recall, mental flexibility and perceptual manipulation tasks, do tend to decline as individuals age[3].

Considerable individual differences exist in terms of aging, and these differences often are first noticed by perimenopausal women. Cognitive functioning falls in a spectrum ranging from impaired to normal to successful at any given point in the aging process. Using the example of normative standards from the Wechsler Memory Scale[1], it is clear that those individuals who performed at the highest levels (99th percentile) in their youth, in a variety of cognitive domains, tend to decline relatively less throughout their life span. Not only do individuals who performed at lower levels (for example, 2nd percentile) when younger exhibit a marked decline as they age, but also the decline seen in lower-functioning individuals is more dramatic than that of individuals in the upper percentile ranges. The individuals at the top of the distribution consistently outperform those at the lower levels by a progressively greater extent as they become older (Figure 1).

The idea that normal adults who perform at higher baseline levels of intellectual function will exhibit little cognitive decline with age is supported by Rowe and Kahn's reports on successful aging[4,5]. These authors define successful aging as including three main components: low probability of disease and disease-related disability, high cognitive and physical functioning, and active engagement with life. Continuing engagement with life has two major elements: maintenance of interpersonal relations and productive activities. Membership of a social network is an

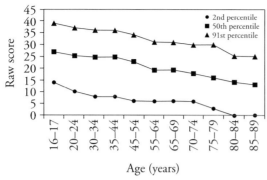

Figure 1 Lifespan changes in delayed recall scores for individuals with different baseline abilities: based on reference 1

important determinant of longevity[6]. Network membership research[7-9] has demonstrated that two types of supportive transactions may be prophylactic in aging: socioemotional and instrumental. Socioemotional transactions include expressions of respect and affection, while instrumental transactions comprise direct giving of services or money. It follows that women who have enjoyed lifelong higher levels of engagement, and who are accustomed to fulfilling and diverse relationships, will be more likely to adjust well to the menopause and ultimately to aging[10].

It is critical in the assessment of aging individuals to take into account the relative nature of observed cognitive deficits: relative, that is, to the patient's own previous levels of functioning. Current functioning, in terms of engagement in life as well as presence/absence of disease and cognitive normalcy, must be viewed against the individual's overall level of previous functioning.

Overall assessment

A history is necessary to establish premorbid levels of functioning in all areas of the individual's life. It should include relevant medical, family, social, occupational, educational, cultural and medication history, as well as substance abuse, if any, and a detailed description of the changes in functioning that precipitated the contact. It is important to establish the nature of the onset of these changes (whether abrupt or insidious), the progression of

these changes (stepwise or steady, worsening versus fluctuating versus improving) and the duration of the changes.

In addition to a thorough medical history, including a review of any diseases, psychiatric or medical, and known neurological disorders, history of head trauma, alcohol or other substance abuse as well as exposure to toxins should be reviewed. Because these and other contributing factors (for example human immunodeficiency virus (HIV), diabetes, urinary tract infection) may affect cognitive functioning, a careful interview documents any illness or infection, past or present. Medication history is an important part of the initial evaluation because drug-induced cognitive changes are among the most easily reversible. All medications, including over-the-counter formulas, could have an effect on cognition, especially in combination.

When performing a physical examination on a menopausal or postmenopausal woman, a brief neurological evaluation, designed to identify lesions, vascular illness and infection, is advisable. Illnesses, such as urinary tract infection or medication toxicity, are assessed in order to rule out or address delirium. The physical examination needs to incorporate a check for signs of contusions that may indicate either accidental injuries or domestic abuse of the patient. Keeping an eye open for such signs is particularly important, given studies showing that at least 28% of couples experience violence at some point and 16% of couples experience violence in a given year[11], and that patients who suffer from domestic abuse tend to seek treatment in primary care, not mental health, settings[12]. These patients will often present with other difficulties in addition to their physical complaints, including psychological and emotional distress, suicidality and substance abuse[13,14].

Family history

A family history of dementia and other conditions (such as Huntington's disease and schizophrenia) should be established, as the genetic component of these illnesses is significant[15-20]. It is important, for example, when evaluating patients who present with psychotic symptoms (i.e. delusions and hallucinations), to weigh family and personal history of schizophrenia in making a decision about the primary disorder in the clinical picture.

Social adaptation

The history taking should include a review of educational level, career and hobbies, along with socioeconomic, ethnic and cultural background. The evaluation should take into account the possibility of either minimization or exaggeration of symptoms. Information on major life events and social supports, and especially recent changes, is necessary, owing to their possible contribution to the individual's performance in tests of cognitive functioning. The frequency of changes in living situations, support systems and resources among elderly patients is common. The impact on a woman's adjustment with regard to changes in family structure as children move out of the home and begin independent lives may be profound[21]; changes for the worse in the marital relationship may be formidable as well.

Psychiatric conditions

Besides evaluating family history of psychiatric conditions, the physician must outline the patient's own psychiatric history[22]. If the patient does have a psychiatric history, the evaluator should ascertain whether the previous episodes were reactive or not, and what types of situations have precipitated onset of symptoms in the past.

Depression

The assessment of depression in patients presenting with cognitive impairment involves some level of sophistication in order to parse the relative contributions of affective, neurological and other medical illness[23]. This is critical because of treatment selection issues; if cognitive impairment is attributed to incipient dementia, a treatable affective disorder may be overlooked. If the patient's cognitive dysfunction can be attributed with some degree of certainty to depression, the clinician has strong reasons to pursue vigorous antidepressant treatment. The failure to treat a primary depression is potentially disastrous for a patient, especially given the fairly good response of depressed patients in general to various treatments[24-26]. How-

ever, if the patient's cognitive impairment is due to a primary dementing illness, then aggressive treatment of depressive symptoms may not substantially improve the quality of the patient's life. Overall, the issue is one of careful assessment of the clinical picture[27].

The differential diagnosis of behavioral and cognitive disorders in aging patients is made more complicated by depression, which can produce symptoms that mimic those of early dementia. This is understandable, given evidence from neuroimaging studies showing that patients with late-onset depression have enlarged ventricles and decreased brain density[28]. Estimates of the incidence of depression in the elderly indicate that it may be slightly higher among persons aged 65 and older than in the younger population[29,30], and it may be the most common emotional problem among elderly patients[31,32]. Depressive symptoms are often precipitated by either a traumatic loss of a family member, or an event such as retirement or poor health. In cases such as these, the depression is reactive, and fits better with the diagnosis of 'adjustment disorder with depressed mood' than with that of 'major depressive disorder'. While a chronic physical illness greatly increases the likelihood of depression in an older patient, making the diagnosis of depression in a physically sick patient is often complicated by the iatrogenic factors. Depressive symptoms may arise either from an illness itself or from medication used to treat it[33,34].

Assessment of depression in the perimenopausal patient usually begins with clinical interview of the patient, and ideally this is supplemented by corroborative information from a family member. The assessment must focus on objective symptoms of depression, including mood, behavior, anxiety and vegetative symptoms such as sleep disturbance, anhedonia, anergia and loss of appetite, as well as the subjective experiences outlined by the individual. The diagnosis of perimenopause-related depression is made in the same way as that for depression at any other time in the life span; however, with the perimenopausal woman, the depression must occur in the context of endocrine evidence of the perimenopause. Major and/or less significant depression may occur in the perimenopause. Women may also present with a mixed anxiety–depressive disorder.

The affective symptoms are often described[35] as having a gradual onset, and sometimes as occurring during hot flushes. It is the relative prominence of the mood and behavioral symptoms compared with the somatic complaints that leads to the diagnosis of a depressive syndrome. One reliable scale frequently used to measure depression is the Beck Depression Inventory-II, in which the patient checks 21 four-choice statements presented on a single page for the choice or choices most appropriate. The statements refer to the following areas: sadness, pessimism/discouragement, sense of failure, dissatisfaction, guilt, expectation of punishment, self-dislike, self-blame, suicidality, tearfulness, irritability, social withdrawal, indecisiveness, unattractiveness, work difficulty, sleep disruption, fatigue, appetite loss, weight loss, somatization and diminished libido[36].

Prevalence of depression in the perimenopause

It remains controversial whether postmenopausal women are more vulnerable to the development of depression. Improvement in mood, attention, concentration and libido in postmenopausal women without depression has been observed with estrogen replacement therapy[37,38]. Because of the number of women entering the menopause at any given time, it is important to understand the nature of the relationship between affective disorders and the perimenopause. Weissman[39] suggests a peak in the onset of depressive illness during the perimenopausal years (ages 45–50). Other writers (for example, reference 40) suggest that the etiology of major depressive illness occurring in the context of the menopause may be related to changes in reproductive hormones that occur at that time. Rather than the direct effects of these hormones, or the absolute levels of the hormones, it may be the rate of change of hormone levels or their indirect effects on neurotransmitter, neuroendocrine or circadian systems that lead to mood alteration[41-44]. In addition to the etiology of depression in perimenopausal women being fundamentally different from that in other patient groups, both the nature of the depression itself and response to treatment may also be unique[35].

Menopause-related depression is defined by the onset of depression (major or minor) in association with changes in an individual's menstrual cycle, and evidence of endocrine changes (for example elevations of plasma follicle stimulating hormone (FSH) levels). Vasomotor or other physiological symptoms associated with the menopause may lead to affective changes, rather than the menopause status itself. Persistent hot flushes may disturb sleep patterns, which can result in fatigue, diminished ability to concentrate and irritability; these symptoms may disrupt daily functioning.

Some investigators have concluded that there is little evidence for a relationship between perimenopause and depression[45-47]. More recently, however, epidemiological studies and clinic-based surveys have reported that as many as 10% of women participating in longitudinal community-based studies have been observed to have perimenopause-related changes in mood[48,49]. Other reports indicate that both perimenopausal and postmenopausal women have a higher prevalence of depressive symptoms than do premenopausal women, and that perimenopausal women are more symptomatic than postmenopausal women[50-52].

Effects of hormone replacement therapy on menopausal depression

Hormone replacement therapy (HRT) has been approved for the prevention of osteoporosis[53,54], cardiovascular disease[55] and postmenopausal genitourinary problems. Early studies have suggested that HRT may be useful for treatment of depression and cognitive changes associated with the menopause. These studies were eagerly anticipated, as women may now reasonably expect to live a third of their lives following the menopause, and preventive interventions potentially improve the quality of those years for millions of women internationally. HRT most commonly consists of estrogen and progesterone administered in a cyclical manner. A number of different estrogen preparations with and without progesterone have been studied in both mood and cognitive disorders. Unfortunately, negative mood symptoms may be associated with cyclical estrogen and progesterone administration, particularly after the introduction of progesterone in the treatment cycle. These effects seem to be dose-related, increasing with the progesterone dose[56,57].

Estrogen acts as a serotoninergic and cholinergic agonist, but also selectively increases norepinephrine in the brain; in addition, administration of estrogen has been shown to decrease dopamine type-2 receptors, and possibly other dopamine receptor subtypes[41]. It has mixed actions on endorphins. It has been suggested that decreases in postmenopausal serotoninergic and noradrenergic functioning are associated with declining levels in estrogen. It is unclear whether HRT decreases the vulnerability caused by this hypofunctioning. Studies have suggested that monoamine oxidase (MAO) activity is decreased by estrogen administration in depressed postmenopausal women[42] and that fluctuations in MAO activity vary with estrogen levels during the menstrual cycle[43]. Recent work suggests that estrogen augmentation to antidepressant medication may benefit women with menopausal depression[44,58,59], although the addition of estrogen supplements to tricyclic antidepressants (TCAs) may induce rapid mood cycling or other undesirable side-effects in some patients[60,61]. Estrogen as a monotherapy does not seem to have impressive antidepressant properties but may be useful for mood stabilization[62,63].

Cognitive changes in the menopause

It has long been suspected that estrogen deficiency may be a cause of memory loss in postmenopausal women[22]. While it has been reported that the female-to-male gender ratio for major depression increases during middle age from approximately 2 : 1 to approximately 3–4 : 1[64,65], one recent large-scale study found weak or absent gender differences in cognitive decline with aging[66]. These findings, known as the Rancho Bernardo Study, do not support the idea that estrogen deficiency is associated with a decline in cognitive functioning among postmenopausal women. A recent review of the literature on estrogen effects on cognition in menopausal women concluded that results are, at best, inconsistent. There are quite a few studies that demonstrate a clear improvement on verbal recall tasks, but no changes in visual recall tasks (for example, references 67–69), while others show no

effects of estrogen treatment on memory[37,70]. A study by Resnick and colleagues[71] demonstrates an improvement in visual memory. In general, the epidemiological evidence for an association between estrogen and cognitive function among postmenopausal women remains controversial[72-74]. Overall, the evidence for a positive relationship comes primarily from randomized clinical trials, which suggest an acute effect on specific verbal memory tasks[75] as well as some tasks that incorporate concept formation and reasoning.

A recent study demonstrates that estrogen in a therapeutic dosage alters brain activation patterns in postmenopausal women during the performance of certain memory tasks, although no significant *performance* differences were found[76]. Some writers have pointed out that the equivocal data on estrogen effects on cognition in menopausal women may be due to the artifacts of group membership. In at least one large-scale, community-based study, ever-users had significantly higher levels of education, and presumably IQ, than never-users[67]. Advanced education may be more protective of cognitive function in later life than HRT, as is demonstrated by a recent large-scale study[77]. Other factors that may contribute towards explaining inconsistencies in the data produced by these studies include concomitant medication use, different types of estrogen preparations and a disparity in psychometric tests used as dependent variables. In summary, although there is some encouraging evidence from observational studies for the beneficial use of estrogen on cognitive function, especially verbal memory, that evidence is rather questionable because of methodological inconsistencies both within and between studies. There is currently inadequate evidence from randomized controlled trials to support the conclusion that HRT improves cognitive function in postmenopausal women.

Rationale for HRT treatment of postmenopausal women with dementia

The rationale for estrogen treatment for Alzheimer's disease is based on preclinical, epidemiological and preliminary treatment studies[78]. Evidence from these studies indicates that estrogen receptors are present in the nucleus basilus of

Meynert[79], hippocampus and hypothalamus[80]. A decline in choline acetyltransferase activity in the frontal cortex and hippocampus can be prevented by the administration of estrogen[81,82]. Estrogen has been shown to mediate neuronal sprouting response to injury and survival. It also potentiates neurite outgrowth, and dendritic spine and synapse formation[83,84]. The changes seen in the estrous cycle are also seen in the hippocampus, an area well known to be associated with memory and learning. Here, the rise in progesterone is associated with involution of neuronal elements in the CA1 region, a phenomenon that is also reversed by estrogen use[85].

A mechanism whereby estrogen affects cognition in Alzheimer's disease is still not well understood. There are several possibilities: Hagino's work with rats[86] demonstrated that early-aging females exhibited a decrease in hippocampal function that was restored with supplemental estradiol administration. Arai and colleagues suggested[87] that estrogen may play a role in the reparative neuronal response to injury. Arimatsu and Hatanaka demonstrated[84] that estrogen enhanced the survival of amygdala neurones in culture. Goldman's work[88] revealed an increase in cerebral blood flow to the frontal cortex, the hippocampus, the basal ganglia and the cerebellum with administration of estrogen to rats, a finding that was more robust in female than in male rats.

The area of the central nervous system responsive to estrogen possesses estrogen receptors, and these areas, including the basal forebrain nuclei and cholinergic neurones, are the ones predominantly affected in Alzheimer's disease[89]. These cholinergic neurones with estrogen receptors also have receptors for nerve growth factor, whose expression is modulated by the hormone. Estrogen also affects norepinephrine and other neurotransmitter systems. Beta-endorphin neurones are lost in the face of chronic estradiol exposure. Female patients with Alzheimer's disease have been reported to have lower serum estrone sulfate levels than non-senile females[79].

Estrogen may affect the progression of Alzheimer's disease via its effects on the metabolism of amyloid precursor protein (APP)[90]. In the cell culture, physiological concentration of 17β-estradiol increases the secretory metabolism of the soluble fragment of APP without increasing the intracellular levels of APP. Hence, the deposition of β-amyloid and plaque formation may be reduced. Estrogen reduces plasma levels of apolipoprotein E[91,92]. Plaque formation may also be reduced by the modification of the inflammatory response by estrogen, via its effects of interleukin 6, a cytokine postulated to participate in plaque formation[93,94]. Estrogen has also been found to have antioxidant properties[95,96] via its action on free radicals. Estrogen prevents platelet aggregation by influencing the production of prostacyclin, which opposes thromboxane. It is thought to do this via cycloxygenase 2 and phospholipase stimulation. Prostaglandins are thought to be possible mediators of histopathological damage in Alzheimer's disease; they inhibit nitric oxide (NO) production and decrease NO synthetase mRNA, whereas estrogen increases NO production by upgrading NO synthetase[97]. This influence is also seen in vessel walls; estrogen may exert antihypertensive effects in premenopausal women; other studies have revealed that it increases both cerebral blood flow and cerebral glucose utilization[98–100].

HRT has been shown to blunt stress-induced cortisol levels; it is known that cortisol levels are elevated in Alzheimer's disease. Stress has detrimental effects on memory and may lead to neuronal damage in the hippocampus. After the menopause, aromatization of androgens provides most estrogen. Studies have demonstrated that higher weights in women with Alzheimer's disease are associated with higher scores on some measures of cognitive testing.

HRT and risk of Alzheimer's disease

The first studies of estrogen therapy effects on cognitive function yielded results suggesting that improvements were found in language comprehension, naming and arithmetic. Ditkoff and colleagues[37], Kampen and Sherwin[101] and Fillet and co-workers[102] reported improvements in cognition with estradiol treatment in postmenopausal women with Alzheimer's disease. This was later confirmed by a placebo-controlled double-blind trial by Honjo and associates[103]. Ohkura's group[104] also demonstrated increases in cerebral blood flow. Four open-label and two double-blind placebo-controlled trials with relatively small patient samples reported improvements in cognition with estradiol treatment in postmenopausal women with Alzheimer's disease. One study showed that the improvement in cognitive scores with estrogen in Alzheimer's disease was independent of possible confounding mood-elevating effects. Three recent epidemiological studies are notable for the inclusion of information about women's use of estrogen prior to the onset of dementia symptoms. Paganini-Hill and Henderson[105] performed a case-controlled study nested within a large prospective cohort of women in a retirement community in southern California. The results showed that ever-users of HRT had a 30% decreased risk of developing Alzheimer's disease compared to never-users, with a positive relationship between dosage and duration. A population based case–control study at the Group Health Cooperative in Seattle, Washington found no relationship between estrogen use and development of Alzheimer's disease[106]. Results from another large-sample longitudinal study[107] of elderly women in New York City indicate that 12.5% of women reported taking estrogen after the menopause. Among this group, the age of Alzheimer's disease onset was significantly later, with a reduced relative risk of 5.8% adjusted for education, ethnic origin and apolipoprotein E genotype, compared with those not taking estrogen. Results also confirmed those of other investigators, that HRT use for more than 1 year in duration was associated with a greater reduction in risk. Barrett-Connor and Kritz-Silverstein[70] did not find an association between the use of estrogen and impaired cognitive function in late life.

Ohkura and colleagues[108] recently published a study of seven patients with mild to moderate dementia of the Alzheimer's type who received long-term low-dose HRT over a period of 5–45 months. Four of the seven showed improvements on a brief cognitive rating scale and on a dementia rating scale over pretreatment levels during HRT; these results decreased when HRT was stopped.

Schneider and associates[109] examined the effects of HRT in response to tacrine in patients with Alzheimer's disease. Results indicated that women taking HRT performed better on measures of cognition and overall functioning than those without. The authors suggested that the improvements may have been related to the increase in choline acetyltransferase activity in the hippocampus.

Conclusions

Although there is currently an enhanced awareness of the prevalence of both mood and cognitive disorders with onset in the menopausal years of a woman's life, it is vital that a comprehensive assessment be performed to maximize potential treatments. In addition to research initiatives focused on HRT, large case-controlled and cohort studies will be required to clarify the impact of other hormonal interventions such as the contraceptive pill, life-style choices and antiestrogenic agents on the risk of developing Alzheimer's disease later in life. A multicenter double-blind trial comparing placebo with two strengths of estrogen preparation is currently under way. Further research continues into the effects of estrogen combined with antioxidants, nerve growth factors, anti-inflammatory agents and cholinergic agents.

Review of the research to date indicates that the evidence for a beneficial effect of HRT on cognition in normal peri- or postmenopausal women is inconclusive. However, there is certainly no evidence that such treatment has any deleterious effects on either emotional or cognitive functioning. Studies that seem to provide evidence of modest cognitive improvements due to HRT have yet to be standardized and replicated. It remains to be clarified whether estrogen has uses as a treatment once Alzheimer's disease has appeared, or simply as a preventive measure. In terms of the utility of HRT as a treatment for depression, there is some evidence that it is effective when used as an augmentation to enhance other psychopharmacological interventions.

References

1. Wechsler D. *Wechsler Memory Scale - III Administration and Scoring Manual*. San Antonio, TX: The Psychological Corporation, 1997

2. Wechsler D. *Wechsler Adult Intelligence Scale - III Administration and Scoring Manual*. San Antonio, TX: The Psychological Corporation, 1997

3. Harvey PD, Dahlman KL. Neuropsychological evaluation of dementia. In Chalev A, ed. *Neuropsychological Assessment of Neuropsychiatric Disorders*. Washington: American Psychiatric Press, 1999: 329–72

4. Rowe JW, Kahn RL. Usual and successful aging. *Science* 1987;237:143–8

5. Rowe JW, Kahn RL. Successful aging. *Gerontologist* 1997;37:433–40

6. House JS, Landis KR, Umberson D. Social relationships and health. *Science* 1988;241:540–5

7. Cassel J. The contribution of social environment to host resistance: the fourth Wade Hampton Frost lecture. *Am J Epidemiol* 1976;104:107–23

8. Kahn RL, Byosiere P. Stress in organizations. In Dunnette MD, Hough LM, eds. *Handbook of Industrial and Organizational Psychology* 2nd edn. Palo Alto, CA: Consulting Psychologists Press, 1992;3:571–650

9. Glass TA, Seeman TE, Herzog AR, Kahn RL, Berkman LF. Changes in productivity in late adulthood: MacArthur Studies of Successful Aging. *J Gerontol Soc Sci* 1995;50B:S65–76

10. Anderson E, Hamburger S, Liu JH, Rebar RW. Characteristics of menopausal women seeking assistance. *Am J Obstet Gynecol* 1987;156:428–33

11. Straus MA, Gelles RJ. Societal change and change in family violence from 1975 to 1985 as revealed by two national surveys. *J Marriage Fam* 1986;48: 465–79

12. Samson AY, Benson S, Beck A, Price D, Nimmer C. Post traumatic stress disorder in primary care. *J Fam Pract* 1999;48:222–7

13. Van Hasselt VB, Morrison RL, Bellack AS, Hersen M. Overview. In Van Hasselt VB, Morrison RL, Bellack AS, Hersen M, eds. *Handbook of Family Violence*. New York: Plenum Press, 1988:3–8

14. Umberson D, Anderson K, Glick J, Shapiro A. Domestic violence, personal control and gender. *J Marriage Fam* 1998;60:442–52

15. Bachman DL, Wolf PA, Linn RT, *et al.* Incidence of dementia and probable Alzheimer's disease in a general population: The Framingham Study. *Neurology* 1993;43:515–19

16. Bierer LM, Silverman JM, Mohs RC, *et al.* Morbid risk to first degree relatives of neuropathologically confirmed cases of Alzheimer's disease. *Dementia* 1992;3:134–9

17. Goldberg TE, Ragland JD, Torrey EF, *et al.* Neuropsychological assessment of monozygotic twins discordant for schizophrenia. *Arch Gen Psychiatry* 1990;47:1066

18. Mayeux R, Ottman R, Tang MX, *et al.* Genetic susceptibility and head injury as risk factors for Alzheimer's disease among community dwelling elderly persons and their first degree relatives. *Ann Neurol* 1993;33:494–501

19. Neale JM, Oltmanns TF. *Schizophrenia*. New York: John Wiley, 1980

20. Schellenberg GD, Bird TD, Wijsman EM, *et al.* Genetic linkage evidence for a familial Alzheimer's disease locus on chromosome 14. *Science* 1992;258:668–71

21. Carter BF, Fink PJ. Psychiatric myths of the menopause. In Eskin B, ed. *The Menopause: Comprehensive Management*, 3rd edn. New York: Field & Wood Medical Publishers, Inc., 1994

22. Sherwin BB. Cognitive assessment of postmenopausal women and general assessment of their mental health. *Psychopharmacol Bull* 1998;34:323–6

23. Schmidt PJ, Roca CA, Block M, Rubinow DR. The perimenopause and affective disorders. *Semin Reprod Endocrinol* 1997;15:91–100

24. Benedict KB, Nacost DB. Dementia and depression: a framework for addressing difficulties in differential diagnosis. *Clin Psychol Rev* 1990;10: 513–37

25. Koenig HG, Blazer DG. Mood disorders and suicide. In Birren JE, Sloane RB, Cohen GD, eds. *Handbook of Mental Health and Aging*, 2nd edn. San Diego, CA: Academic Press, 1992: 379–407

26. Salzman C, Nevis-Olesen J. Psychopharmacologic treatment. In Birren JE, Sloane RB, Cohen GD, eds. *Handbook of Mental Health and Aging*, 2nd edn. San Diego, CA: Academic Press, 1992:722–62

27. Paquette I, Ska B, Joanette Y. Delusions, hallucinations, and depression in a population-based, epidemiological sample of demented subjects. In Bergener M, Finkel SI, eds. *Treating Alzheimer's and Other Dementias*. New York: Springer Publishing Co., 1995:172–83

28. Alexopoulous GS, Young RC, Abrams RC, *et al.* Chronicity and relapse in geriatric depression. *Biol Psychiatry* 1989;26:551–64

29. Blazer D. The epidemiology of late life depression. *J Am Geriatr Soc* 1982;30:587–92

30. Marcopulos BA. Pseudodementia, dementia and depression: test differentiation. In Hunt T, Lindley CJ, eds. *Testing Older Adults: A Reference Guide for Geropsychological Assessments*. Austin, TX: Pro-Ed, 1989:70–91

31. Hassinger M, Smith G, LaRue A. Assessing depression in older adults. In Hunt T, Lindley CJ, eds. *Testing Older Adults: A Reference Guide for Geropsychological Assessments*. Austin, TX: Pro-Ed, 1989: 92-121

32. Thompson LW, Gong V, Haskins E, Gallagher D. Assessment of depression and dementia during the late years. In Schaie KW, ed. *Annual Review of Gerontology and Geriatrics*. New York: Springer, 1987:295-324

33. Jenike MA. Depression and other psychiatric disorders. In Albert MS, Moss M, eds. *Geriatric Neuropsychology* New York: Guilford Press, 1988: 115-44

34. Greenblatt DJ, Harmatz JS, Shapiro L, Engelhardt N, Gouthro TA, Shader RI. Sensitivity to triazolam in the elderly. *N Engl J Med* 1991;324:1691-8

35. Schmidt PJ, Roca CA, Rubinow DR. Clinical evaluation in studies of perimenopausal women: position paper. *Psychopharmacol Bull* 1998;34: 309-11

36. Beck AT, Steer RA. *Beck Depression Inventory Manual*. San Antonio, TX: Psychological Corporation, 1993

37. Ditkoff EC, Crary WG, Cristo M, Lobo RA. Estrogen improves psychological function in asymptomatic postmenopausal women. *Obstet Gynecol* 1991;78:991-5

38. Furuhjelm M, Fedor-Freybergh P. The influence of estrogens on the psyche in climacteric and post-menopausal women. In Van Keep, PA, Greenblatt RB, Albeaux-Femet, MM, eds. *Consensus on Menopause Research*. Baltimore, MD: Baltimore University Park Press, 1976:84-93

39. Weissman MW. Epidemiology of major depression in women. Women and the controversies in hormonal replacement therapy. Presented at the *American Psychiatric Association Annual Meeting*, New York, 4 May 1996

40. Haynes P, Parry BL. Mood disorders and the reproductive cycle: affective disorders during the menopause and premenstrual dysphoric disorder. *Psychopharmacol Bull* 1998;34:313-18

41. Halbreich U. Role of estrogen in postmenopausal depression. *Neurology* 1997;48(Suppl 7):516-19

42. Holsboer F, Benkert O, Demisch L. Changes in MAO activity during estrogen treatment of females with endogenous depression. *Mod Probl Pharmacopsychiatry* 1983;19:321-6

43. Belmaker RH. The lessons of platelet monoamine. *Psychol Med* 1984;14:249-53

44. Schneider LS, Small GW, Hamilton SH, Bystritsky A, Nemeroff CB, Meyers BS, the Fluoxetine Collaborative Study Group. Estrogen replacement and response to fluoxetine in a multi-center geriatric depression trial. *Am J Geriatr Psychiatry* 1997;5:97-106

45. Weissman MM. The myth of involutional melancholia. *J Am Med Assoc* 1979;242:742-4

46. Winokur G. Depression in the menopause. *Am J Psychiatry* 1973;130:92-3

47. Winokur G, Cadoret R. The irrelevance of the menopause to depressive disease. In Sachar EJ, ed. *Topics in Psychoendocrinology*. New York: Grune and Stratton, 1975:59-66

48. Hunter H. The South-East England longitudinal study of the climacteric and menopause. *Maturitas* 1992;14:117-26

49. Matthews KA. Myths and realities of the menopause. *Psychosom Med* 1992;54:1-9

50. Dennerstein L, Smith AMA, Morse C, *et al*. Menopausal symptoms in Australian women. *Med J Aust* 1993;159:232-6

51. Hay AG, Bancroft J, Johnstone EC. Affective symptoms in women attending a menopause clinic. *Br J Psychiatry* 1994;164:513-16

52. Stewart DE, Boydell K, Derzko C, Marshall V. Psychologic distress during the menopausal years in women attending a menopause clinic. *Int J Psychiatry Med* 1992;22:213-20

53. Belchetz P. Hormonal treatment of postmenopausal women. *N Engl J Med* 1994;330:1062-71

54. Lindsay R. Why do oestrogens prevent bone loss? *Baillière's Clin Obstet Gynaecol* 1991;5:837-52

55. Stampfer MJ, Colditz GA, Willett WC, *et al*. Postmenopausal estrogen therapy and cardiovascular disease: ten year follow up from the Nurses' Health Study. *N Engl J Med* 1991;325: 756-62

56. Magos AL, Collins WP, Studd JW. Management of the premenstrual syndrome by subcutaneous implants of estradiol. *J Psychosom Obstet Gynaecol* 1984;3:93-9

57. Magos AL, Brewster E, Singh R, O'Dowd T, Brincat M, Studd JW. The effects of norethisterone in postmenopausal women on estrogen replacement therapy: a model for the premenstrual syndrome. *Br J Obstet Gynaecol* 1986; 93:1290-6

58. Klaiber EL, Broverman DM, Vogel W, Kobayashi Y. Estrogen therapy for severe persistent depressions in women. *Arch Gen Psychiatry* 1979;36:550-4

59. Stahl SM. Role of hormone therapies for refractory depression. Presented at the *American Psychiatric Association Annual Meeting* New York, 4 May 1996

60. Oppenheim G. A case of rapid mood cycling with estrogen: implications for therapy. *J Clin Psychiatry* 1984;45:34-5

61. Shapira B, Oppenheim G, Zohar J, Segal M, Malach D, Belmaker R. Lack of efficacy of estrogen supplementation to imipramine in resistant female depressives. *Biol Psychiatry* 1985;20:570-83

62. Stahl SM. Augmentation of antidepressants by estrogen. *Psychopharmacol Bull* 1998;34:319-21

63. Schneider MA, Brotherton PL, Hailes J. The effect of exogenous oestrogens on depression in menopausal women. *Med J Aust* 1977;2:162-3

64. Kessler RC, McGonagle KA, Swartz M, *et al.* Sex and depression in the National Comorbidity Survey. I. Lifetime prevalence, chronicity and recurrence. *J Affect Disord* 1993;29:85–96

65. Weissman MM, Leaf PJ, Tischler GL, *et al.* Affective disorders in five United States communities. *Psychol Med* 1988;18:141–53

66. Barrett-Connor E, Kritz-Silverstein D. Gender differences in cognitive function with age: The Rancho Bernardo Study. *J Am Geriatr Soc* 1999;47: 159–64

67. Jacobs DM, Tang MX, Stern Y, *et al.* Cognitive function in nondemented older women who took estrogen after menopause. *Neurology* 1998;50: 368–73

68. Sherwin BB, Philips S. Estrogen and cognitive functioning in surgically menopausal women. *Ann NY Acad Sci* 1990;592:474–5

69. Philips S, Sherwin BB. Effects of estrogen on memory function in surgically menopausal women. *Psychoneuroendocrinology* 1992;17:485–95

70. Barrett-Connor E, Kritz-Silverstein D. Estrogen replacement therapy and cognitive function in older women. *J Am Med Assoc* 1993;269:2637–41

71. Resnick SM, Metter EJ, Zonderman AB. Estrogen replacement therapy and longitudinal decline in visual memory: a possible protective effect? *Neurology* 1997;49:1491–7

72. Birge SJ. The role of estrogen in the treatment of Alzheimer's disease. *Neurology* 1997;48(Suppl 7): S36–41

73. Haskell SG, Richardson ED, Horwitz RI. The effect of estrogen replacement therapy on cognitive function in women: a critical review of the literature. *J Clin Epidemiol* 1997;50:1249–64

74. Henderson VW. The epidemiology of estrogen replacement therapy and Alzheimer's disease. *Neurology* 1997;48(Suppl 7):S27–35

75. Sherwin BB. Estrogen and/or androgen replacement therapy and cognitive functioning in surgically menopausal women. *Psychoneuroendocrinology* 1988;13:345–57

76. Shaywitz SE, Shaywitz BA, Pugh KR, *et al.* Effect of estrogen on brain activation patterns in postmenopausal women during working memory tasks. *J Am Med Assoc* 1999;281:1197–202

77. Matthews KA, Cauley J, Kristine Y, Zmuda JM. Estrogen replacement therapy and cognitive decline in older community women. *J Am Geriatr Soc* 1999;47:518–23

78. Kawas C, Resnick S, Morrison A, *et al.* A prospective study of estrogen replacement therapy and the risk of developing Alzheimer's disease: the Baltimore Longitudinal Study of Aging. *Neurology* 1997;48:1517–21

79. Luine V, McEwen BS. Sex differences in cholinergic enzymes of diagonal band nuclei in the rat preoptic area. *Neuroendocrinology* 1983;36: 475–82

80. Gould E, Wooley C, Franfurt M, McEwen BS. Gonadal steroids regulate dendritic spine density in hippocampal pyramidal cells in adulthood. *N Neurosci* 1990;10:1286–91

81. Singh M, Meyer EM, Huang FS, *et al.* Ovariectomy reduces CHAT activity and NGF mRNA levels in the frontal cortex and hippocampus of the female Sprague-Dawley rat. *Abstr Soc Neurosci* 1993;19:1254

82. Singh M, Meyer EM, Simpkins JW. The effect of ovariectomy and estradiol replacement on brain derived neurotrophic factor messenger ribonucleic acid expression in cortical and hippocampal brain regions of female Sprague-Dawley rats. *Endocrinology* 1995;136:2320–4

83. Simpkins JW, Meharvan S, Bishop J. The potential role for estrogen replacement therapy in the treatment of the cognitive decline and neurodegeneration associated with Alzheimer's disease. *Neurobiol Aging* 1994;15:195–7

84. Arimatsu Y, Hatanaka H. Estrogen treatment enhances survival of cultured amygdala neurons in a defined medium. *Dev Brain Res* 1986;26: 151–9

85. Woolley CS, McEwan BS. Estradiol mediates fluctuation in hippocampal synapse density during the estrous cycle in the adult. *J Neurosci* 1992;12: 2549–54

86. Hagino N. Aged limbic system: interactions of estrogen with catecholaminergic and peptidergic synaptic transmissions. *Biomed Res* 1981;2: 85–108

87. Arai Y, Matsumoto A, Nishizuka M. Synaptogenic action of estrogen on the hypothalamic arcuate nucleus (ARCN) of the developing rat brain and of the deafferented adult brain in female rats. In Dorner G, Kawakami M, eds. *Hormones and Brain Development* North Holland: Elsevier, 1978:43–8

88. Goldman H, Skelley EB, Sandman CA, *et al.* Hormones and regional blood flow. *Pharmacol Biochem Behav* 1976;5(Suppl 1):165–9

89. Toran-Allerand CD, Miranda RC, Betham WDL, *et al.* Estrogen receptors co-localize with low-affinity nerve growth factor receptors in cholinergic neurons of the basal forebrain. *Proc Natl Acad Sci USA* 1992;89:4668–72

90. Jaffe AB, Toran-Allerand CD, Greengard P, Gandy SE. Estrogen regulates metabolism of Alzheimer amyloid beta precursor protein. *J Biochem* 1994;269:13065–8

91. Honjo H, Tanaka K, Kashiwagi T, *et al.* Senile dementia – Alzheimer's type and estrogen. *Horm Metab Res* 1995;27:204–7

92. Applebaum-Bowden D, McClean P, Steinmetz A, *et al.* Lipoprotein, apolipoprotein, and lipolytic enzyme changes following estrogen administration in post menopausal women. *J Lipid Res* 1989;30:895–906

93. Bauer J, Ganter U, Strauss S, *et al*. The participation of interleukin-6 in pathogenesis of Alzheimer's disease. *Res Immunol* 1992;43:650–7

94. Ershler WB. Interleukin-6: a cytokine for gerontologists. *J Am Geriatr Soc* 1993;41:176–81

95. Niki E, Nakano M. Estrogens as antioxidants. *Meth Enzymol* 1990;186:330–3

96. Mooradian AD. Antioxidant properties of steroids. *J Steroid Biochem Mol Biol* 1993;45:509–11

97. Gambassi G, Landi F, Bernabei R. Oestrogen and Alzheimer's disease [Letter]. *Lancet* 1996;348:1029

98. Ohkura T, Isse K, Akazawa K, *et al*. Evaluation of estrogen treatment in female patients with dementia of the Alzheimer's type. *Endocr J* 1994; 41:361–71

99. Belfort MA, Saade GR, Snabes M, *et al*. Hormonal status affects the reactivity of the cerebral vasculature. *Am J Obstet Gynecol* 1995;172:1273–8

100. Bishop J, Simpkins JW. Role of estrogens in peripheral and cerebral glucose utilization. *Rev Neurosci* 1992;3:121–37

101. Kampen DL, Sherwin BB. Estrogen use and verbal memory in healthy postmenopausal women. *Obstet Gynecol* 1994;83:979–83

102. Fillet H, Weinraub H, Cholst L, *et al*. Observations in a preliminary open trial of estradiol therapy for senile dementia – Alzheimer's type. *Psychoneuroendocrinology* 1986;11:337–45

103. Honjo H, Ogino Y, Tanaka K, *et al*. An effect of conjugated estrogen to cognitive impairment in women with senile dementia – Alzheimer's type: a placebo controlled double blind study. *J Menopause Soc* 1993;1:167–71

104. Ohkura T, Isse K, Akazawa K, *et al*. Low dose estrogen replacement therapy for Alzheimer's disease in women. *Menopause* 1994;1:125–30

105. Paganini-Hill A, Henderson VW. Estrogen replacement therapy and risk of Alzheimer's disease. *Arch Intern Med* 1996;156:2213–17

106. Brenner D, Kukull WA, Stergachis A, *et al*. Postmenopausal estrogen replacement therapy and the risk of Alzheimer's disease: a population-based case-controlled study. *Am J Epidemiol* 1994;140: 262–7

107. Tang MX, Jacobs D, Stern Y, *et al*. Effects of estrogen during menopause on risk and age of onset of Alzheimer's disease. *Lancet* 1996;348:429–32

108. Ohkura T, Isse K, Akazawa K, *et al*. Long term estrogen replacement therapy in female patients with dementia of the Alzheimer's type: 7 case reports. *Dementia* 1995;00:99–107

109. Schneider LS, Farlow MR, Henderson VW, Pogoda JM. Effects of estrogen replacement therapy on response to tacrine in patients with Alzheimer's disease. *Neurology* 1996;46:1580–4

17

Nutritional aspects of the menopause

Mona R. Sutnick

Nutritional requirements

Nutrition plays a vital role in the health of women of all ages. An extensive body of literature documents the role of diet and nutrients during growth and development and during pregnancy and lactation. There is less information about the nutritional needs of women beyond the child-bearing years. This situation is improving as a result of two trends: the aging of the American population has stimulated interest in changes in nutritional needs in adulthood while concern about osteoporosis is focusing particular attention on certain of the nutritional needs of women during the peri- and postmenopausal periods.

Nutritional requirements

The recommended dietary allowances (RDAs) are the standards most often employed in evaluating American diets. Because the are used so commonly, a word about the RDAs is in order. Historically, the RDAs go back to 1943 when the first edition, listing ten nutrients, was published. The intent of those recommendations was to provide guidance in determining military rations and feeding of groups of people during wartime conditions. In the years since the first edition, the guide has been periodically revised and updated, with the tenth edition having appeared in 1989[1]. This remains the most recent version of the RDAs. Emerging concepts of optimal nutrition and the recognition that nutrients may play health-promoting roles in quantities larger than those required to prevent deficiencies complicate efforts to produce a new set of standards.

The tenth edition of the RDAs lists recommended levels of energy, protein, 11 vitamins and seven minerals. The RDAs for vitamin K and selenium are included for the first time. Ranges of safe and adequate intakes are given for two additional vitamins and five trace elements, for which there is insufficient information to recommend specific allowances. A separate table lists estimated minimum requirements for sodium, chloride and potassium for healthy persons.

The levels of nutrients recommended in the RDAs are defined as '... levels of intake of essential nutrients that, on the basis of scientific knowledge, are judged by the Food and Nutrition Board to be adequate to meet the known nutrient needs of practically all healthy persons'[1]. Except for energy and electrolytes, they are not 'requirements' but recommendations that are set at about two standard deviations above the mean requirement. This generosity of the RDAs ensures that the allowance will be adequate for persons whose individual needs are higher than average. It follows, too, that an intake below the RDA is not necessarily deficient.

Like the first edition, the current RDAs are intended to be applied to groups of people. They are the basis for standards for programs such as school lunch, meals for the elderly and food assistance. While recognizing that the RDAs are not intended to designate amounts of nutrients needed by individuals, researchers and clinicians still use them for that purpose for want of a better standard. Because of the day to day variability of any individual's nutrient intake, if the RDAs are to be used to assess risk of a nutritional deficiency, it is essential that they be applied to average intakes over a period of time, and not to food consumption on a single day.

The RDAs for adult women are summarized in Table 1, the estimated safe and adequate daily dietary intakes of selected vitamins and minerals in

Table 2, and the estimated minimum requirements of sodium, chloride and potassium in Table 3.

The RDAs for women aged 25–50 and 51 plus are similar. The only major difference is the

Table 1 Recommended dietary allowances for adult women. Adapted from reference 1

Nutrient	25–50 years	51+ years
Vitamin A (μg RE*)	800	800
Vitamin D (μg)	5	5
Vitamin E (mg α-TE†)	8	8
Vitamin K (μg)	65	65
Vitamin C (mg)	60	60
Thiamin (mg)	1.1	1.0
Riboflavin (mg)	1.3	1.2
Niacin (mg NE‡)	15	13
Vitamin B_6 (mg)	1.6	1.6
Folate (μg)	180	180
Vitamin B_{12} (μg)	2.0	2.0
Calcium (mg)	800	800
Phosphorus (mg)	800	800
Magnesium (mg)	280	280
Iron (mg)	15	10
Zinc (mg)	12	12
Iodine (μg)	150	150
Selenium (μg)	55	55

*1 RE (retinol equivalent) = 1 g retinol or 6 g β-carotene;
†1 α-TE (tocopherol equivalent) = 1 mg α-tocopherol;
‡1 NE (niacin equivalent) = 1 mg niacin or 60 mg dietary tryptophan

Table 2 Estimated safe and adequate daily dietary intake of selected vitamins and minerals for adults. Adapted from reference 1

Vitamins		Trace elements	
Biotin (μg)	30–100	copper (mg)	1.5–3.0
Pantothenic acid	4–7	manganese (mg)	2.0–5.0
(mg)		fluoride (mg)	1.5–4.0
		chromium (μg)	50–200
		molybdenum (μg)	75–250

Table 3 The estimated sodium, chloride and potassium requirements of healthy adults. Adapted from reference 1

Electrolyte	
Sodium (mg)	500
Chloride (mg)	750
Potassium (mg)	2000

reduced iron level recommended for the older group who no longer have menstrual losses to replace. Recommended amounts of several B vitamins are linked to caloric intake. Since the caloric needs and intakes of women over 50 are lower than those of younger women, RDAs for these vitamins are also decreased.

It is also important to recognize that the RDAs are 'amounts intended to be consumed as part of a normal diet', and not formulas for vitamin and mineral supplements. Supplements do not supply the full range of nutrients and other beneficial substances, known and possibly unrecognized, which are obtained from a varied diet.

Nutrition concerns

Weight control

Weight control is a preoccupation of a majority of American women. In a culture which equates slenderness with attractiveness, 60% of adult women 'go on a diet' and spend billions of dollars in pursuit of slimness each year[2]. Despite their efforts at weight loss, women are obese more often than men. The prevalence of overweight in white women increases from 18% among those aged 25–34 to 37% in the 65–74-year-olds[3]. Among black women, the comparable figures are 18% and 61%[4]. Recent surveys document the increasing prevalence of obesity among all age and sex groups in the USA and other countries[5].

Body mass index (BMI), a measure of relative weight calculated as weight (kg) divided by height squared (m^2) is a useful replacement for height–weight tables, as it converts height and weight to a single number, enabling standards to be defined independently of height. The BMI can also be calculated from pounds and inches using the formula BMI = [weight (lb)/height (in)^2] $\times$ 703. An Expert Panel of the National Heart, Lung and Blood Institute has set the following standards for BMI: underweight, < 18.5; normal weight, 18.5–24.9; overweight, 25.0–29.9; and obese, > 30.0[6].

Weight or BMI is only one consideration in assessing the importance of a woman's weight status. Waist circumference and overall risk status should also be assessed. Excessive abdominal fat is an independent predictor of risk factors and morbidity. A cut-off level of > 88 cm (> 35 in) has been recommended to identify increased relative risk of disorders associated with obesity in adult women. The presence of other risk factors, including smoking, hypertension, low high-density lipoprotein (HDL) cholesterol, elevated fasting glucose and family history of premature coronary heart disease, should be considered when making decisions about weight control interventions[6].

Middle-aged women often find, to their dismay, that they tend to gain weight more rapidly and have to work harder to lose it than had been the case in earlier years. While there is a common tendency to look at eating habits to explain weight gain, the difficulty experienced by these women may be more closely related to changes in energy intake. Resting energy needs decrease by about 2% per decade throughout adulthood[7]. If not compensated for, this fairly small decline can lead to a gain of 2–3 lb per year, or 20–30 lb per decade. Furthermore, the decline in metabolic rate is often accompanied by a decrease in physical activity, the most important and controllable variable in determining energy need. While individuals will, of course, differ in their energy need, the average energy intake recommended for women over 50 (1900 kcal) is about 14% lower than the calories suggested for women from 25 to 50 (2200 kcal)[1]. An excess intake of 300 kcal per day, if maintained over a year, can result in a weight gain of over 30 lb.

The two ways to counter the tendency to gain weight are to reduce caloric intake and to maintain or increase physical activity.

Dietary control is a necessary part of weight control. The approximate rate of weight loss can be predicted based on the value of 3500 kcal per lb of adipose tissue. A deficit of 500 kcal per day will produce a loss of 1 lb per week. Using the RDA figure of 1900 kcal per day, a 51-year-old woman who made no changes in her physical activity would have to reduce her daily intake to about 1400 kcal to lose 1 lb per week. Since there is no evidence that requirements for protein and most vitamins and minerals decrease with age, there is less room in the diet for high-calorie, low-nutrient foods and women would be instructed about food choices. For some women, the support of a weight-loss group or consultation with a registered dietitian can be very helpful in making dietary changes.

Behavior therapy, employing strategies such as self-monitoring, stimulus control, stress management and social support can also increase women's abilities to manage their eating[6].

With our national penchant for dieting, it is equally important to emphasize the role of exercise in maintaining weight and health[8]. In an hour of brisk walking, a 60-kg woman will use 200 kcal, in addition to the benefits of exercise for cardiopulmonary conditioning and maintenance of bone mass. And, if more persuasion is needed, we should note that when intakes are held too low – below 1000–1200 kcal – it is difficult to obtain adequate amounts of essential nutrients[9].

Drug therapy may be a useful adjunct but should be reserved for patients whose BMI is > 30 or > 27 with concomitant risk factors or diseases, including hypertension, dyslipidemia, coronary heart disease, type 2 diabetes and sleep apnea. Even for these selected patients, the combination of dietary and behavioral therapy with physical activity should be tried for 6 months before beginning a drug regimen[6].

Panelists at a National Institutes of Health Technology Assessment Conference on Methods for Voluntary Weight Loss and Control concluded that '. . . most people who achieve weight loss . . . regain weight. For many overweight persons, achieving and maintaining a healthy weight is a lifelong challenge', and emphasized the need for more research into the biological and social influences on weight and weight control[10].

Whatever combination of physical activity and modification of food consumption is used for weight loss, the approach should stress the need for permanent adjustment of eating and exercise habits to maintain desirable weight over the long term.

Osteoporosis

Changes in calcium metabolism leading to a negative calcium balance, bone loss and osteoporosis are well known concomitants of the menopause. Since the etiology and hormonal aspects of osteoporosis are reviewed elsewhere in this book, the emphasis here is on nutritional factors and dietary strategies to prevent or minimize bone loss.

Although the precise mechanism by which calcium intake influences the genesis and progression of osteoporosis remains to be clarified, there is ample evidence to support recommendations for increased dietary calcium and/or the use of calcium supplements. Markovic and colleagues studied bone mass and fracture rates in two regions of Yugoslavia where life-styles were similar but diets differed in the use of milk and dairy products[11]. Mean calcium intake was calculated as 445 mg per day for women aged 40–42 and 343 mg per day for those from 70 to 72 years in the low-calcium region. (These are just slightly lower than the calcium intakes found in surveys of American women[12].) In the high-calcium region, mean intakes were 940 and 812 mg per day for the same age groups. Women in the high-calcium group had significantly more bone mass and, after age 65, fewer fractures than those who consumed less calcium. In the USA, Sandler and co-workers[13] have shown a significant relationship between calcium intake in adolescence and bone mass after the menopause. Heaney and associates[14] have shown in several studies of perimenopausal women that intakes in the order of 1–1.5 g per day are required to maintain calcium equilibrium.

These and other reports[15,16] led participants in a 1984 National Institutes of Health Consensus Conference on Osteoporosis to conclude that intakes of 1000–1500 mg of calcium per day are needed to prevent osteoporosis[17].

More recently, Dawson-Hughes and co-workers[18] showed that women ingesting less than one-half of the RDA for calcium lost bone more rapidly than those whose calcium intake was equal to or greater than the RDA, and Polley and others[19] demonstrated a slowing of bone loss when daily calcium intake was increased from 700 to 1400 mg. Ulrich and co-workers[20], in a study of 25 mother–daughter pairs, found no significant correlation between milk consumption and bone mineral density but did find significantly higher bone mineral density in women who regularly took calcium supplements. Tranquilli and colleagues[21] also observed a correlation between calcium intake and bone mineral content in postmenopausal women.

A study by Riis and co-workers in Copenhagen[22] compared the effect on bone loss of calcium carbonate, estrogen and placebo. They found that estrogen was the most effective, but that calcium supplementation was significantly more effective than placebo in maintaining forearm bone mass. A similar, but non-significant trend was seen for the entire skeleton. Although the authors did not estimate habitual calcium consumption of the experimental group, they had previously reported that Danish women similar to their subjects consume from 430 to 2350 mg per day, considerably more than their American counterparts. The impact of additional calcium on these women might, therefore, be different from that on women whose diets contain less calcium.

The panel which drafted the tenth edition of the RDAs, however, declined to change the recommended level of calcium for adult women from the 800 mg of earlier editions; however, they did make one change[1]. In previous editions, a higher RDA, 1200 mg, was advised for adolescent females up to the age of 18. The tenth edition extends this recommendation to 25 years based on studies showing that mineralization continues for some years after longitudinal growth is completed. They also point out that their recommendations 'do not address the possible increased needs of persons who may have osteoporosis . . .'.

Dietary surveys of American women indicate usual intakes of 450–550 mg, barely or less than half the amount needed to maintain bone mass, and that milk[21,23] and diary products supply 5% of the calcium in US diets. To double her calcium intake, then, a woman must increase her use of diary products, preferably skim or low-fat milk and low-fat yogurt and cheeses. Other food also supply calcium, as shown in Table 4. Based on reports of typical diets, an American woman gets about 200–300 mg of calcium from foods other than diary products. Careful selection of other foods can raise that somewhat, but 0.5–1 g or more of calcium will still need to be provided by milk and its products or by supplements.

There may be an advantage in using milk as the main source of calcium as it has been shown to lead to less suppression of remodelling than does calcium carbonate[24]. In addition, reliance on food sources of nutrients promotes a sound diet while ensuring against the risk of nutritional imbalance[25]. Realistically, however, not all women can be expected to add a pint or more of milk or its equivalent to their diets, and women who are at high risk of osteoporosis may need to add calcium supplements.

A variety of calcium salts and calcium-fortified products are on the market and being promoted to

Table 4 Calcium value of selected foods

	Amount	Calcium (mg)
Dairy products		
Milk, whole, low-fat or skim	1 cup	300
Yogurt, with added milk solids	1 cup	400
Cheese, hard	1 oz	200
cottage	1 oz	25
cream	1 oz	20
Ice cream	½ cup	75
Vegetables		
High: broccoli, kale, mustard, collard, turnip, dandelion greens (note: beet greens and spinach contain calcium but it is not absorbed)	½ cup	175
All others	½ cup	20
Fruits		
Juices	½ cup	10–30
Fruits	1 piece or ½ cup	10–30
Meats		
Canned salmon and sardines (with bones)	3 oz	200
All other meat and fish	3 oz	5–20
Eggs	1	25
Legumes		
All	1 cup	100
Nuts		
Almonds, Brazil nuts	1/4 cup	80
All others	1/4 cup	25
Peanut butter	1 tbsp	10
Starches		
Bread	1 slice	20
Rice, pasta	½ cup	10
Cereals	½ cup	10
Miscellaneous		
Bacon	2 slices	5
Cake	1 slice	85
Candy, chocolate	1 oz	60
Molasses	1 tbsp	60
Pie, fruit	1 slice	10
custard	1 slice	160
Soup, bean	1 cup	95
made with milk	1 cup	215
other	1 cup	15–50

women. (The percentage of calcium in several common supplements is given in Table 5). When advising patients about supplementary calcium, it is important to clarify the difference between the total weight of the tablet and the weight of elemental calcium it contains. For foods such as orange juice which have been fortified with calcium, the nutrition facts panel on the package states the amount of calcium in a serving as a percentage of the daily value. The daily value for calcium is set at 1000 mg, so the commonly seen '35% of daily value' equals 350 mg of calcium.

Another precaution concerns the 'natural' products dolomite and bone meal. Both are sold by health food distributors as calcium supplements. Samples of both products have been shown to be contaminated with lead and other heavy metals, and cases of toxicity have been reported[26]. Patients need to be apprised of this risk in any discussion about the choice of calcium products.

Other components of the diet have been shown to affect calcium balance. Adequate vitamin D is needed for calcium absorption. The dietary requirement for vitamin D is variable, as the vitamin can be synthesized in the skin from 7-dehydrocholesterol with exposure to ultraviolet light. Individuals who lack such exposure have a greater need for exogenous vitamin D than those who synthesize more of the vitamin. The RDA for vitamin D for women 51 years and older is set at 5 g of cholecalciferol (equivalent to 200 IU of vitamin D) per day[1].

Chapuy and colleagues[27] have recently shown that a regimen of 1200 mg calcium and 800 IU vitamin D_3 (cholecalciferol) resulted in increased bone density and decreased hip fractures in older (69–106 years) postmenopausal women.

Naturally occurring food sources of vitamin D are limited to fish oils, eggs and butter, but nearly all milk sold in the USA is fortified with vitamin D at a level of 400 IU per quart. Other food products,

Table 5 Calcium content of common supplements

Calcium salt	Elemental calcium (%)
Calcium carbonate	40
Calcium gluconate	9
Calcium lactate	13
Calcium phosphate, dibasic	23.3

especially breakfast cereals, may be fortified with vitamin D. The vitamin is also added to many calcium supplements and is found in multivitamin preparations. Women who take supplements should be instructed about the potential for toxicity of vitamin D. Prolonged ingestion of excess vitamin D can cause hypercalcemia and hypercalcinuria[28]. While the amount of vitamin D from any one of the usual sources is no more than the RDA, a combination of milk, a highly fortified cereal, a multivitamin and a combined calcium and vitamin D supplement is quite possible, and would add up to excessive levels of this vitamin. A reasonable recommendation to patients is that they take no more than one supplementary source of vitamin D.

Other minerals have also been shown to influence bone density. Magnesium and phosphorus intakes correlate with bone density[21]. Nielsen demonstrated that calcium excretion was increased on a low-boron diet[29]. Understanding the practical significance of this observation awaits further research. At present it reinforces the importance of a well-balanced diet, as fruits and vegetables are the best sources of this mineral.

Diet and disease prevention

Nutritional factors have been identified as risk factors for other diseases, including coronary heart disease[30,31] and cancer at several sites[32].

Women lag about 10 years behind men in the incidence of coronary heart disease. After the menopause, the incidence increases so that women as well as men should benefit from measures that will reduce this risk[23]. Obesity, abdominal adiposity and high intakes of saturated fat and trans fatty acids have been associated with elevated serum cholesterol levels and increased risk of cardiovascular disease[33,34]. Ample consumption of folate and fiber from fruits, vegetables and whole grains, regular inclusion of fish in the diet and moderate, but not heavy, consumption of ethanol have been associated with a decreased risk of coronary heart disease[35-42]. Supplements of folate and vitamin E also appear to reduce the risk of coronary disease[43]. While there is no unequivocal proof of the effectiveness of dietary change in preventing atherosclerosis, there is a body of data which supports controlling calorie, fat and cholesterol intakes as a means of reducing cardiovascular risk. The American Heart Association[44] advises a diet with no more than 30% of calories from fat, distributed equally among saturated and mono- and polyunsaturated fats. The National Cholesterol Education Program has recommended a similar regimen[45].

Research into the role of diet in cancer is more recent, and much more investigation is needed to define the mechanisms and importance of the associations that have been observed. Aromatic hydrocarbons and nitroso compounds in smoked and cured foods have been associated with cancer of the esophagus and stomach[32,46]. Investigations of meat and animal fat in relation to colon cancer have had inconsistent results[47,48]. Fruits and vegetables and dietary fiber consistently appear to be protective for both colon and breast cancer[49,50]. Obesity and high dietary fat consumption, which often go together, appear to increase the risk of breast cancer in postmenopausal women[51]. Alcohol may also increase this risk, although one large study found an increased risk among women who had taken estrogen but not among these who had never taken the hormone[52]. Dietary fiber has been associated with a lower risk of breast cancer[32,46].

Although current knowledge is inadequate to resolve debates over nutrient supplementation or fortification programs, diets containing liberal amounts of fruits and vegetables are clearly protective and should be encouraged. The Five a Day program, a collaborative public information and education effort of the National Cancer Institute and the Produce for Better Health Foundation has the goal of persuading all Americans to consume more fruits and vegetables[53].

In 1982, The National Academy of Science Committee on Diet, Nutrition and Cancer, while acknowledging the preliminary nature of the evidence, offered interim dietary guidelines for cancer risk reduction and good nutrition[46]:

(1) Reduce total fat from current 40% to 30% of calories;

(2) Include whole grains, fruits and vegetables in the daily diet, especially citrus fruits and carotene-rich (dark green and deep yellow) and cruciferous (cabbage family) vegetables;

(3) Minimize the consumption of salt-cured and smoked foods;

(4) If alcoholic beverages are consumed, it should be done in moderation.

Hot flushes

Hot flushes are one of the most common annoyances associated with the perimenopause. They are not a nutritional problem but this author has encountered many women who report that their hot flushes are relieved by eliminating caffeine, sugar and alcohol from their diets. The evidence, such as it is, is purely anecdotal, but the measure is simple and safe and can be offered to patients for a trial.

Vitamins E and B_6 also appear in the folklore concerning menopausal symptoms. Again, the evidence is mostly anecdotal. One study of vitamin E in breast cancer survivors showed a statistically significant but clinically marginal benefit from the vitamin[54]. Dosing with vitamins, however, is not innocuous, so one should be cautious in advising it. Being fat-soluble, vitamin E is stored in the body and, theoretically, could reach toxic levels. In fact, vitamin E is readily available and is often promoted in the popular literature with few, if any, reports of toxicity.

Vitamin B_6, on the other hand, is water-soluble so would be expected to be easily excreted. But in 1983, Schaumberg and colleagues[55] reported peripheral neuropathies in women who had been taken doses of 2–6 g daily for months. Subsequent reports have attributed peripheral neuropathies to doses of 500 mg and doses closer to 100 mg[56]. Clearly, women should be warned about self-medicating with megadoses of vitamin B_6.

Herbs and alternatives

The use of herbal and other alternative therapies is becoming increasingly common in North America. An estimated 42% of American consumers have tried some type of alternative therapy in 1997, compared with 33.8% in 1990[57]. At an Iowa State University conference on herbal remedies,

Greg Kitzmiller reported a survey of grocery shoppers, which found that over two-thirds acknowledged using supplements and 29% herbal products. Herbs are big business, with an estimated $US5.1 billion spent in 1997, a sum expected to grow to about $US25 billion by 2010.

Seidl and Stewart conducted intensive interviews with 13 perimenopausal women who acknowledged using alternative therapies, mainly herbal preparations[58]. The found that women perceived the alternatives as 'natural' and, therefore, safe. They liked the sense of personal control that they felt in using alternatives, contrasted with what they felt was 'pressure' from their physicians to use hormone replacement therapy. The same authors reviewed scientific and lay literature on alternative treatments, and concluded that the strongest evidence emerging is in favor of phytoestrogens, plant components which have estrogen-like activity[59].

Alternative modalities that have been recommended for perimenopausal women include nutrient supplements, herbs, acupuncture, relaxation techniques, massage and chiropractic. It is difficult to find reliable evidence on acupuncture, massage and chiropractic. Practitioners speak of energy and balance and offer anecdotal evidence, but controlled trials still need to be conducted[59].

There are more data on phytoestrogens and herbal products. Phytoestrogens, lignans and isoflavones, are converted in the intestine to heterocyclic phenols with structures similar to estrogens, but their estrogenic activity is far lower than that of synthetic estrogens[60]. Lignans are widely distributed in grains, fruits and vegetables, with flaxseed having a particularly high concentration. Isoflavones are found in all legumes, with the highest concentrations in soy[61]. The observation that women in Asian countries, who consume larger amounts of soy foods than do Americans, report fewer hot flushes[62] led to trials of isolated soy protein in postmenopausal women. Murkies and colleagues[63] supplemented subjects' diets with either soy or wheat flour and found decreases in hot flushes in both groups, with the soy group having a more rapid response. Albertazzi and co-workers[64] compared isolated soy protein with placebo; both groups reported a decrease in hot flushes, with the soy group having a significantly greater improvement. Soy protein may also improve cardiovascular risk profiles by decreasing the ratio of total to HDL cholesterol[65], although this finding is not consistent[66], and by maintaining arterial elasticity[66]. There are some indications that soy protein may also be effective in decreasing bone loss; more, and longer, trials are needed to clarify this possibility[61]. It has also been suggested that soy consumption may play an important role in the well-known lower rate of breast cancer among Japanese women, compared to Americans[61,67].

A variety of herbal therapies has been recommended for alleviation of menopausal symptoms: black cohosh, vitex agnus castelli, rehmannia, Siberian ginseng, dong quoi, fo ti, wild yam and St John's wort[68,69]. Herbs are regulated as food supplements, not drugs, and as such are not subjected to review for safety and efficacy or regulation by the Food and Drug Administration. There is relatively little, good scientific literature on the use of herbal remedies available in English. Two reliable references are *The Honest Herbal: A Sensible Guide to the Use of Herbs and Related Remedies*[70] and *Herbs of Choice: The Therapeutic Use of Phytomedicinals*[71] both by Varro E. Tyler, PhD, Distinguished Professor of Pharmacognosy at Purdue University. He offers the following information:

Black cohosh (*Cimicifuga racemosa*) has been shown to suppress hot flushes. It is usually administered in an alcoholic extract equivalent to 40 mg daily. Because of the lack of long-term toxicity studies, Tyler recommends that it be used for no longer than 6 months.

Chaste tree berry (*Vitex agnus-castus*) appears to inhibit the secretion of prolactin and needs to be evaluated for its effectiveness in treating menopausal symptoms.

Dong quai (*Angelica polymorpha*) contains several coumarin derivatives and lacks evidence supporting its effectiveness.

Evening primrose oil (*Oenothera biennis*) lacks evidence supporting its use.

Fo ti (*Polygonum multiforum*) is effective only as a laxative with undetermined side-effects.

Practical applications

Dietary assessment

Recommendations for dietary change should be individualized based on an evaluation of the patient's health status and her current dietary practices as well as on principles of nutrition. Comprehensive evaluation of nutritional status is beyond the scope of this chapter; several books on the subject are available. Suggestions are offered here for a simple approach to dietary evaluation that can be used in the routine care of healthy women. This can be accomplished by adding questions about diet to the history and, of course, bearing nutritional considerations in mind when interpreting clinical and laboratory data.

One can begin by asking a patient whether she restricts her diet in any way. Economic or cultural factors may influence food choices and availability, and should be considered along with health and medical concerns. More detailed information can be obtained by asking the patient to recall her consumption of food and beverages during the past 24 h or by having her keep a record of her intake for several days prior to the next office visit. Although it will be imprecise – food consumption is highly variable and difficult to quantitate – the general adequacy of a day's intake can be assessed by comparing it with recommended servings from the food groups listed below.

Another approach is to inquire about the frequency with which specific foods or food groups are used. For example, one can ask a patient whether she drinks milk, how often she drinks it and how often she eats cheese or yogurt, to estimate calcium intake, or about the use of whole grains, legumes and fresh fruits and vegetables, to estimate fiber in the diet. Information about the use of nutritional supplements should also be obtained, to ensure that the patient is meeting her needs and is not at risk for vitamin toxicity.

Dietary guidance

To be effective, dietary guidance should build, as indicated above, on each woman's needs and status. The bases for recommendations to ensure nutritional adequacy and reduce the risk of disease have been presented. The body of evidence relating diet to health promotion and disease risk reduction has been reviewed by expert panels from the National Academy of Science's Food and Nutrition Board[72] and Committee on Diet, Nutrition and Cancer[46], the Public Health Service[73] and other health agencies. While their recommendations vary in some particulars, creating a stir in the media and confusion for the public, there is a consensus around a dietary pattern with lower fat, especially saturated fat and cholesterol, and more complex carbohydrate. Those who address alcohol consumption indicate that if one consumes alcohol it should be done in moderation, usually interpreted as no more than one or two drinks per day. Energy intake and expenditure should be balanced to maintain desirable weight.

Nutrition and Your Health: Dietary Guidelines for Americans[74], a joint publication of the US Departments of Agriculture and Health and Human Services, summarizes healthful eating in seven recommendations:

(1) Eat a variety of foods;

(2) Balance the food you eat with physical activity – maintain or improve your weight;

(3) Choose a diet with plenty of grain products, vegetables and fruits;

(4) Choose a diet low in fat, saturated fat and cholesterol;

(5) Choose a diet moderate in sugars;

(6) Choose a diet moderate in salt and sodium;

(7) If you drink alcoholic beverages, do so in moderation.

This author would add one more guideline: eat foods that you like and enjoy them. The medical and nutrition communities, with the media, have done such an energetic job of proclaiming the health values of food that eating has, too often, become 'medicalized'. Women need to understand how to balance appropriate amounts of all food to make meals a source of pleasure as well as health.

These suggestions can be translated into practical guidance by recommendations of food groups as depicted in Figure 1, the food guide pyramid.

Grains and cereals Six or more servings of cereal products should be used, emphasizing whole grains, as refined products lack trace minerals and fiber. One slice of bread, 1 oz of cold cereal or one half-cup of cooked cereal, rice or pasta is a serving. Women often restrict starches in an effort to cut calories. They may be reminded that these foods are excellent sources of nutrients and that 'starchy' foods are not excessively high in calories unless fat is added, i.e. it is the butter, not the bread, which is 'fattening'.

Fruits and vegetables These foods should be used liberally, two to four servings of fruit and three to five of vegetables each day. A serving is one medium piece of fruit or one half-cup of cut raw or cooked fruit or vegetable. The only restriction is the avoidance of excess calories; even fresh fruits and juices can contribute to obesity if consumed in excessive amounts. Certain fruits and vegetables should be emphasized: citrus fruits, berries, melons, tomatoes, peppers and cabbage for vitamin C; dark green vegetables such as broccoli and kale for calcium; the same vegetables and deep yellow vegetables and fruits, such as winter squash, carrots and apricots for vitamin A; and cruciferous vegetables, including cabbage, broccoli, cauliflower, Brussels sprouts and rutabaga.

Milk and dairy products Two to three cups of milk or the equivalent in other dairy products will supply ample calcium to menopausal women. A cup of yogurt, 1.5 oz of natural cheese or 2 oz of processed cheese is equivalent to one cup of milk. Skim or low-fat milk and yogurt and low-fat cheese are preferable to full-fat products. The latter should be used only in limited amounts. Lactose-intolerant women who must avoid milk can often tolerate yogurt, buttermilk and hard cheeses. They can also purchase products which have been enzymatically treated to hydrolyze the lactose, and are labelled low-lactose or reduced-lactose.

Protein foods Two 2–3-oz servings per day, or a total of 5–7 oz per day, of lean meat, fish or poultry are sufficient. One half-cup of cooked dried beans or peas can replace an ounce of meat. Visible fat on meat should be removed before cooking. Poultry

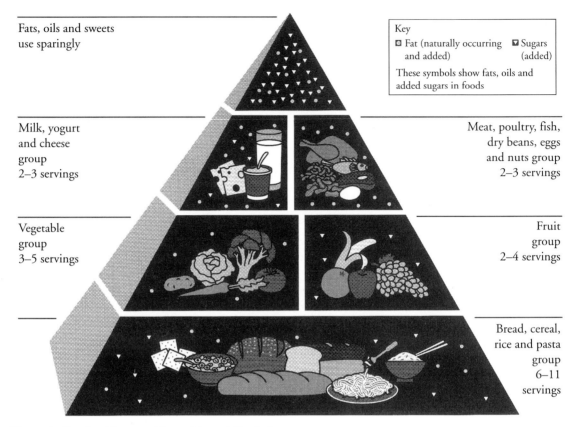

Figure 1 Food guide pyramid: a guide to daily choices

skin is also high in fat and can be removed to reduce the fat and calorie value of the food. Eggs are a good source of protein and other nutrients.

Other foods are:

Fats As stated above, fats should be limited. This includes butter, margarine, oils, salad dressings, cream, fried foods, chips and pastries. A point worth noting is that butter and margarine have the same fat and calorie value. Margarine, a vegetable product, does not contain cholesterol, but many women mistakenly think that it is lower in fat as well. With the proliferation of low- and reduced-fat products on the market, it is good practice to check the nutrition information of the food package to be certain of the product's composition.

Sweets Nutritionally, sugar is sugar regardless of its source. 'Natural sugar' has the same calorie value and effect on dental caries as refined sugar.

Foods in which sugar occurs naturally, such as fruits and juices, however, are usually higher in nutrient density than foods, such as confections and soft drinks, to which sugar has been added. Sweetened foods tend to be high palatable and highly caloric and should be limited as needed to maintain desirable weight.

Salt Excessive salt should be avoided by limiting the use of table-salt, salty condiments and highly salted commercially prepared foods.

Alcohol If alcoholic beverages are consumed, they should be used in moderation, no more than one to two drinks per day.

Caffeine Coffee, tea and soft drinks that contain caffeine should be limited to about two or three per day. Decaffeinated coffee and tea, herb teas, fruit juices and water should be used instead.

Summary

Good nutrition is important in maintaining the health of menopausal women. Dietary advice should include the liberal use of low-fat dairy products, fresh fruits and vegetables, whole grains and moderate amounts of lean meat, poultry and fish. Unless the diet includes two to three cups of milk or its equivalent per day, calcium supplementation should be considered.

References

1. Subcommittee on the Tenth Edition of the RDAs. Food and Nutrition Board, Commission on Life Sciences, National Research Council. *Recommended Dietary Allowance*, 10th edn. Washington, DC: National Academy Press, 1989

2. Mahan LK. Fad diets and weight control. In *Proceedings of Nutrition Concerns of Women: A Symposium for Health Professionals*. Seattle: University of Washington, 1983:5-10

3. Abraham S, Johnson CL, Najar MF. *Weight and Height of Adults 18-74 Years of Age, United States, 1971-74*. DHEW Publication No. (PHS) 75-1659, Center for Health Statistics, Hyattsville, MD, 1979

4. Van Itallie TB. Health implications of overweight and obesity in the United States. *Ann Int Med* 1985;103:983-8

5. Flegal KM, Carroll MD, Kuczmarski RJ, Johnson CL. Overweight and obesity in the United States: prevalence and trends, 1960-1994. *Int J Obesity Relat Metab Disord* 1998;22:39-47

6. The National Heart, Lung and Blood Institute Expert Panel on the Identification, Evaluation, and Treatment of Overweight and Obesity in Adults. Executive summary of the clinical guidelines on the identification, evaluation, and treatment of overweight and obesity in adults. *J Am Dietet Assoc* 1998;98:1178-91

7. Dumin JUCA, Passmore R. *Energy, Work and Leisure*. London: Heinemann Educational Books, 1967

8. Pi-Sunyer FX. Exercise in the treatment of obesity. In Frankle R, Yang M-U, eds. *Obesity and Weight Control*. Rockville, MD: Aspen Publishers, Inc., 1988:

9. Robinson CH, Lawler MR, Chenowith WL, Garwick AE. *Normal and Therapeutic Nutrition*, 17th edn. New York: Macmillan Publishing Co. 1986

10. *National Institutes of Health Technology Assessment Conference Statement: Methods for Voluntary Weight Loss*. Office of Medical Applications of Research, National Institutes of Health, Bethesda, MD, 1992

11. Markovic V, Kostial K, Simonovic I, Buzina R, Brodarec A, Nordin BEC. Bone status and fracture rates in two regions of Yugoslavia. *Am J Clin Nutr* 1979;32:540-9

12. US Department of Agriculture. *Nationwide Food Consumption Survey. Continuing Survey of Food Intakes of Individuals. Women 19-50 Years and Their Children 1-5 Years, 4 Days, 1986*. Report No. 86-3, Nutrition Monitoring Division, Human Nutrition Information Service, Hyattsville, MD, 1988

13. Sandler RB, Slemendra CW, LaPorte RE, *et al.* Postmenopausal bone density and milk consumption in childhood and adolescence. *Am J Clin Nutr* 1985;42:270-4

14. Heaney RP, Recker RR, Savile PP. Calcium balance and calcium requirements in middle aged women. *Am J Clin Nutr* 1977;30:1603-11

15. Heaney RP, Recker RR, Savile PP. Menopausal changes in calcium balance performance. *J Lab Clin Med* 1978;92:953-63

16. Aloia JF, Naswani AN, Yeh JK, Ross P, Ellis K, Cohn S. Determinants of bone mass in menopausal women. *Arch Intern Med* 1983;143:1700-4

17. Office of Medical Applications of Research, National Institutes of Health. Osteoporosis. *J Am Med Assoc* 1984;252:72

18. Dawson-Hughes B, Jacques P, Shipp C. Dietary calcium intake and bone loss from the spine in healthy postmenopausal women. *Am J Clin Nutr* 1987;46:685-7

19. Polley KJ, Nordin BE, Baghurt PA, Walker CJ, Chatterton BE. Effect of calcium supplementation on forearm bone mineral content in postmenopausal women: a prospective, sequential controlled trial. *J Nutr* 1987;117:1929-35

20. Ulrich CM, Georgio CC, Snow-Herter CM, *et al.* Bone mineral density in mother–daughter pairs: relations to lifetime exercise, lifetime milk consumption, and calcium supplements. *Am J Clin Nutr* 1996;63:72-9

21. Tranquilli AL, Lucino E, Garzetti GG, Romani C. Calcium, phosphorus and magnesium intakes correlate with bone mineral content in postmenopausal women. *Gynecol Endocrinol* 1994;8:55-8

22. Riis B, Thomsen K, Christiansen C. Does calcium supplementation prevent postmenopausal bone loss? *N Engl J Med* 1987;316:173-7

23. Committee on Diet and Health, Food and Nutrition Boards, National Research Council. *Diet and Health: Implications for Reducing Chronic Disease Risk*. Washington, DC: National Academy Press, 1989

24. Recker RR, Heaney RP. The effect of milk supplements on calcium metabolism, bone metabolism and calcium balance. *Am J Clin Nutr* 1985;41:254-63

25. Heaney RR. The role of nutrition in prevention and management of osteoporosis. *Clin Obstet Gynecol* 1987;50:833-46

26. Food and Drug Administration. Advice on limiting intake of bone meal. *FDA Drug Bull* 1982;12:5-6

27. Chapuy MC, Arlot ME, Duboeuf F, *et al*. Vitamin D_3 and calcium to prevent hip fractures in elderly women. *New Engl J Med* 1992;327:1637-42

28. Food and Nutrition Board. Hazards of overuse of vitamin D. *Nutr Rev* 1975;33:61-2

29. Nielsen FH. Effect of dietary boron on mineral, estrogen and testosterone metabolism in postmenopausal women. *FASEB J* 1987;1:394-7

30. Atherosclerosis Study Group, Intersociety Commission for Heart Disease Research. Optimal resources for primary prevention of atherosclerotic diseases. *Circulation* 1954;70:153A-205A

31. Stamler J. Diet-related risk factors for human atherosclerosis: hyperlipidemia, hypertension, hyperglycemia. Current status. *Adv Exp Med Biol* 1975;60:125-58

32. Doll R, Peto R. The causes of cancer, quantitative estimates of available risks of cancer in the United States today. *J Natl Cancer Inst* 1981;66:1191-308

33. Manson JE, Colditz GA, Stampfer MJ, *et al*. A prospective study of obesity and risk of coronary heart disease in women. *N Engl J Med* 1990;322:882-9

34. Rexrode KM, Carey VJ, Hennekens CH, *et al*. Abdominal adiposity and coronary heart disease in women. *J Am Med Assoc* 1998;280:1843-8

35. Willett W, Stampfer MJ, Manson JE, *et al*. Intake of trans fatty acids and risk of coronary heart disease among women. *Lancet* 1993;341:581-5

36. Stampfer MJ, Hennekins CH, Manson JE, *et al*. Vitamin E consumption and the risk of coronary disease in women. *N Engl J Med* 1993;328:1444-9

37. Kushi LH, Folsom AR, Prineas RJ, *et al*. Dietary antioxidant vitamins and death from coronary heart disease in postmenopausal women. *N Engl J Med* 1996;334:1156-62

38. Knekt P, Reunanen A, Jarvinen R, *et al*. Antioxidant vitamin intake and coronary mortality in a longitudinal population study. *Am J Epidemiol* 1994;139:1180-9

39. Bianchi C, Negri E, La Vecchia C, Francheschi S. Alcohol consumption and the risk of acute myo-cardial infarction in women. *Epidemiol Community Health* 1993;4:308-11

40. Rimm EB, Klaatsky A, Grobbe D, *et al*. Review of moderate alcohol consumption and reduced risk of coronary heart disease: is the effect due to beer, wine or spirits. *Br Med J* 1996;312:731-6

41. Stampfer MJ, Colditz GA, Willett WC. A prospective study of moderate alcohol consumption and the risk of coronary disease and stroke in women. *N Engl J Med* 1988;319:267-73

42. Gramenzi A, Gentile A, Fasoli M, *et al*. Association between certain foods and risk of acute myocardial infarction in women. *Br Med J* 1990;300:771-3

43. Rimm EB, Willett WC, Hu FB, *et al*. Folate and vitamin B_6 from diet and supplements in relation to risk of coronary heart disease in women. *J Am Med Assoc* 1998;279:359-64

44. American Heart Association. *Dietary Treatment of Hypercholesterolemia. A Handbook for Counselors*. Dallas, TX: American Heart Association, 1988

45. National Cholesterol Education Program. Second report of the Expert Panel on Detection, Evaluation, and Treatment of High Blood Cholesterol in Adults. Summary Report. *J Am Med Assoc* 1993;269:3015-23

46. Committee on Diet, Nutrition and Cancer, Assembly of Life Sciences, National Research Council. *Diet, Nutrition, and Cancer*. Washington, DC: National Academy Press, 1982

47. Goldbohm RA, van den Brandt PA, van't Veer P, *et al*. A prospective cohort study on the relation between meat consumption and the risk of colon cancer. *Cancer Res* 1994;54:718-23

48. Willett WC, Stampfer MJ, Colditz GA, *et al*. Relation of meat, fat and fiber intake to the risk of colon cancer in a prospective study among women. *N Engl J Med* 1990;323:1664-72

49. Steinmetz KA, Kushi LH, Bostick RM, *et al*. Vegetables, fruit and colon cancer in the Iowa Women's Health Study. *Am J Epidemiol* 1994;139:1-15

50. Rohan TE, Howe GR, Friedenreich CM. Dietary fiber, vitamins A, C, and E and risk of breast cancer. *Cancer Causes Control* 1993;4:29-37

51. Barrett-Connor E, Friedlander NJ. Dietary fat, calories, and the risk of breast cancer in postmenopausal women: a prospective population-based study. *J Am Coll Nutr* 1993;12:390-9

52. Gapstur SM, Potter JD, Sellers TA, *et al*. Increased risk of breast cancer with alcohol consumption in postmenopausal women. *Am J Epidemiol* 1992;136:541-2

53. Produce for Better Health Foundation. *Five a Day for Better Health*, Newark, DE: 1991

54. Barton DL, Loprinzi CL, Quella SK, *et al*. Prospective evaluation of vitamin E for hot flashes in breast cancer survivors. *J Clin Oncol* 1998;16:495-500

55. Schaumberg H, Kaplan J, Windebank N, *et al*. Sensory neuropathy from pyridoxine abuse. *N Engl J Med* 1983;309:445-8

56. Dalton K, Dalton MJT. Characteristics of pyridoxine overdose neuropathy syndrome. *Acta Neurol Scand* 1987;76:8–11

57. Eisenberg D, Davis RB, Ettner SL, *et al*. Trends in alternative medicine use in the United States. 1990-1997; results of a follow-up national survey. *J Am Med Assoc* 1998;280:1569–75

58. Seidl MM, Stewart DE. Alternative treatments for menopausal symptoms. *Can Fam Physician* 1998;44: 1271–6

59. Seidl MM, Stewart DE. Alternative treatments for menopausal symptoms: systematic review of scientific and lay literature. *Can Fam Physician* 1998;44: 1299–1308

60. Adlercreutz H, Mazur W. Phyto-oestrogens and western diseases. *Duodecim Ann Med* 1997;29: 95–120

61. Murkies AL, Wilcox G, Davis S. Clinical review; phytoestrogens. *J Clin Endocrinol Metab* 1998;83: 297–303

62. Knight PC, Edden JA. Phytoestrogens – a short review. *Maturitas* 1995;22:167–75

63. Murkies AL, *et al*. Dietary flour supplementation decreases post-menopausal hot flushes: effect of soy and wheat. *Maturitas* 1995;21:189–95

64. Albertazzi P, Pansini F, Bonaccorsi G, *et al*. The effect of dietary soy supplementation on hot flushes. *Obstet Gynecol* 1998;91:6–11

65. Baum JA, Teng H, Erdman JW, *et al*. Long-term intake of soy protein improves blood lipid profiles and increases mononuclear cell low-density lipoprotein receptor messenger RNA in hypercholesterolemic, postmenopausal women. *Am J Clin Nutr* 1998;68:545–51

66. Nestel PJ, Yamashita T, Sasahara T, *et al*. Soy isoflavones improve systemic arterial compliance but not plasma lipids in menopausal and perimenopausal women. *Atherosc Thromb Vasc Biol* 1997;17:3392–8

67. Shimizu H, Ross RK, Bernstein L, *et al*. Cancers of the prostate and breast among Japanese and white immigrants to Los Angeles County. *Br J Cancer* 1991;63:963–6

68. Mayo JL. A natural approach to menopause. *Clin Nutr Insights* 1997;5:1–8

69. Northrup C. Menopause. *Compl Altern Ther Primary Care* 1997;24:921–48

70. Tyler V. *The Honest Herbal: A Sensible Guide to the Use of Herbs and Related Remedies*, 3rd edn. Binghamton, NY: Pharmaceutical Products Press

71. Tyler V. *Herbs of Choice: The Therapeutic Use of Phytomedicinals*. Binghamton, NY: Pharmaceutical Products Press, 1994

72. National Research Council. *Diet and Health: Implications for Reducing Chronic Disease Risk*. Report of the Committee on Diet and Health, Food and Nutrition Board, Commission of Life Sciences, National Academy Press, Washington, DC, 1989

73. US Department of Health and Human Services. *The Surgeon General's Report on Nutrition and Health*. DHHS (PHS) Publ. No. 88–50210, Public Health Service, US Department of Health and Human Services, Washington, DC, 1988

74. US Department of Agriculture, US Department of Health and Human Services. *Nutrition and Your Health: Dietary Guidelines for Americans*. Home and Garden Bulletin No. 232, 4th edn, Washington, DC, 1995

Section IV
Therapy of the menopause

18

Pharmacology of hormonal therapeutic agents

Bhagu R. Bhavnani

In this chapter, the pharmacology of estrogens and progestins used for hormone replacement therapy (HRT) and estrogen replacement therapy (ERT) in postmenopausal women is discussed. The structures of some of the estrogens and progestins are shown in Figures 1 and 2. The emphasis is on estrogens and on factors such as rate of absorption, enterohepatic circulation, route of administration and serum transport via serum binding proteins, and how these factors influence the bioavailability of these steroids. The genomic mechanism of action involved in estrogen and progestin effects is described. Differences between various preparations, and the impact these may have clinically, are presented. The antioxidant properties of various estrogens are discussed in the context of cardiovascular disease and Alzheimer's disease in postmenopausal women. The most frequently and widely prescribed estrogen preparation for postmenopausal estrogen replacement is conjugated equine estrogen (CEE). This preparation contains a number of components that are also used individually, and therefore the pharmacology of this preparation is dealt with in detail.

Introduction

Natural menopause is a normal physiological process that occurs in healthy Caucasian women at a median age between 50 and 55 years[1]. Current smokers reach the menopause an average of 1.5–2 years earlier[1]. The menopause is associated with a cessation of ovarian function and menstrual bleeding. This physiological change generally takes place over a period of time (years) and is roughly divided into three phases[2]: the perimenopause is the phase during which, in most women, ovarian function generally declines, and may result in irregular and anovulatory menstrual cycles; the menopause is the absence of menstrual flow for 12 months, characterized by low serum 17β-estradiol and high follicle stimulating hormone (FSH) levels, and during this phase, all of the ovarian follicles have been depleted or the follicles are unresponsive to gonadotropin stimulation; the postmenopausal years are the continuation of the changes that have occurred at menopause for the rest of the woman's life. Although during the postmenopausal years the ovary does not secrete estrogens, its stromal cells continue to produce small amounts of androstenedione. The importance of this ovarian androgen secretion is discussed in subsequent sections.

Some authors refer to the three phases collectively as the 'climacteric', while others refer to the transitional period between the perimenopause and actual menopause as the climacteric. In contrast to natural menopause, which occurs gradually over a period of time, removal of ovaries in a young woman results in a very rapid and perhaps unexpected entry into menopause.

During the past century, the world population and, more importantly, the elderly population has been increasing at a rapid rate[3]. Thus, in 1900, the world population was around 1.7 billion people; by the year 2000, the United Nations project it to be 6.2; and in the year 2020, 7.9 billion[3]. The elderly (above 65 years) will have increased from 5.1% in 1950 to 8.8% by the year 2020, and this represents an elderly population of 796 million people. Moreover, nearly 124 million are expected to be 80 years and over. The majority of this elderly population will be postmenopausal women[3]. It is estimated that the average life expectancy of women in the next millennium is going to be over 81 years in the USA and Canada. Thus, most

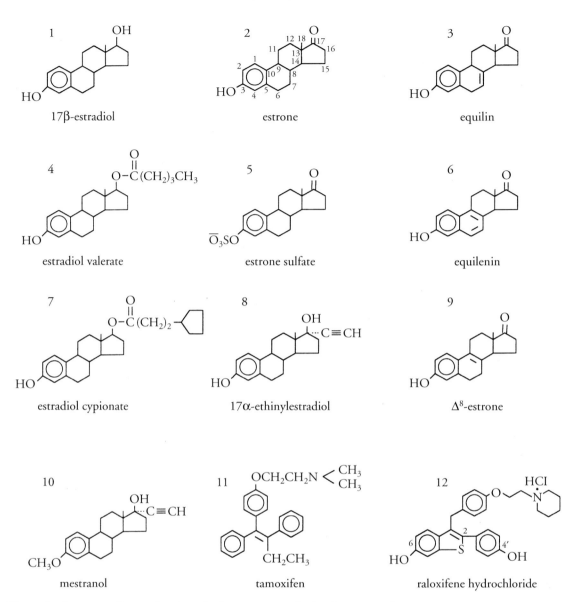

Figure 1 Structure of natural and synthetic estrogens and related compounds

women can expect to live more than one-third of their lives in the postmenopausal years. The demographic health, socioeconomic and ethical implications of the soaring elderly population have been recently reviewed[3].

Since normal aging is associated with increasing health problems, such as osteoporosis, cardiovascular disease, neurodegenerative diseases and cancer, it is essential that we strive to develop preventive and interventional strategies that will assist postmenopausal women to maintain a healthy and productive quality of life.

Estrogen and progesterone production during menopause

During the premenopausal reproductive years, the human ovaries utilize the classical pathway of steroidogenesis to biosynthesize both estrogens and progesterone from simple precursors such as

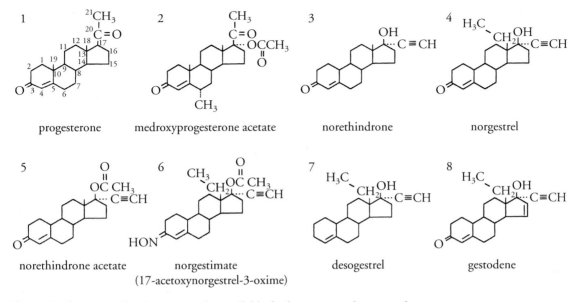

Figure 2 Structure of various progestins available for hormone replacement therapy

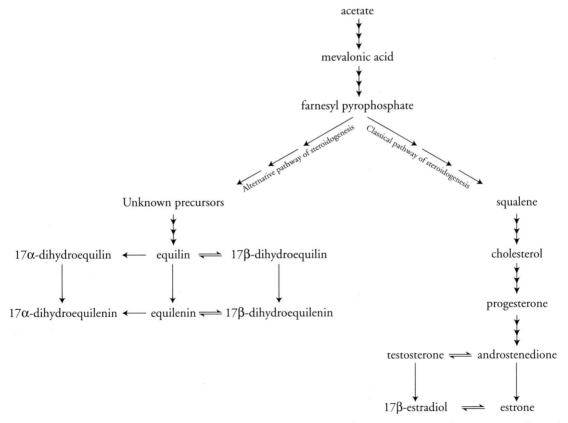

Figure 3 Biosynthesis of classical estrogens estrone and estradiol and ring B unsaturated estrogens equilin and equilenin

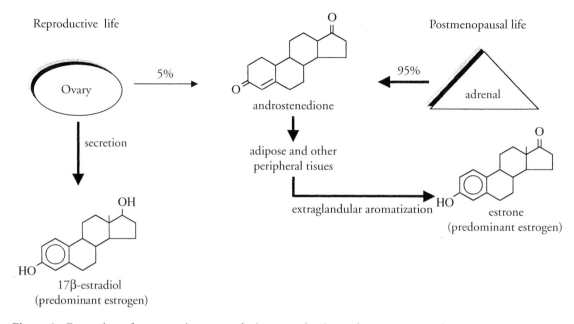

Reproductive life

Ovary

5%

androstenedione

Postmenopausal life

95%

adrenal

secretion

adipose and other
peripheral tisues

OH

17β-estradiol
(predominant estrogen)

HO

extraglandular aromatization

estrone
(predominant estrogen)

Figure 4 Formation of estrogens in women during reproductive and postmenopausal years

acetate (Figure 3). In this pathway, cholesterol is the obligatory intermediate, and several enzymes and cofactors are involved[4]. In contrast to this classical pathway of steroidogenesis, an alternative pathway where cholesterol is not an obligatory precursor has been described for the biosynthesis of unique ring B unsaturated estrogens[4]. These estrogens are components present in the most frequently used drug (conjugated equine estrogens, CEEs) for ERT. In premenopausal women, estrogen is produced by two pathways, and the precursors needed arise from the ovary and the adrenal (Figure 4). The predominant estrogen during the premenopause is 17β-estradiol, and this is secreted by the ovary. The serum levels range from 40 pg/ml in the early proliferative (follicular) phase to 250 pg/ml at mid-cycle and 100 pg/ml during the mid-secretory (mid-luteal) phase[5]. The total amount of 17β-estradiol secreted varies from 20–40 μg/day during the early proliferative and late secretory phases of the menstrual cycle to 600–1000 μg/day just prior to ovulation[6]. During premenopause, along with 17β-estradiol, a small amount of estrone is produced by the peripheral or extraglandular aromatization of adrenal androstendione. This extraglandular formation of estrone does not vary during the menstrual cycle, and approximately 45 μg/day of estrone is pro-

duced from this source[6]. In contrast, in postmenopausal women, the predominant estrogen is estrone, produced almost exclusively by extraglandular aromatization (Figure 4). The androgen precursor needed for this aromatization is circulating androstenedione, secreted mainly (95%) by the adrenal cortex and perhaps to a lesser extent (5%) by the ovarian stroma. The primary site of peripheral aromatization is the adipose tissue, although tissues such as muscle, bone, brain and hair follicles may also be involved[7]. Obesity is associated with higher levels of circulating estrogens, which arise from peripheral aromatization[8].

During the perimenopausal phase and with cessation of menstruation, the 17β-estradiol secretion declines to low levels (Table 1) during the first year, and these low levels (20–40 pg/ml) are maintained over the postmenopausal years[9]. During the menopause, there is a decline in the ovarian secretion of androgens, particularly that of androstenedione[9,10], yet during the transition from perimenopause to postmenopause, the levels of androgens do not decline significantly. As a result of the declining levels of estrogen during the menopause, the negative feedback effect on the hypothalamic–pituitary axis is lost, and the levels of gonadotropins (Table 1), particularly that of FSH, increase several-fold[9].

232

Table 1 Concentrations of 17β-estradiol and follicle stimulating hormone (FSH) in peri- and postmenopausal women. Values are expressed as mean ± SEM. Data from reference 9

Months from last menses	17β-estradiol (pg/ml)	FSH (mIU/ml)
< 3	108 ± 19	27 ± 4
9–12	26 ± 4*	84 ± 16*
12–24	19 ± 4*	97 ± 18*
> 24	14 ± 1*	69 ± 9*

*$p < 0.05$, compared to value at < 3 months

Although the levels of testosterone in post-menopausal women do not significantly decline[9], peripheral aromatization of testosterone to 17β-estradiol or estrone is minimal. In contrast to premenopausal women, the principal source of 17β-estradiol in postmenopausal women is from the peripheral conversion of estrone by 17β-hydroxysteroid dehydrogenase[11].

It has been estimated that the conversion of androstenedione to estrone in peripheral tissues is about 2–3% and, based on the androstenedione production rate of 1500 μg per day in healthy menopausal women, approximately 30–45 μg of estrone per day is produced by this mechanism. This amount of estrone represents essentially the total amount found in these women, and therefore nearly all of the estrone is derived from the peripheral mechanism. There is no evidence for direct secretion of estrogens by either the ovary or the adrenal[6,8]. In obese postmenopausal women, the amount of androstenedione secreted by the adrenal is the same, but the percentage conversion to estrone is over 11%. This then accounts for the higher level (120–130 μg/day) of estrone found in those women[12]. Since the amount of progesterone found in postmenopausal women is extremely low, the extraglandular estrogen is considered to be unopposed estrogen, and a correlation between this estrogen and increased risk of endometrial cancer has been proposed[12].

In vivo transport of estrogens and progestins

The binding of steroid hormones to serum proteins such as sex hormone-binding globulin (SHBG) and corticosteroid-binding globulin (CBG) plays an important role in the transport and distribution of hormones. In the human circulation, estrogens and progestins are primarily bound non-specifically and with low affinity to albumin, and specifically with high affinity to SHBG or CBG[13,14]. Only a small fraction of these hormones circulates in the unbound or free form[13,14]. It is generally accepted that only the free steroid hormone can readily enter the target cell to exert its biological effect, or be further metabolized and excreted. There is evidence that the protein-bound form of some steroids can also enter the cell[15], but the physiological significance of this remains to be established.

The levels of SHBG and CBG regulate the free hormone concentration, and the protein-bound hormones constitute a readily available pool of hormones. Since steroid hormones bind to serum albumin with low affinity and are easily dissociable to the free hormones, the albumin-bound hormone can also be considered, to some extent, to be available for biological action and metabolism.

The extent and degree of binding of estrogens to serum proteins therefore determines the bioavailability of the estrogen. In premenopausal women, approximately 60% of the 17β-estradiol in circulation is loosely (i.e. with low affinity) bound to albumin, and 38% is bound to SHBG with relatively high affinity[16]. The relative affinity constants for various estrogens and androgens: estrone, equilin, 17β-dihydroequilin, 17β-estradiol, testosterone and 5α-dihydrotestosterone are: 0.07, 0.15, 0.22, 0.29, 2.70 and 4.53×10^9 M^{-1}, respectively[17]. Although the 17β-reduced estrogens have a relatively higher affinity for SHBG than the corresponding 17-ketones, these relative binding affinities are much lower than those observed with androgens[17,18]. In contrast to the unconjugated estrogens, the sulfate esters of estrogens do not bind to SHBG but instead bind to serum albumin[17,19] with relatively high affinity ($0.9–1.1 \times 10^5$ M^{-1}). Between 60 and 90% of estrogen sulfates are bound to albumin, and this is the main circulating form of estrogen sulfates in postmenopausal women. These estrogen sulfates serve as reservoirs from which the unconjugated estrogens are being continuously formed.

Oral administration of estrogen is associated with an increase in SHBG levels, which results in a greater percentage of estrogen bound to SHBG, and therefore a lesser amount of the free hormone is available for biological action. Levels of SHBG are also increased during pregnancy, hyperthyroidism and cirrhosis. In contrast, obesity, androgen excess and hypothyroidism lower the level of SHBG and can result in an increase in the free fraction of estrogens[8]. The extent and degree of binding of estrogen to serum proteins not only determines the amount of estrogen available for biological action, but also plays an important role in the metabolic clearance rate (MCR) of estrogens, and this aspect is discussed in subsequent sections.

Like estrogens, progestins (Figure 2) also circulate primarily in a bound form. Approximately 20% of progesterone is bound to CBG[14], and the rest to albumin. Similarly, over 90% of medroxyprogesterone is bound to albumin[20]. Progesterone and medroxyprogesterone do not appear to bind to SHBG to any significant extent; however, binding of progesterone to other proteins, particularly in some species, has been noted[13]. In contrast to progesterone and medroxyprogesterone acetate, 19-norprogestins bind in substantial amounts to SHBG. Thus, the amount of norethindrone, levonorgestrel, desogestrel (3-ketodesogestrel) and gestodene bound to SHBG is 35, 47, 32 and 75%, respectively[21,22]. Approximately 0.6–3.7% of these progestins is present in the free form, and the remainder is bound to albumin[21,22]. Norgestimate is a 3-oximo-17-acetoxy derivative of norgestrel (levonorgestrel), and since it is metabolized to levonorgestrel[23,24], essentially all of its biological effects are most probably a result of its first metabolism to norgestrel and/or norgestrel acetate. Its distribution in serum has not been well documented, and will essentially be similar to that of levonorgestrel[21].

Genomic mechanism of steroid hormone action

The basic genomic mechanism of steroid hormone action has been known for more than three decades, and excellent detailed reviews are available[25–30]. In the following section, the genomic mechanism of action of steroid hormones with emphasis on estrogens is briefly outlined.

As discussed above, in the human, estrogens circulate in the blood bound mostly to serum proteins; the free (unbound) hormone enters the target tissues and interacts with estrogen receptors (ERs) as shown in Figure 5. The estrogen receptor belongs to a superfamily of ligand-dependent transcription factors[25] that regulate estrogen-responsive genes, and it is by this process that the main biological effects of estrogens are exerted. Until 1995, only one specific estrogen receptor, ERα, located in the target cell nuclei had been described. However, now another gene that codes for a second estrogen receptor, ERβ, has been identified[31]. These two receptors are similar (Figure 6), and even though the ERβ is considerably smaller, it binds with estrogens with similar affinity. In the absence of estrogen, the ER resides in a transcriptionally inactive (latent) form associated with heat shock proteins (HSPs) in the cell nuclei (Figure 5).

The mechanism of estrogen hormone action involves a series of molecular steps that are schematically depicted in Figure 5. Briefly, the unbound (free) estrogen is lipophilic, and readily enters target tissue cells by passive diffusion through the cell membrane and binds to its specific receptor in the nuclear compartment. This estrogen–receptor complex undergoes a series of concerted steps that include phosphorylation, homodimerization and allosteric conformational changes. This 'activated' estrogen–receptor complex then binds to a specific region of DNA called the estrogen response element (ERE; or hormone response element, HRE; or steroid response elements, SREs), located near the promoter of the target gene (Figure 5). The receptor complex then stimulates or induces transcription by yet to be defined mechanisms. The process appears to involve interaction with accessory transcription factors that are needed for RNA polymerase II to bind to the promoter and, thereby, initiate transcription. The pre-mRNA formed is processed and the mRNA is exported to the cytoplasm where it is translated in the ribosomes to new protein. It is via the newly synthesized protein(s) that the biological effects of estrogens are expressed via autocrine, paracrine and endocrine mechanisms (Figure 5).

Although the above mechanism of estrogen action is based on a substantial body of evidence

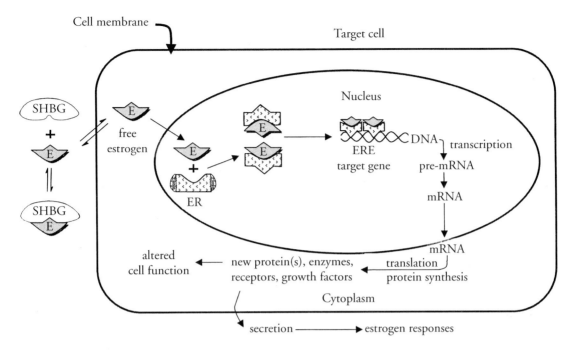

Figure 5 Simplified model of estrogen action. In this model estrogen (E) in the unbound form enters the target cell by diffusion. In the absence of estrogen (ligand), the estrogen receptor (ER) resides in the nucleus associated with heat shock proteins (HSPs). Upon interaction with estrogen, a series of molecular events are initiated (removal of HSP, phosphorylation, dimerization, recruitment of adapters) that permit the estrogen–receptor complex to bind to specific DNA response elements (EREs) and allow transcription to proceed. The new mRNA synthesized after processing is exported to the cytoplasm where it is translated into a new protein(s) (enzymes, growth factors) that result in altered cell function. The effects by these newly synthesized proteins are expressed by autocrine, paracrine or endocrine mechanisms[29]. SHBG, sex hormone-binding globulin

and has gained general acceptance, it however does not explain how different target cells distinguish between different estrogens, i.e. how different estrogens that interact with the same ER display different activities in different cells[30]. The original concept proposed that first, the main determinant of selectivity and efficacy was the binding affinity of the specific estrogen for the estrogen receptor, second, all estrogens function in the same manner in any cell that has an ER and third, no other cellular factors were required. In this model, the biological activity of an estrogen was believed to be directly proportional to its binding affinity[32]. Similarly, the above general mechanism does not explain tissue-selective effects of estrogens and antiestrogens, for example tamoxifen's differential effect on the uterus, bone and breast. In all three tissues, tamoxifen's action is mediated by the same

estrogen receptor(s), yet the effects are profoundly different.

Three distinct mechanisms for steroid hormone selectivity for nuclear receptors at the tissue, the cell and the gene have been proposed[26] and are: ligand-based selectivity; receptor-based selectivity; and effector-based selectivity. To understand these mechanisms better, knowledge of the receptor structure and its interaction with DNA and the general transcription apparatus is essential and is briefly described here.

The ER protein and other members of this family have a modular structure[25,29], and are made up of six distinct domains that are termed A/B, C, D, E and F domains. In Figure 6, these domains along with the amino and carboxy termini of the protein are depicted. These domains[29] have the following functions: regions A/B and E contain

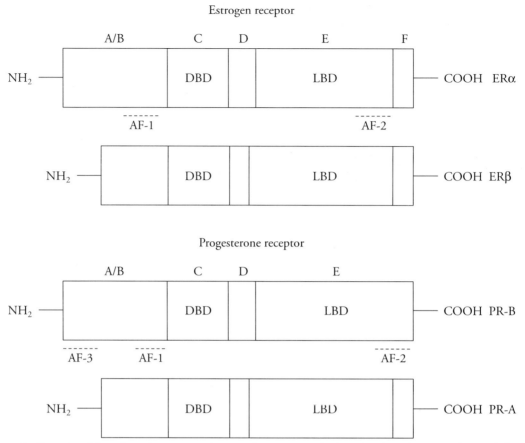

Figure 6 Functional domains of estrogen and progestin receptors: six domains A, B, C, D, E and F are defined in text. AF, activation function; DBD, DNA-binding domain; LBD, ligand-binding domain; ER, estrogen receptor; PR, progesterone receptor

hormone-independent transactivation function AF-1 (or TAF-1) and the hormone-dependent transactivation function AF-2 (or TAF-2)[33]; region C contains two type II zinc fingers that are involved in DNA binding (DBD) and dimerization of the receptor; region D or the 'hinge' region contains a nuclear localization signal sequence (NLS) for receptors; the DNA-binding domain (DBD) also contains specific binding sequences termed steroid response elements (SREs); region E is the ligand (hormone)-binding domain (LBD) and AF-2, and is important for the hormone specificity of the receptor; region F present in the ER but absent in the progesterone-receptor (PR) has minimal function[29]. The ER functions as a ligand-dependent transcription activator through the concerted action of the activation functions AF-1 and AF-2 in a tissue- and promoter-specific manner[34,35]. It has

further been shown that in most cell environments both AF-1 and AF-2 participate and stimulate ER transactivation of gene expression[36]; however, in some contexts individual activation functions can act independently. Estrogens such as 17β-estradiol act as ER agonists in cells where either or both AFs are required. Compounds such as tamoxifen and its active metabolite *trans*-4-hydroxy tamoxifen function as partial agonists (bone, uterus) in cells where AF-1 alone is required. In tissue where only the hormone-dependent AF-2 is required, these triphenylethylene derivatives act as antagonists and inhibit the activity of the AF-2[30,36]. In contrast, pure estrogen antagonists such as ICI-164 384 and ICI-182 780 inhibit the activity of AF-1 and AF-2, and this completely blocks the ER's transcriptional activity[36]. This mechanism provides a rational explanation not only of how some estrogenic compounds may have both agonist and antagonist activity, but more importantly how compounds such as tamoxifen, raloxifene and other selective estrogen receptor modulators (SERMs) can manifest specific activities in different target tissues.

It has also been proposed[28,29], and recently confirmed experimentally[37], that different estrogens which interact with ERs produce a unique conformational form (shape) of the receptor. This specific conformation of the receptor is able to recruit a distinct protein(s) termed the co-activator (adapter) protein, which then allows contact with the target gene control region and promotes transcription[26,29,36,38,39]. In Figure 7, two different estrogens (estrogen A and estrogen B), after interaction with ER and dimerization, result in a specific estrogen–receptor configuration that can only be

recognized by a specific adapter protein present in that target cell. Since several adapter proteins have been identified[29,39], it is now possible to envision that, in the presence of two ERs and different estrogens, the estrogen–receptor complexes generated will have conformations that can be recognized differentially in various target cells, depending on the presence or absence of a specific adapter protein. Thus, depending on which estrogen (agonist, partial agonist or antagonist) binds to the ER (ERα or ERβ or both), the receptor complex can associate with a specific co-activator which positively interacts with the gene transcription apparatus to activate target gene transcription. Since estrogens such as 17β-estradiol appear to be active in all estrogen target tissues, it is likely that the receptor conformation induced is recognized by co-activators in all target cells. Alternatively, if the

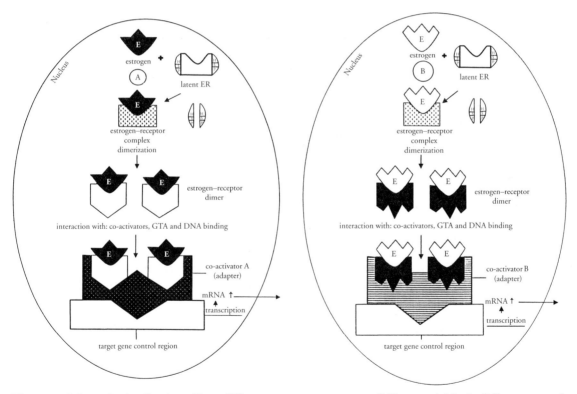

Figure 7 Schematic visualization of how different estrogens can express different activities in different target tissues. Each estrogen (E) induces a distinct conformational form (shape) in the estrogen receptor (ER). In this overly simplified figure, two different estrogens A and B and the conformations these induce in the ER are shown (black/white). Each form of ER is then able to recruit a specific adapter protein or co-activator (A and B), and the complex is then able to interact with the transcription apparatus, which ultimately results in the stimulation of transcription. Each adapter protein recognizes only specific estrogen–receptor configurations[26–29]. GTA, general transcription apparatus; HSP, heat shock protein

conformation of ER generated can only recruit a co-repressor protein, this will have a negative impact on gene transcription[36], and the estrogen analog acts as an antiestrogen.

In the above model, the relative binding affinity of an estrogen for ERs is not the sole determinant of biological activity or potency, yet binding of the estrogen or antiestrogen with the ER is a prerequisite. It therefore appears that all three mechanisms proposed[26] are involved in the overall mechanism of steroid hormone action. The ligand-based selectivity also takes into consideration the pharmacokinetics of each estrogen; thus, the same receptor in different target tissues or cells is exposed to a different group of hormones and, hence, mediates responses in a tissue-selective manner[26]. Similarly, the receptor-based selectivity is plausible as different target tissues, or cells exposed to the same hormones, may react in a specific manner because they have a different composition of receptors, for example the amount of ERα and ERβ, or the A and B subtypes of the PR. Although these two mechanisms are important, the evidence discussed above strongly suggests that to explain the tissue-selective actions of agonists, partial agonists and antagonists, the effector site-based selectivity is perhaps the most important. The cell-specific factors (co-activators, co-repressors) play a key role in the overall pharmacology of steroid hormones such as estrogens and progestins[26].

Progesterone's effects are also mediated by its nuclear receptor, and two receptor isoforms PR-A and PR-B (Figure 6), which are encoded by a single gene, have been identified[40]. Recent evidence indicates that these two forms are functionally different, and the ratio of PR-A to PR-B may modulate the cellular activity. The form PR-B appears to be a more potent activator of target genes, while PR-A acts as a dominant repressor of PR-B[40]. Since different progestins can interact with the two receptors differentially, all progestins, just like the various estrogens, may not have the same effects in different progesterone target tissues.

Although substantial evidence in support of effector site-based selectivity is based on *in vitro* transient transfection assay techniques, and the transfected gene constructs may not fully mimic the normal physiological conditions *in vivo*, recent demonstration that nuclear receptor corregulator complexes do exist *in vivo*[41], that steroid receptor co-activator-1 (SRC-1) is a histone acetyltransferase[42] and that similar proteins can play a functional role *in vivo* strongly support the concept discussed above.

Conjugated equine estrogens (CEEs) preparation is the single most prescribed drug for ERT for treatment of vasomotor symptoms and vaginal dryness, for prevention of osteoporosis and for reducing the risk of cardiovascular disease, Alzheimer's disease and colon cancer. The clinical aspects of these are dealt with in other sections of this book. The drug CEEs is a complex 'natural' extract of pregnant mares' urine, and contains at least ten different estrogens in their sulfate ester forms[4,43]. All ten of these estrogens in their unconjugated form have been shown to bind with estrogen receptors in human endometrial and rat uterine preparations[44]. The relative binding affinities[44–46] have the following order of activity: 17β-dihydroequilin ≥ 17β-estradiol > 17β-dihydroequilenin > estrone > equilin > 17α-dihydroequilin > 17α-estradiol > Δ8-17β-estradiol > 17α-dihydroequilenin > equilenin > Δ8-estrone. The Δ8-17β-estradiol has not yet been shown to be present in CEEs, but is an *in vivo* metabolite of Δ8-estrone in postmenopausal women[46]. Based on the mechanism of action of steroid hormones discussed, it would appear that each individual component of CEEs can result in a specific estrogen–receptor conformation that can potentially have different or selective effects in different estrogen target tissues, i.e. act as SERMs. Therefore, the overall biological and clinical effects observed in postmenopausal women treated with CEEs are the result of the sum of the individual activities of all of its estrogenic components. This is in keeping with observations that all of these estrogens are biologically active and have varying degrees of uterotropic activity[44,45].

Most of the estrogen and progestin actions can be explained by the above genomic mechanism; however, some extremely rapid effects of 17β-estradiol and other steroids are observed within minutes (acute effects) and these suggest the existence of what has been termed the 'non-genomic' mechanism of steroid hormone action. These non-genomic actions appear to be mediated by cell-membrane receptors and involve calcium, cyclic adenosine monophosphate (cAMP) and other second messengers[47–49]. The physiological and clinical relevance of this mechanism, and the likelihood of 'cross-talk' between these two mechanisms, remain to be established.

Natural and synthetic estrogens and progestins for ERT and HRT

Estrogens and progestins used for ERT and HRT have, for simplicity, been divided into three types: natural, native/synthetic and synthetic (Figure 8). The term 'natural' implies that the substance exists in nature in that form, and that it can be formulated into a drug with minimal processing and requires no chemical modification, for example CEEs. Native/synthetic means that the steroid exists in nature, for example 17β-estradiol, but for it to be formulated as a drug, it has to be synthesized (several chemical steps) from a natural starting material such as Mexican yams or soy beans. It is important to note that steroid hormones such as 17β-estradiol, estrone sulfate or progesterone are not found in Mexican yam or the soy bean, but can

be prepared from sterols and sapogenins present in these plants. For more than 50 years, most of the currently available steroid hormones have been synthesized from these plant sources[50].

Although the steroid hormones synthesized from these plants are chemically and biologically the same as those produced by humans or animals, there is no scientific evidence to date which indicates that the ingestion or application of topical creams containing Mexican yams, or soy beans, leads to the formation of 17β-estradiol, estrone, progesterone, etc. The human body lacks the necessary enzymes to transform plant sterols and sapogenins biochemically into active steroid hormones.

The term 'synthetic' means that these steroids do not exist in nature and are designed and chemically synthesized by man. Like the native/synthetic steroids, these can also be synthesized from the same plant sources[50]. A wide variety of these drugs is currently available, and some of the oral and parenteral forms of estrogens used for replacement therapy are given in Table 2. The active components and their concentrations are also indicated.

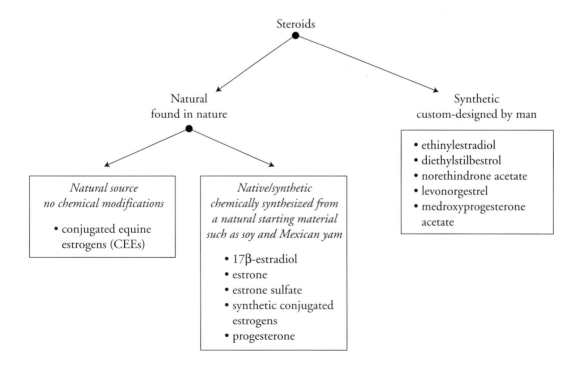

Figure 8 Examples of natural and synthetic estrogens and progestins

Table 2 Examples of various estrogen preparations (concentration of active estrogens)

Brand name	Active components (concentration)	Available dose(s)
Estrace®	micronized 17β-estradiol (100%)	1 mg, 2 mg
Ogen®	piperazine estrone sulfate (100%)	0.625 mg, 1.25 mg, 2.5 mg, 5 mg
Premarin®	mixture of at least ten conjugated equine estrogens (CEEs): sulfate esters of estrone (50%), equilin (22%), 17α-dihydroequilin (14%), 17α-estradiol (4.5%), Δ⁸-estrone (3.5%), equilenin (2%), 17β-dihydroequilin (1.7%), 17α-dihydroequilenin (1.2%), 17β-estradiol (1%), 17β-dihydroequilenin (0.5%)	0.3 mg, 0.625 mg, 0.9 mg, 1.25 mg, 2.5 mg
Estratab®	estrone sulfate (75–85%), equilin sulfate (6–15%)	0.625 mg
Estinyl®	ethinylestradiol (100%)	0.02 mg, 0.05 mg, 0.5 mg
Estraderm®	transdermal 17β-estradiol (100%)	0.025 mg, 0.05 mg, 0.1 mg
Premarin® vaginal cream	mixture of ten estrogens – CEEs (see Premarin)	0.625 mg/g cream
Estring®	vaginal ring containing 17β-estradiol (100%)	2 mg/90 days (7.5 μg/day release)
Del estrogen®	17β-estradiol valerate (100%)	10 mg/ml sesame oil for im administration

im, intramuscular

Pharmacokinetics of various estrogens: effect of route of administration

Absorption and metabolic changes

For an estrogen to exert its biological effects, it must first be absorbed, then reach and interact with its receptors in target tissues. The rates at which these events occur depend on the route of administration. The overall metabolic fate of an estrogen (or progestin) in the human body is schematically depicted in Figure 9 (for details see reference 51).

The oral route of administration is the most frequently used method, and appears to be the route preferred by a majority of postmenopausal women. As depicted in Figure 9, the route and dose of administration of an estrogen can have distinct and divergent effects in postmenopausal women. Oral estrogen by virtue of the first-pass effect results in marked alterations in hepatic metabolism, such as increases in angiotensinogen, SHBG, CBG, high-density lipoprotein (HDL) cholesterol, triglycerides and clotting factors, and a decrease in low-density lipoprotein (LDL) cholesterol and total cholesterol levels. These changes in plasma proteins and lipids are a consequence of the initial high concentrations of estrogens in the liver after oral administration. These metabolic changes can have important clinical implications, particularly

for cardiovascular disease in postmenopausal women[52,53], and these aspects are discussed in other parts of this book.

Routes of administration whereby the liver is bypassed, such as transdermal and parenteral administration (Figure 9), do not undergo the first-pass effect, and either the changes in serum proteins and lipids are not observed or the effects are blunted[54-58]. A comparison of the effects of oral and transdermal administration on hepatic parameters is given in Table 3. The improvements in lipid profiles observed with oral estrogens have recently been confirmed in a prospective prevention trial[59]. Another factor that may have an important role in cardiovascular disease is plasminogen activator inhibitor type 1 (PAI-1), which is an important inhibitor of fibrinolysis[58]. Changes in PAI-1 levels are the result of the first-pass effect seen with oral estrogens (Table 3). The increase in triglycerides seen with oral estrogens is not observed with transdermal estrogens[54-56]. Although triglycerides are considered to be a separate risk factor for cardiovascular disease, the modest increases seen with oral estrogens in normal healthy postmenopausal women do not appear to have a negative impact[52,53,59].

Apart from differences between oral and nonoral estrogens, there are important differences between different oral estrogens. In general, oral

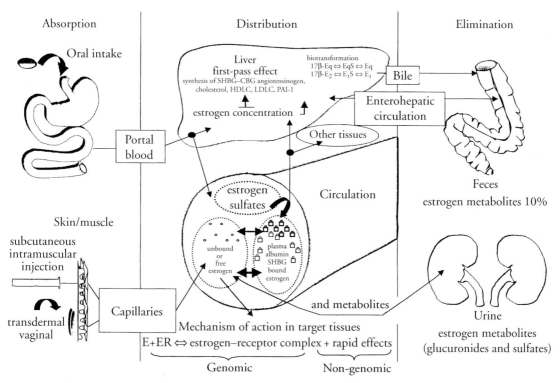

Figure 9 Effect of route of administration on metabolic fate of estrogens. SHBG, sex hormone-binding globulin; CBG, corticosteroid-binding globulin; HDLC, high-density lipoprotein cholesterol; LDLC, low-density lipoprotein cholesterol; PAI, plasminogen activator inhibitor; 17β-Eq, 17β-dihydroequilin; EqS, equilin sulfate; Eq, equilin; 17β-E$_2$, 17β-estradiol; E$_1$S, estrone sulfate; E$_1$, estrone; E, estrogen; ER, estrogen receptor

Table 3 Effect of oral and transdermal estrogens on hepatic parameters

Hepatic parameter	Oral estrogens	Transdermal estradiol
SHBG	↑	→
CBG	↑	→
Renin substrate (angiotensinogen)	↑	→
IGF-I	↓	↓
Total cholesterol	↓	↓
HDL cholesterol	↑	→↓
LDL cholesterol	↓	↓
Triglycerides	↑	→↓
PAI-1	↓	→

↑, increase; ↓, decrease; →, no effect; SHBG, sex hormone-binding globulin; CBG, corticosteroid-binding globulin; IGF, insulin-like growth factor; HDL, high-density lipoprotein; LDL, low-density lipoprotein; PAI, plasminogen activator inhibitor

estrogen sulfates, for example equilin sulfate (a major ring B unsaturated component of CEEs), after oral administration are directly absorbed to some extent from the gastrointestinal tract without prior hydrolysis[60]. However, a substantial portion of the ingested estrogen sulfate is absorbed after the removal of the sulfate ester by hydrolysis[60]. The unconjugated estrogen after absorption is rapidly resulfated as the result of the first-pass effect (Figure 9). The estrogen sulfates such as estrone sulfate and equilin sulfate are the main (> 90%) circulating forms of estrogens in postmenopausal women taking ERT[60-62]. Similarly, ingestion of 10 mg of CEEs containing approximately 4.5 mg of estrone sulfate and 2.5 mg of equilin sulfate results in maximum levels of equilin (560 pg/ml) and estrone (1400 pg/ml) after 3 and 5 h, respectively. Plasma levels decline gradually, and only small amounts of both estrogens are detectable after 24 h[63]. Similar rates of appearance and disappearance of estrogens are also observed when smaller doses of CEEs are administered. In contrast, intravenous administration of 10 mg of CEEs results in maximum concentrations of equilin (4000 pg/ml) and estrone (11 200 pg/ml) within 10 min[63]. Oral administration of estrone sulfate also results in the rapid appearance of unconjugated 17β-estradiol and estrone in the blood[64,65]. Oral administration of micronized 17β-estradiol (Estrace®) has also been shown to be efficacious[66], provided sufficiently high doses are administered. Although oral micronized 17β-estradiol is absorbed, a substantial amount of it is metabolized in the gastrointestinal tract prior to it reaching the liver, where it is further metabolized and inactivated (Figure 9). The main metabolites that enter the circulation are estrone and estrone sulfate. These observations indicate that not only are estrogen sulfates highly water-soluble and easily absorbable, but also that the sulfation protects the estrogen from rapid metabolism in the gastrointestinal tract.

The synthetic estrogens such as ethinylestradiol are infrequently used in North America for ERT, and are also readily absorbed from the gastrointestinal tract. Peak serum levels are observed between 1 and 4 h[67]. This estrogen, because of its structure (17-ethinyl group), is not readily deactivated in the liver, and therefore it has a profound and prolonged effect on hepatic protein synthesis (Table 4).

Although all oral estrogens undergo the first-pass effect, the amounts bioavailable are quite variable, and this is reflected in their potencies. Comparison of the relative potencies of four oral estrogens, piperazine estrone sulfate, micronized estradiol, CEEs and ethinylestradiol, in terms of suppression of serum FSH and increase in hepatic protein synthesis (Table 4), indicates that on a weight basis, ethinylestradiol is far more potent than the other three oral estrogens. The CEEs are up to three times more potent in inducing hepatic proteins than micronized estradiol and estrone sulfate[68]. As discussed above in 'In vivo transport of estrogens and progestins', the significantly higher levels of SHBG will result in a lower level of the physiologically active free form of estrogen available for biological action.

A recent, large prospective study of postmenopausal women showed a significant association between a lower percentage of endogenous 17β-estradiol bound to SHBG, or in other words, an increase in the percentage of free 17β-estradiol, and a higher risk for breast cancer[69]. Thus, estrogen formulations for ERT or HRT that increase the levels of SHBG to a greater extent may be preferable. Even though, as discussed above, ethinylestradiol compared to other oral estrogens stimulated the synthesis of SHBG by over 600 times (Table 4), this estrogen may not be an ideal estrogen for ERT (at least in concentrations used in oral contraceptives); it does not bind to SHBG, and therefore most of it is essentially in a bioavailable form, and this is reflected in its much higher stimulatory hepatic activity.

The notion that dosages of various estrogens which result in comparable serum levels of unconjugated 17β-estradiol, or the assumption that all of the estrogenic effects of natural estrogens are solely dependent on levels of 17β-estradiol, is not supported by firm scientific data. On the contrary, a recent prospective study[70] of menopausal women

Table 4 Differences in relative potency of oral estrogens according to some serum parameters of estrogenicity. Data derived from reference 68

Estrogen preparation	SHBG-BC	CBG-BC	Angiotensinogen	FSH
Ogen® (piperazine estrone sulfate)	1.0	1.0	1.0	1.1
Estrace® (micronized estradiol)	1.0	1.0	0.7	1.3
Premarin® (conjugated equine estrogens)	3.2	2.5	3.5	1.4
Estinyl® (ethinylestradiol)	614	1000	232	80–200

SHBG-BC, sex hormone-binding globulin binding capacity; CBG-BC, corticosteroid-binding globulin binding capacity; FSH, follicle stimulating hormone

compared the effects of CEEs, micronized estradiol and transdermal 17β-estradiol on serum SHBG, and correlated this with serum levels of 17β-estradiol, estrone and free 17β-estradiol. The data indicated that the levels of unconjugated 17β-estradiol were the lowest after CEE therapy (4 months), yet the levels of SHBG were the highest. In contrast, levels of 17β-estradiol following administration of micronized estradiol and transdermal estradiol were significantly higher, yet compared to CEEs, the effect on SHBG was only 50% and 14%, respectively. The increase in SHBG levels following CEEs was associated with a corresponding decrease in the free form of 17β-estradiol. Therefore, the estrogenic effects of various ERT modalities are dependent on factors besides serum levels of unconjugated estradiol[70]. Moreover, the same drug in different formulations can give rise to differences in the rate of absorption and biological effects. For example, vaginal CEE cream is rapidly absorbed, but the serum levels of estrogens attained are approximately one-quarter of those obtained with similar oral doses[71,72]. However, even though the serum levels of estrogens following 0.3 mg vaginal CEEs are low, this dose is sufficient to provide physiological replacement to the vaginal epithelium, but no effects on hepatic proteins are observed[72]. In contrast, after 25 mg vaginal CEEs, systemic effects comparable to those with 0.625 mg oral CEEs are observed[72,73]. Similarly, comparison of the rate and extent of absorption following administration of 0.625 mg CEEs or 0.625 mg of a mixture of estrone sulfate and equilin sulfate (Estratab®) indicates significant differences in the relative bioavailability of estrogens[74,75]. Since osteoporosis and coronary heart disease are silent diseases, it seems prudent to require at least some clinical evidence of efficacy for each different estrogen formulation.

Metabolic clearance rate of conjugated and unconjugated estrogens

The metabolic clearance rate (MCR) of a steroid is defined as the volume of plasma (blood) from which the steroid is totally and irreversibly cleared in unit time (liters per day or liters per day/m^2), and provides information regarding the overall *in vivo* metabolic fate of the steroid[76]. The MCRs of some sulfate-conjugated and unconjugated estrogens have been reported (Table 5). The elimination from plasma of equilin sulfate, 17β-dihydroequilin sulfate and estrone sulfate is described as a function of two exponentials, and examples of these are shown in Figure 10[77,78]. The initial fast component for the three estrogens has a half-life ($t_{1/2}$) of 3–5 min, while the $t_{1/2}$ of the slower component of equilin sulfate, 17β-dihydroequilin sulfate and estrone sulfate is 190 ± 23, 147 ± 15 and 300–500 min, respectively[61,62,77,78]. The initial volume of distribution (V_1) for equilin sulfate, 17β-dihydroequilin sulfate and estrone sulfate is 12.4 ± 1.6, 6.0 ± 0.5 and 7.2 ± 0.6, respectively. The V_1 of estrogen sulfates depend on their relative binding affinities to plasma proteins. However, since the apparent V_1 is higher than the plasma volume, these sulfates bind to plasma proteins such as albumin with relatively low affinity, as has been discussed[17]. The MCR of estrone sulfate (80–105 l/day/m^2), equilin sulfate (170–176 l/day/m^2) and 17β-dihydroequilin sulfate (376–460 l/day/m^2) (Table 5) indicates that ring B unsaturated

Table 5 Metabolic clearance rate (MCR) of estrogens. Values are expressed as mean $\pm$ SEM

Estrogen	MCR (l/day/m^2)	Reference(s)
Estrone sulfate	$80 \pm 10^*$; 105 ± 20	61, 62
Equilin sulfate	$176 \pm 44^*$; 170 ± 18	77, 79
17β-Dihydroequilin sulfate	$376 \pm 53^*$; 460 ± 60	78, 80
Estrone	1050 ± 70	81, 82
17β-Estradiol	580 ± 30	81, 82
Equilin	2641^*	77
17β-Dihydroequilin	$1252 \pm 103^*$	78
Δ^8-Estrone	$1711 \pm 252^*$	46

*MCR measured by the single injection technique

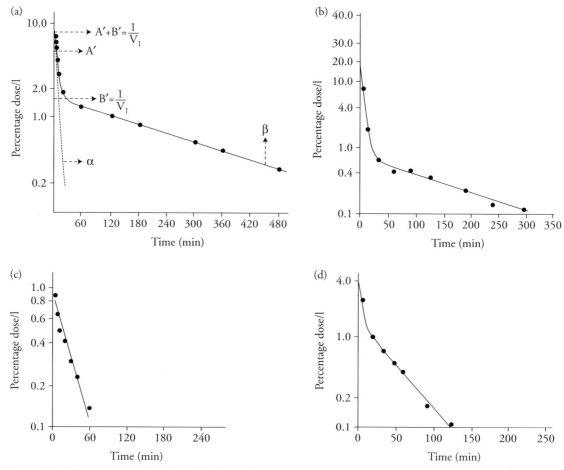

Figure 10 Disappearance of radioactivity from plasma as [³H]equilin sulfate (a), [³H]17β-dihydroequilin sulfate (b), [³H]equilin (c) and [³H]17β-dihydroequilin (d) plotted as percentage of administered dose versus time of blood sampling[77,78]

estrogens are cleared from the circulation at a faster rate than the ring B saturated estrogen, estrone sulfate[61,62,77-81]. The MCRs of these sulfates, compared to their unconjugated forms, are low (Table 5), and this is due to their relatively higher binding affinity for serum albumin, compared to unconjugated forms[16-19]. The ionic nature of the steroid sulfates may also play a role in the overall clearance of the estrogen sulfates. The low MCR can also result if only a small fraction of these estrogen sulfates is being metabolized. This appears to be the case, as only 11, 16 and 35% estrone sulfate, equilin sulfate and 17β-dihydroequilin sulfate is metabolized, respectively[61,62,75-79]. The 2–5-fold higher MCR of 17β-dihydroequilin sulfate, compared to equilin sulfate and estrone

sulfate, is in keeping with its higher rate of metabolism[78].

The MCRs of unconjugated equilin (2641 l/day/m²), 17β-dihydroequilin (1252 l/day/ m²), estrone (1050 l/day/m²) and 17β-estradiol (580 l/day/m²) are several-fold higher than those of their corresponding sulfate forms (Table 5). The pattern of disappearance of equilin (Figure 10) and estrone is consistent with a one-component model[77,81], whereas those of 17β-dihydroequilin and Δ⁸-estrone exhibit two components[46,78]. The 17β-reduced estrogens such as 17β-estradiol and 17β-dihydroequilin have a much higher affinity for SHBG, and therefore are cleared more slowly (two times) than their corresponding 17-keto forms, estrone and equilin.

244

The pharmacokinetics of estrogen sulfates compared with their unconjugated (non-sulfated) forms further indicate that the sulfate-conjugated forms of estrogens are cleared from the circulation at a much slower rate (Table 5). These data support the general hypothesis that sulfate-conjugated steroids act as reservoirs from which the unconjugated steroids are being formed as needed.

Interconversions between estrogens under steady state conditions

In postmenopausal women, estrone Δ^8-estrone and equilin are metabolized to circulating 17β-estradiol, Δ^8-17β-estradiol and 17β-dihydro-equilin, respectively[46,61,62,77,78]. The precise conversion ratios for the formation of some of these metabolites have been determined under steady state conditions (Figure 11). The transfer constants (ρ values) for the conversion of equilin sulfate to equilin and 17β-dihydroequilin are 0.25 and 0.15, respectively[79]. The corresponding ρ values for the conversion of estrone sulfate to estrone and 17β-estradiol are 0.15–0.21 and 0.014–0.03, respectively[61,62] (Figure 11). Recent data[46] also indicate that, like equilin sulfate and estrone sulfate, the main circulating forms of Δ^8-estrone are Δ^8-estrone sulfate and Δ^8-17β-estradiol sulfate. Moreover, the amounts of these Δ^8-metabolites are almost equal[46]. This pattern of metabolism, i.e. formation of equal amounts of 17-oxidized and 17β-reduced

metabolites, is not observed with other estrogens. The oxidative pathway is generally preferred, compared to the reductive pathway[82]. The 17β-reduced estrogens are considered to be the active metabolites, and the activation by 17β-reduction is several-fold higher for the ring B unsaturated estrogens, compared to the ring B saturated estrogens. These types of metabolic differences between various estrogens may impact on the overall biological and clinical activity of different estrogens. The increased estrogenicity (Table 4) associated with CEEs may in part be due to the higher level of 17β-activation.

Estrogen metabolism

Apart from metabolic interconversions, estrogens ultimately undergo irreversible metabolism primarily in tissues such as the liver and kidney, and to some extent in target tissues such as the endometrium and brain[66]. The major irreversible metabolic transformations of estrogens occur in the A and D ring, yielding mainly the 2-, 4- and 16α-hydroxylated metabolites (Figure 12). The 16α-hydroxylated metabolites are discussed separately under urinary excretion of estrogens.

Catechol estrogens

Both 2- and 4-hydroxy estrogen metabolites (catechol estrogens) are formed in the human, and

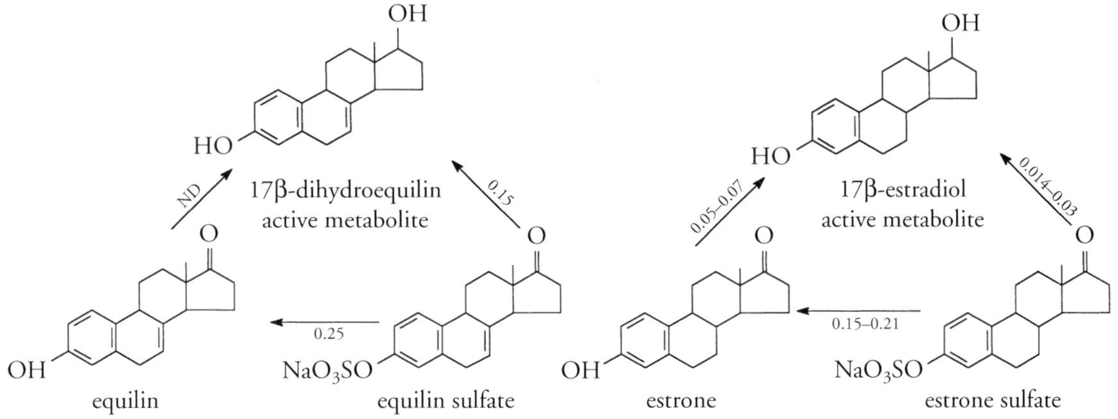

Figure 11 Extent of *in vivo* activation of two main components of conjugated equine estrogens by 17β-hydroxysteroid dehydrogenase: values shown are transfer constants (ρ values). ND, not determined

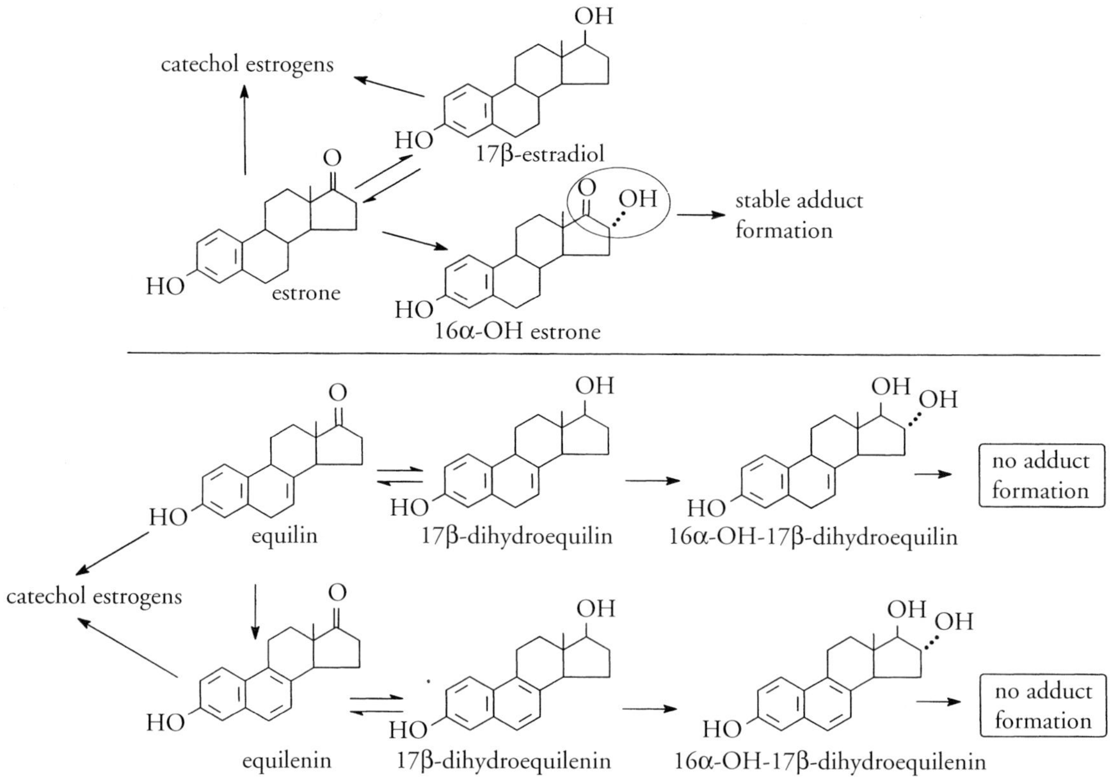

Figure 12 *In vivo* and *in vitro* metabolism of estrone and equilin via catechol estrogen and 16α-hydroxylation. The potential for adduct formation with macromolecules is indicated. The α-ketol structure is circled[45]

it has been suggested that the oncogenic potential of endogenous estrogens, estrone and 17β-estradiol, and synthetic estrogens depends on the extent of their metabolism to catechol estrogens[83,84]. Thus, in the Syrian hamster kidney model, 17β-estradiol, estrone and equilin induced kidney tumors in the majority of animals; however, 2-hydroxyestrone and 2-hydroxy-17β-estradiol were inactive, while the corresponding 4-hydroxylated metabolites, 4-hydroxyestrone and 4-hydroxy-17β-estradiol, induced tumors in 100% of the animals[85,86]. In contrast, 4-hydroxyequilenin was devoid of any carcinogenic activity in the hamster kidney[85,86]. Conflicting data have been reported by the same group of investigators[85,86], and the relevance of these observations in post-menopausal women taking exogenous estrogens has not been established.

In the human endometrium, equilin forms mostly 2-hydroxyequilin and small amounts of 4-hydroxyequilin[87]. In contrast, 2-hydroxy-17β-estradiol and 4-hydroxy-17β-estradiol are formed in equal amounts by the proliferative human endometrium[88]. Thus, the extent of 2- and 4-hydroxylation depends on the structure of the estrogen. The role of catechol estrogen formed *in vivo* by the endometrium in postmenopausal women is not known. Whether the catechol derivatives of ring B unsaturated estrogens serve as substrates for redox cycling, and generate free radicals that may subsequently cause cell damage in a manner proposed for the classical estrogens, remains to be established. Alternatively, catechol equilin derivatives and those of other estrogens can play a protective role in the endometrium and other estrogen target tissues as free radical scavengers and antioxidants[45]. Moreover, the formation of these types of catechol estrogen metabolites can also decrease the amount of active estrogens available for metabolism to the more potent 17β-reduced products (Figure 12).

Urinary excretion of ring B unsaturated estrogens

In postmenopausal women, ring B unsaturated estrogens equilin sulfate, equilin, 17β-dihydroequilin sulfate and 17β-dihydroequilin are extensively metabolized. Approximately 50% of the administered dose is excreted in the urine[43,45,89] and, of this, approximately 60–75% is in the form of glucuronides and 16–17% as sulfate metabolites. Only 1–2% is excreted as unconjugated metabolites. These data indicate that, although estrogens circulate mainly in the form of estrogen sulfates in postmenopausal women, before excretion these estrogens are further metabolized to the corresponding glucuronides. In the urine of women, small amounts of equilin, equilenin, 17β-dihydroequilin and 17β-dihydroequilenin are excreted following administration of equilin or equilin sulfate[43,45,89].

In postmenopausal women and men, the bulk of equilin metabolites formed and excreted in the urine following administration of equilin or equilin sulfate or 17β-dihydroequilin sulfate, are two extremely polar metabolites[4,43,45,89]. These metabolites were recently[45,90] identified as being 16α-hydroxy-17β-dihydroequilin and 16α-hydroxy-17β-dihydroequilenin (Figure 12). The corresponding 17-keto metabolites 16α-hydroxyequilin and 16α-hydroxyequilenin were not identified (or present) in the urine.

Earlier studies[91,92] with classical estrogens indicate the potential involvement of 16α-hydroxylated estrogens in the oncogenic process. The hypothesis is based on the demonstration that 16α-hydroxyestrone, a major urinary metabolite of 17β-estradiol and estrone, can form stable covalent adducts with macromolecules (proteins, DNA). The authors propose[93] that the covalent adduct formation (Figure 12) between 16α-hydroxyestrone, a major urinary metabolite of estrone can lead to the formation of stable covalent adducts with macromolecules (proteins, DNA) involved in diseases such as breast cancer[94]. They further propose[93] that the covalent adduct formation (Figure 12) between 16α-hydroxyestrone and macromolecules occurs because of the presence of the D ring α-ketol (i.e. 16α-hydroxy-17-ketone structure, Figure 12, circled). These investigators[95] have

further suggested that metabolism favoring 16α-hydroxylation leads to an increased cancer risk in postmenopausal women. Based on the observation that 16α-hydroxyestrone is a potent estrogen while 2-hydroxyestrone is relatively inactive, they further propose that the ratio of urinary 2-hydroxyestrone to 16α-hydroxyestrone is a predictor of cancer risk, and that this ratio is inversely correlated with risk for breast and cervical cancer[95]. A recent[96] pilot study did not find a significant correlation between the ratio of urinary 2-hydroxyestrone and 16α-hydroxyestrone in postmenopausal women with and without breast cancer. Careful analysis of these data indicates that the association observed previously[95] is most likely an 'artifact' of subgroup analysis, or a result of the disease process itself or the treatment the women with breast cancer received. Further studies are required either to confirm or to refute this hypothesis.

Interestingly, the two 16α-hydroxylated metabolites of ring B unsaturated estrogens isolated from the human urine lack the α-ketol structure (Figure 12); it is therefore highly unlikely that these 16α-hydroxylated metabolites of equilin can form the potentially carcinogenic stable adducts, by the proposed mechanism[91-94]. The absence of 17-keto-16α-hydroxylated derivatives of equilin in human urine following administration of equilin, equilin sulfate, 17β-dihydroequilin and 17β-dihydroequilin sulfate supports the previous conclusions that 17β-reduction occurs at a much higher extent with ring B unsaturated estrogens than with the classical estrogen estrone (Figure 11). Based on these observations, it appears that 17β-reduction of ring B unsaturated estrogens occurs not only at a higher rate, but prior to 16α-hydroxylation as depicted in Figure 12. Whether these differences in metabolism between various estrogens determine if an estrogen has a potential for carcinogenicity in the human remains to be investigated.

The facts that some of those estrogens (CEEs) have been in use for more than five decades, and the increased risk for breast cancer in women taking these estrogens is barely detectable argue against the hypothesis that exogenous estrogens or their catechol or 16α-hydroxylated metabolites play a significant role in the etiology of breast cancer.

Pharmacokinetics of progestins

The doses of estrogen used for ERT to prevent bone loss can result in endometrial hyperplasia in 15–30% of non-hysterectomized postmenopausal women[59]. Various progestins are available to prevent endometrial hyperplasia and thus reduce or eliminate the risk for endometrial adeno-carcinoma[97,98]. Uterine protection requires that progestin be given in sufficient amounts for 10–14 days per month (sequential estrogen–progestin) or with each dose of estrogen (continuous combined). The former regimen causes monthly bleeding and the latter may result in spotting or bleeding for the first few months of therapy. All progestins attenuate some of the estrogens' favorable effects on lipoproteins[59]. Progesterone and hydroxypro-gesterone derivatives appear to have a less negative impact than the more androgenic 19-nortestos-terone derivatives (Figure 2).

There are few published pharmacokinetic data relating to the use of various progestins in post-menopausal women. Most of the pharmacokinetic data regarding progestins are derived from studies of oral contraceptives in young women. Moreover, these data are based on studies where the pharma-cokinetics of the progestin were determined in the presence of a relatively high dose of an extremely potent oral estrogen ethinylestradiol. This estrogen has profound effects on hepatic protein synthesis which can have a major impact on the amount of bioavailable progestin, as discussed above. The 'ideal' progestin, i.e. a progestin that can selectively antagonize the effect of estrogen only at the endo-metrium, is not yet available: however, a number of progestins have been shown to be effective in protecting the endometrium[97-99]. Medroxy-progesterone acetate (MPA) is the most frequently used progestin in North America, while others such as norethindrone acetate, norethisterone and norgestrel are also used, more frequently in Europe. More recently, micronized progesterone has become available, and has been shown also to be effective in protecting the endometrium[59].

Medroxyprogesterone acetate is readily absor-bed after oral administration, and peak levels (3–5 ng/ml) are observed between 1 and 4 h. Its MCR is approximately 21 l/day/kg, and it has a $t_{1/2}$ of 24 h[20,100,101]. Over 90% of MPA circulates bound to serum albumin and is metabolized to 3-, 6- and 20-hydroxy-5α- and 5β-reduced com-pounds. These metabolites are excreted in urine in the form of glucuronides[100]. The usual effective dose when given over the last 10–14 days of each monthly cycle is 10 mg; however, 2.5 mg given daily in combination with estrogen is as effective in protecting the endometrium in most postmenopausal women[59,97-99].

Oral crystalline progesterone is poorly absorbed, and is rapidly inactivated in the gastro-intestinal tract and during the first pass through the liver. However, sufficient amounts of micro-nized progesterone (200 mg) are absorbed and escape the first-pass hepatic metabolism such that levels of approximately 4–12 ng/ml are observed within 4 h. This dose of micronized progesterone is sufficient to protect the endometrium, and does not appear to reduce the benefits of estrogens on lipids[59]. Progesterone circulates primarily bound to albumin, and approximately 20% is bound to CBG. Progesterone is rapidly metabolized to its 3-, 5- and 20-reduced (α and β) metabolites, which are excreted mainly as glucuronides.

The detailed pharmacokinetics of synthetic progestins such as norethindrone, levonorgestrel, norgestimate, desogestrel and gestodene have been determined in young cycling women and usually in combination with ethinylestradiol. The comparative data indicate that the plasma half-life of these progestins is between 8 and 12 h. Maxi-mum plasma levels are attained within 1–2 h. Gestodene is cleared at a slower rate (48 ml/h/kg), compared to levonorgestrel (105 ml/h/kg), 3-keto-desogestrel (174 ml/h/kg) and norethindrone (355 ml/h/kg)[102-105].

Studies are needed to determine the pharmaco-kinetics, the efficacy and the minimum doses of these progestins that are required to protect against endometrial hyperplasia in postmenopausal women taking ERT. Long-term comparative trials of these progestins versus progesterone and medroxyprogesterone acetate are also needed to determine whether there are any advantages in using these C_{19}-nortestosterone derivatives.

Antioxidant properties of estrogens

Low-density lipoprotein (LDL) cholesterol is a risk factor for atherogenesis[106]. Several observational studies indicate that ERT and HRT in post-menopausal women are cardioprotective[59,107–110]. However, clinical trials are still needed to confirm these important observations. The mechanism(s) by means of which these estrogens exert their beneficial effects is not known. An earlier hypothesis proposed that changes in total cholesterol, LDL cholesterol and HDL cholesterol are key factors. Recent observations suggest that these types of lipid changes account for only 25–35% of the cardioprotective benefits associated with ERT[107]. Recent studies suggest that excess free radicals may initiate atherosclerosis by damaging blood vessel walls, and that oxidized LDL which can be formed *in vivo* is more atherogenic than native LDL[111]. Inhibition of this free radical-initiated LDL oxidation can be one of the mechanisms by means of which antioxidants such as vitamin E and phenolic compounds such as estrogens exert their beneficial effects. Indeed, *in vivo* and *in vitro* studies have demonstrated that estrogens can inhibit oxidation of LDL[112–117]. *In vitro* studies[115] have demonstrated that all estrogens are potent antioxidants (Figure 13) with Δ^8-estrone, 17β-dihydroequilenin and 17α-dihydroequilenin being the most potent. The dose–response data regarding the quantity of each compound required to double the length of the lag phase of LDL oxidation indicated that the minimum dose of Δ^8-estrone, 17β-dihydroequilenin and 17α-dihydroequilenin was 0.47 nmol, of Δ^8-17β-estradiol and equilenin was 0.7 nmol, of 17β-dihydroequilin and 17α-dihydroequilin was 0.9 nmol, and of equilin, estrone, 17β-estradiol and 17α-estradiol was 1.3 nmol. In comparison with estrogens, antioxidants such as two red-wine components *trans*-resveratrol (4,3′,5′-trihydroxystilbene) and quercetin (3,3′,4′,5,7-pentahydroxyflavone), vitamin E and a serum cholesterol-lowering drug probucol are, with the exception of quercetin, much weaker antioxidants (Figure 13).

All of the estrogens tested appear to act directly, as no metabolism of any of these estrogens to more potent antioxidants occurred under the conditions used. These results further indicate that all of

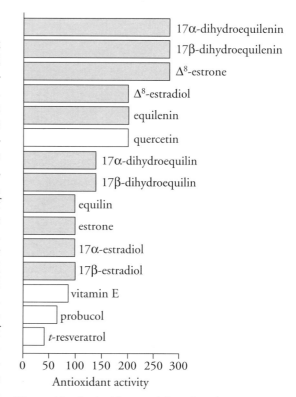

Figure 13 Antioxidant activity of various estrogens and other phenolic compounds

the estrogenic components of CEEs are potent antioxidants[115]. Interestingly, the most potent estrogenic antioxidants are relatively weak uterotropic agents[45]. These types of weak estrogens can serve as models for development of selective estrogens that may be useful in reducing the risk of cardiovascular disease not only in postmenopausal women, but also in men. Since the cardioprotective effects are to some extent due to the ability of these estrogens to protect LDL against oxidative modification(s), the mechanism involved is most likely non-genomic.

The ability of these estrogens to protect *in vivo* the oxidation of LDL in postmenopausal women has also been demonstrated, both when given individually (Δ^8-estrone sulfate) and after long-term (> 1 year) treatment of postmenopausal women with CEEs[116,117]. Addition of medroxyprogesterone acetate in the long-term study did not reduce the antioxidant effect of estrogens[116]; however, in the short term (30 days), the addition of a progestin given either continuously or in a cyclic manner caused the effect of CEEs on LDL oxidation to be blunted or absent[117].

The precise mechanism(s) by which estrogens inhibit LDL oxidation remains to be established; however, a number of potential mechanisms can be proposed: estrogens may become incorporated into the LDL particle in a manner similar to that described for the incorporation of vitamin E into LDL. This incorporation of estrogen may change the conformation of LDL such that it is protected from oxidation. Alternatively, estrogens can function as free radical scavengers, and thereby inhibit the lipid peroxidation process. Estrogens may also act by directly sequestering endogenous metal ions such as copper and iron, or by donating a proton to reduce the peroxyl free radical[118]. Estrogens may also function synergestically with endogeneous antioxidants associated with LDL. Along with the above, a number of other possible mechanisms involving effects of estrogens on arachidonic acid-induced DNA damage have been proposed and recently reviewed[119,120].

Recent observational studies also indicate that ERT in postmenopausal women significantly reduces the risk, or delays the onset, of Alzheimer's disease[121-123]. A number of mechanisms such as increase in cerebral blood flow, prevention of neuronal and vascular injury from oxidative stress, and inhibition of the cytotoxicity of amyloid β-proteins have been proposed to explain the neuroprotective effect of estrogens. Recently, it was demonstrated that LDL is transported to the brain[124,125], and oxidative stress in the brain can result in the oxidation of LDL. Several studies have suggested that oxidative stress may be involved in the pathogenesis of Alzheimer's disease[126,127]. Similarly, β-amyloid is thought to play a role in the neurodegenerative process occurring in Alzheimer's disease by inducing lipid peroxidation via free radical-mediated mechanisms[128]. Since both oxidized LDL and β-amyloid are extremely cytotoxic, inhibition of the oxidative stress by estrogens may be an important mechanism by means of which estrogens express their neuroprotective effects.

Summary and future directions

Most menopausal women can expect to live more than one-third of their lives in the postmenopausal years. This period of life is associated with an estrogen- and progesterone-deficient state and, as a result, women often experience a series of menopausal symptoms. The most frequent early symptoms are hot flushes, dyspareunia, atrophic vaginitis, insomnia and mood disturbances. Some of the long-term and potentially fatal consequences of estrogen loss are osteoporosis, cardiovascular disease and Alzheimer's disease. Estrogen replacement or estrogen–progestin replacement can ameliorate and/or decrease the risk of these debilitating disorders.

Both the structure of the estrogen and route of administration play important roles in the absorption, metabolism and type of pharmacological effects observed. Currently, several types of estrogen preparations such as oral preparations, transdermal patches, percutaneous gels, subcutaneous implants, vaginal rings and impregnated pessaries are available. At equivalent doses, these estrogens are effective in controlling vasomotor symptoms and some, such as the oral (CEEs) and transdermal (Estraderm) forms, prevent osteoporosis.

Regarding cardiovascular disease, different types of estrogens administered by different routes, for example oral versus transdermal, can have profoundly different effects on lipid metabolism and othe risk factors. Most of the long-term studies showing a reduced risk for cardiovascular disease were in postmenopausal women who had used oral estrogens, in particular CEEs.

Although a number of observational studies had also shown a beneficial effect of ERT in postmenopausal women with established coronary artery disease, a recent randomized, blinded placebo-controlled secondary prevention trial (Heart Estrogen/progestin Replacement Study, HERS) did not confirm the earlier observational data. On the contrary, HERS[129] reported that in the first year of HRT, women had a higher relative risk (1.52; 95% confidence interval (CI) 1.01–2.29) of secondary events, compared with the placebo groups. The relative risk, however, decreased after the first year of HRT (year 5, 0.67; 95% CI 0.43–1.04). In the HERS trial, CEEs and medroxyprogesterone acetate were administered daily, and the study did not include an estrogen arm. It is therefore difficult to ascertain whether the initial negative impact in coronary artery disease was a result of the estrogen or the continuous administration of the progestin. Results from a recent animal study[130] indicate that medroxyprogesterone acetate given continuously antagonizes the atheroprotective effect of CEEs. In view of these results, future studies with different types of progestins either administered sequentially or given continuously in women with established coronary disease may be ethically challenging, but are needed.

There is overwhelming evidence that unopposed estrogen is associated with a significant increase in endometrial cancer. However, these cancers have a much better prognosis than those that arise in women who have not taken exogenous estrogens[131]. Addition of a progestin to ERT has been shown to reduce the risk of endometrial cancers to almost undetectable levels[97,98]. However, in view of the potentially negative impact of progestins or HRT on coronary artery disease risk, the use of progestins in hysterectomized women has no advantage, nor is it required.

The recent developments regarding the mechanism of estrogen action indicate that different estrogens appear to exhibit varying degrees of activity in different tissues, and that the potency and efficacy of an estrogen can vary in different target tissues. Understanding of those molecular mechanisms explains not only how different estrogens act, but also how antiestrogens and SERMs exert their selective effects.

SERMs such as tamoxifen and raloxifene are being considered as alternatives to HRT. Raloxifene has recently been approved for use only in the prevention of osteoporosis. Although raloxifene has some advantages over tamoxifen and ERT in that it appears to act as an antagonist in tissues such as the uterus, like estrogen and tamoxifen it has agonist activity in the bone. Raloxifene's cardiovascular benefit has not been examined in clinical trials. Moreover, it is associated with a number of adverse effects such as hot flushes, leg cramps, blood clotting disorders and vaginal dryness, to name a few. Long-term consequences of raloxifene use have not been determined, as most of the studies have been carried out for less than 5 years. Similarly, there are no data regarding the effect of this SERM in women who are at high risk of developing breast cancer. However, studies have been initiated to answer these important questions.

All these data clearly indicate that the currently approved SERMs are not appropriate as alternatives to ERT or HRT in the majority of healthy postmenopausal women who are not at risk for breast cancer. However, based on what we now know about the structure–activity relationship, and the mechanisms by means of which SERMs express their selective effects, it is not premature to anticipate the development of more effective and safer tissue-selective estrogens and progestins in the very near future, i.e. designer estrogens and progestins are on their way. Availability of such SERMs and/or specific estrogens which have positive effects on the cardiovascular system may provide a means of reducing the risk of cardiovascular disease, not only in postmenopausal women, but also in men.

In the meantime, large clinical trials to address some of the questions have been initiated. One such trial is the Women's Health Initiative which is assessing the effect of ERT and HRT in women with and without documented heart disease, as well as other outcomes such as breast cancer, Alzheimer's disease, osteoporosis, colon cancer, eye disease and tooth loss. The results of this study will be available within the next 10 years or so.

Overall, during the past decade the benefits associated with the use of estrogens have been increasing rapidly, while the previously recognized serious negative side-effects such as endometrial cancer and possibly breast cancer have remained essentially unchanged, and no new contraindications have been identified. It is anticipated that a greater number of postmenopausal women will start using ERT/HRT as new benefits are recognized and appreciated by both the woman and the clinician.

Acknowledgements

The work in the author's laboratory was supported by the Medical Research Council of Canada Grant MT-11929 and by a basic research grant from

Wyeth-Ayerst, Philadelphia, USA. I would like to express my sincere thanks to Mrs Francine Bhavnani for the preparation of the figures and manuscript.

References

1. Shier MR, Strickler R. The ovaries and related reproductive endocrinology. In Ezrin C, Godden JO, Volpe R, eds. *Systemic Endocrinology*. New York: Harper and Row, 1979:258-331
2. McKinlay SM. The normal menopause transition: an overview. *Maturitas* 1996;23:137-45
3. Diczfalusy E, Benagiano G. Women and the third and fourth age. *Int J Gynecol Obstet* 1997;58:177-88
4. Bhavnani BR. The saga of the ring B unsaturated equine estrogens. *Endocr Rev* 1988;9:396-416
5. Kletzky OA, Nakamura RM, Thorneycroft IH, Mishell DR Jr. Log normal distribution of gonadotropins and ovarian steroid values in the normal menstrual cycle. *Am J Obstet Gynecol* 1975;121:688-94
6. Siiteri PK, MacDonald PC. Role of extraglandular estrogen in human endocrinology. In Greep RO, Astwood EB, eds. *Handbook of Physiology*. Washington, DC: American Physiological Society, 1963;Section 7:615-29
7. Casey ML, MacDonald PC. Origin of estrogen and regulation of its formation in postmenopausal women. In Buchsbaum HJ, eds. *The Menopause*. New York: Springer-Verlag, 1983:1-8
8. Siiteri PK. Adipose tissue as a source of hormones. *Am J Clin Nutr* 1987;45:277-82
9. Longcope C, Franz C, Morello C, Baker R, Johnston CC Jr. Steroid and gonadotropin levels in women during the peri-menopausal years. *Maturitas* 1986;8:189-96
10. Longcope C. Adrenal and gonadal androgen secretion in normal females. *Clin Endocrinol Metab* 1986;15:213-28
11. Judd HL, Shamozki IM, Frumar AM, Lagasse LD. Origin of serum estradiol in postmenopausal women. *Obstet Gynecol* 1982;59:680-6
12. Siiteri PK. Non glandular production of estrogen. In Givens JR, ed. *Gynecologic Endocrinology*. Chicago: Year Book Medical Publishers, Inc., 1977:171-82
13. Siiteri PK, Murai JT, Hammond GL, Nisker JA, Raymoure WJ, Kuhu RW. The serum transport of steroid hormones. *Recent Prog Horm Res* 1982;38:457-510
14. Westphal U. *Steroid-Protein Interactions II*. New York: Springer-Verlag, 1986

15. Partridge WM. Transport of protein-bound hormones into tissues *in vivo*. *Endocr Rev* 1981;2:103-23
16. Wu CH, Motohashi T, Abdel-Rahman HA, Flickinger GL, Mikhail G. Free and protein bound plasma 17β-estradiol during the menstrual cycle. *J Clin Endocrinol Metab* 1976;43:436-45
17. Pan CC, Woolever CA, Bhavnani BR. Transport of equine estrogens: binding of conjugated and unconjugated equine estrogens with human serum proteins. *J Clin Endocrinol Metab* 1985;61:499-507
18. Dunn JF, Nisula BC, Rodbard D. Transport of steroid hormones: binding of 21 endogenous steroids to both testosterone-binding globulin and corticosteroid-binding globulin in human plasma. *J Clin Endocrinol Metab* 1981;53:58-68
19. Rosenthal H, Pietrzak E, Slaunwhite WR Jr, Sandberg AA. Binding of estrone sulfate in human plasma. *J Clin Endocrinol Metab* 1972;34:805-13
20. Mathrubutham M, Fotherby E. Medroxyprogesterone acetate in human serum. *J Steroid Biochem* 1981;14:783-6
21. Hammond GL, Lahteenmaki PL, Luukkainen P, Luukkainen T. Distribution and percentages of non-protein bound contraceptive steroids in human serum. *J Steroid Biochem* 1982;17:375-80
22. Kuhnz W, Pteffer M, Al-Yacoub G. Protein binding of the contraceptive steroids gestodene, 3-keto-desogestrel and ethinyl estradiol in human serum. *J Steroid Biochem* 1990;35:313-18
23. Alton KB, Hetyei NS, Shan C, Patrick JE. Biotransformation of norgestimate in women. *Contraception* 1984;29:19-29
24. McGuire JL, Phillips A, Hahn DW, Tolman EL, Flor S, Kafrissen ME. Pharmacologic and pharmacokinetics characteristics of norgestimate and its metabolites. *Am J Obstet Gynecol* 1990;163:2127-31
25. Evans RM. The steroid and thyroid hormone receptor superfamily: transcriptional regulators of development and physiology. *Science* 1988;240:889-95
26. Katzenellenbogen JA, O'Malley BW, Katzenellenbogen BS. Tripartite steroid hormone receptor

pharmacology: interaction with multiple effector sites as a basis of the cell- and promoter-specific action of these hormones. *Mol Endocrinol* 1996;10: 119–31

27. Beato M, Sanchez-Pacheco A. Interaction of steroid hormone receptor with the transcription initiation complex. *Endocr Rev* 1996;17:587–609

28. Vegeto E, Wagner BL, Imhof MO, McDonnell DP. The molecular pharmacology of ovarian steroid receptors. *Vitam Horm* 1996;52:99–128

29. Shibata H, Spencer TE, Onate SA, *et al*. Role of co-activators and co-repressors in the mechanism of steroid/thyroid receptor action. *Recent Prog Horm Res* 1997;52:141–65

30. McDonnell DP, Norris JD. Analysis of the molecular pharmacology of estrogen receptor agonists and antagonists provides insights into the mechanism of action of estrogens in bone. *Osteoporosis Int* 1997;7(Suppl 1):S29–34

31. Kuiper GGJM, Enmark E, Pelto-Huiko M, Nilsson S, Gustafsson JA. Cloning of a novel estrogen receptor expressed in rat prostate and ovary. *Proc Natl Acad Sci USA* 1996;93:5925–30

32. Clark JH, Peck EJ. *Female Sex Steroids: Receptors and Function*. Berlin: Springer, 1979;14

33. Tora L, White J, Bron C, *et al*. The human estrogen receptor has two independent nonacidic transcriptional activation functions. *Cell* 1989;59: 477–87

34. Berry M, Metzger D, Chambon P. Role of the two activating domains of the estrogen receptor in the cell-type and promoter-context dependent agonistic activity of the anti-oestrogen 4-hydroxy tamoxifen. *EMBO J* 1990;9:2811–18

35. Norris JD, Fan D, Wagner BL, McDonnell DP. Identification of the sequences within the human C3 promoter required for estrogen responsiveness provides insight into the mechanism of tamoxifen mixed agonist's activity. *Mol Endocrinol* 1996; 10:1605–16

36. Smith L, Nawaz Z, O'Malley BW. Coactivator and corepressor regulation of the agonist/antagonist activity of the mixed antiestrogen, 4-hydroxy-tamoxifen. *Mol Endocrinol* 1997;11:657–66

37. Paige LA, Christensen GH, Norris JD, *et al*. Estrogen receptor (ER) modulators each induce distinct conformational changes in ER alpha and ER beta. *Proc Natl Acad Sci USA* 1999;90:3999–4004

38. McInerney EM, Tsai M-J, O'Malley BW, Katzellenbogen BS. Analysis of estrogen receptor transcriptional enhancement by a nuclear hormone receptor coactivator. *Proc Natl Acad Sci USA* 1996;93:10069–73

39. Onate S, Boonyartanakorkit V, Spencer TE, *et al*. The steroid receptor coactivator-1 contains multiple receptor interacting and activation domains that cooperatively enhance the activation function 1 (AF-1) and AF-2 domains of steroid receptors. *J Biol Chem* 1998;273:12101–8

40. Graham JD, Clarke CL. Physiological action of progesterone in target tissues. *Endocr Rev* 1997;18: 502–19

41. McKenna N, Nwaz Z, Tsai SY, Tsai MJ, O'Malley BW. Distinct steady-state nuclear receptor corregulator complexes exist *in vivo*. *Proc Natl Acad Sci USA* 1998;95:11697–702

42. Spencer TE, Jenster G, Burcin ME, *et al*. Steroid receptor co-activator-1 is a histone acetyl transferase. *Nature (London)* 1997;389:194–8

43. Bhavnani BR, Woolever CA. The metabolism of equilin in normal men. *J Steroid Biochem* 1982;17: 217–23

44. Bhavnani BR, Woolever CA. Interaction of ring B unsaturated estrogens with estrogen receptors of human endometrium and rat uterus. *Steroids* 1991;56:201–9

45. Bhavnani BR. Pharmacokinetics and pharmacodynamics of conjugated equine estrogens: chemistry and metabolism. *Proc Soc Exp Biol Med* 1998;217:6–16

46. Bhavnani BR, Cecutti A, Gerulath A. Pharmacokinetics and pharmacodynamics of a novel estrogen Δ_8-estrone in postmenopausal women and men. *J Steroid Biochem Mol Biol* 1998;67:119–31

47. Wehling M. Specific, nongenomic actions of steroid hormones. *Annu Rev Physiol* 1997;59:365–93

48. Revelli A, Massobrio M, Tesarik J. Nongenomic action of steroid hormones in reproductive tissues. *Endocr Rev* 1998;19:3–17

49. Norman AW, Wehling M. Proceedings of the first international meeting on rapid responses to steroid hormones. *Steroids* 1999;64:3–168

50. Bradlow LH. A history of steroid chemistry. Part II. *Steroids* 1992;57:577–664

51. Kalant H, Roschlau WHE. *Principles of Medical Pharmacology*. Toronto: BC Decker, Inc., 1989

52. Gerhard M, Ganz P. How do we explain the clinical benefits of estrogen? *Circulation* 1995;92:5–8

53. Sullivan JM. Hormone replacement therapy in cardiovascular disease: the human model. *Br J Obstet Gynaecol* 1996;103(Suppl 13):50–67

54. Chetkowski RJ, Meldrum DR, Judd HL. Biological effects of transdermal estradiol. *N Engl J Med* 1986;314:1615–20

55. DeLignieres B, Basdevant A, Thomas G. Biological effects of estradiol-17β in postmenopausal women: oral versus percutaneous administration. *J Clin Endocrinol Metab* 1986;62:536–41

56. Crook D, Cust MP, Gamger KF. Comparison of transdermal and oral estrogen–progestin replacement therapy; effects on serum lipids and lipoproteins. *Am J Obstet Gynecol* 1992;166: 950–5

57. Friend KE, Hartman ML, Pezzoli S. Both oral and transdermal estrogens increase growth hormone release in postmenopausal women. A clinical research center study. *J Clin Endocrinol Metab* 1996;81:2250–6

58. Koh KK, Mincemoyer R, Minh RN. Effect of hormone-replacement therapy on fibrinolysis in postmenopausal women. *N Engl J Med* 1997; 336:683–90

59. The writing group for the PEPI trial. Effects of estrogen or estrogen/progestin regimens on heart disease risk factors in postmenopausal women. *J Am Med Assoc* 1995;273:199–208

60. Bhavnani BR, Woolever CA, Pan CC. Metabolism of [³H]equilin, [³⁵S]sulfate and [³H]equilin sulfate after oral and intravenous administration in normal postmenopausal women and men. *J Clin Endocrinol Metab* 1989;68:757–65

61. Ruder HJ, Loriaux DL, Lipsett MB. Estrone sulfate: production rate and metabolism in man. *J Clin Invest* 1972;51:1020–33

62. Longcope C. The metabolism of estrone sulfate in normal males. *J Clin Endocrinol Metab* 1972;34: 113–22

63. Bhavnani BR, Sarda IR, Woolever CA. Radioimmunoassay of plasma equilin, and estrone in postmenopausal women after the administration of Premarin. *J Clin Endocrinol Metab* 1981;52: 741–7

64. Englund DE, Johansson EDB. Plasma levels of oestrone, oestradiol and gonadotrophins in postmenopausal women after oral and vaginal administration of conjugated equine oestrogens (Premarin). *Br J Obstet Gynaecol* 1978;85:957–64

65. Anderson ABM, Sklovsky E, Soyers L, Steele P, Turnbull AC. Comparison of serum oestrogen concentrations in postmenopausal women taking oestrone sulphate and oestradiol. *Br Med J* 1978;1: 140–2

66. Quirk JG, Wendel GD. Biologic effects of natural and synthetic estrogens. In Buchsbaum HJ, ed. *The Menopause*. New York: Springer-Verlag, 1983: 55–75

67. Bhavnani BR. Analytical methodology for estimation of ethinyl estradiol following ingestion of oral contraceptives. *Adv Contracept* 1991;7(Suppl 3):116–39

68. Mashchak CA, Lobo RA, Dozono-Takano R. Comparison of pharmacodynamic properties of various estrogen formulations. *Am J Obstet Gynecol* 1982;144:511–18

69. Toniolo PG, Levitz M, Zeleniuch JA, *et al*. A prospective study of endomenous estrogens and breast cancer in postmenopausal women. *J Natl Cancer Inst* 1995;87:190–7

70. Nachtigal L, Raju U, Banergee S, Wan L, Levitz M. Comparative effects of three common estrogen replacement therapies (ERT) on serum sex hormone binding globulin (SHBG) levels in menopausal women: lack of association with unconjugated estradiol (E₂) and estrone (E₁). *J Soc Gynecol Invest* 1999;6(Suppl 1):164A

71. Deutsch S, Ossowski R, Benjamin I. Comparison between degree of systemic absorption of vaginally and orally administered estrogens at different dose levels in postmenopausal women. *Am J Obstet Gynecol* 1981;139:967–8

72. Mandel FP, Geola FL, Meldrum DR, *et al*. Biological effects of various doses of vaginally administered conjugated equine estrogens in postmenopausal women. *J Clin Endocrinol Metab* 1983;57: 133–9

73. Lobo RA. Absorption and metabolic effects of different types of estrogens and progestogens. *Obstet Gynecol Clin North Am* 1987;14:143–67

74. Troy SM, Hicks DR, Parker VD, Jusko WJ, Rofsky HE, Porter DJ. Differences in pharmacokinetics and comparative bioavailability between Premarin and Estratab in healthy postmenopausal women. *Curr Ther Res* 1994;55:359–72

75. Bhavnani BR, Cecutti A. Estratab, Estratest, and Premarin are not bioequivalent. *Am J Obstet Gynecol* 1993;169:235–6

76. Tait JF, Burstein S. *In vivo* studies of steroid dynamics in man. In Pincus G, Thimann KU, Astwood EB, eds. *The Hormones*. New York: Academic Press, 1964:441–557

77. Bhavnani BR, Woolever CA, Benoit H, Wong T. Pharmacokinetics of equilin and equilin sulfate in normal postmenopausal women and men. *J Clin Endocrinol Metab* 1983;56:1048–56

78. Bhavnani BR, Cecutti A. Pharmacokinetics of 17β-dihydroequilin sulfate and 17β-dihydroequilin in normal postmenopausal women. *J Clin Endocrinol Metab* 1994;78:197–204

79. Bhavnani BR, Cecutti A. Metabolic clearance rate of equilin sulfate, and its conversion to plasma equilin, conjugated and unconjugated equilenin, 17β-dihydroequilin, and 17β-dihydroequilenin in normal postmenopausal women and men under steady state conditions. *J Clin Endocrinol Metab* 1993;77:1269–74

80. Bhavnani BR, Cecutti A, Gerulath AH. 17β-dihydroequilin sulfate dynamics in postmenopausal women and man under steady state conditions. *J Soc Gynecol Invest* 1997;4(Suppl 1): 177

81. Longcope C. Metabolic clearance and blood production rates of estrogens in postmenopausal women. *Am J Obstet Gynecol* 1971;111:778–81

82. Baird DT, Horton R, Longcope C, Tait JF. Steroid dynamics under steady-state conditions. *Recent Prog Horm Res* 1969;25:611–44

83. Purdy RN. Active metabolites and carcinogenesis. In Merriam YR, ed. *Catechol Estrogens* New York: Raven Press, 1983:123–40

84. Zhu BT, Roy D, Liehr JY. The carcinogenic activity of ethinyl estrogens is determined by both their hormonal characteristics and their conversion to catechol metabolites. *Endocrinology* 1993;132:577–83

85. Li JJ, Li SA. Estrogen carcinogenesis in hamster tissues. *Endocr Rev* 1990;11:524–31

86. Li JJ, Li SA, Oberley TD, Passon JA. Carcinogenic activities of various steroidal and non-steroidal estrogens in the hamster kidney. Relation to hormonal activity and cell proliferation. *Cancer Res* 1995;55:4347-51

87. Bhavnani BR, Lau A, Cecutti A, Gerulath A. Demonstration of 2 and 4 hydroxylation of equilin by normal proliferative and secretory human endometrial microsomal preparations. *J Soc Gynecol Invest* 1995;2:424

88. Reddy WR, Hanjani P. Synthesis of catechol estrogens by human uterus and leiomyoma. *Steroids* 1981;37:195-9

89. Bhavnani BR, Cecutti A. Metabolism of [³H]17β-dihydroequilin and [³H]17β-dihydroequilin sulfate in normal postmenopausal women. *Steroids* 1994;59:389-94

90. Bhavnani BR, Cecutti A. Identification of a novel 16α-hydroxylated ring B unsaturated estrogen following administration of equilin to postmenopausal women and men. *J Soc Gynecol Invest* 1996; 3(Suppl 2):365

91. Schneider J, Kinne D, Fraechia A, *et al.* Abnormal oxidative metabolism of estradiol in women with breast cancer. *Proc Natl Acad Sci USA* 1982;79:3047-51

92. Bradlow HL, Hershcopp RJ, Marthtucii CP, Fishman J. Estradiol 16α-hydroxylation in the mouse correlates with mammary tumor incidence and presence of marine mammary tumor virus: a possible model for the hormonal etiology of breast cancer in human. *Proc Natl Acad Sci USA* 1985;82:6295-9

93. Yu SC, Fishman J. Interaction of histones with estrogens: covalent adduct-formation with 16α-hydroxy-estrone. *Biochemistry* 1985;24:8017-21

94. Swaneck GE, Fishman J. Covalent binding of the endogenous estrogen 16α-hydroxy estrone to estradiol receptor in human breast cancer cells: characterization and intranuclear localization. *Proc Natl Acad Sci USA* 1988;85:7831-5

95. Kabat GC, Chang CJ, Sparaho JA, *et al.* Urinary estrogen metabolites and breast cancer: a case-control study. *Cancer Epidemiol Biomarkers Prev* 1997;6:505-9

96. Ursin G, London S, Stanczyk FZ, *et al.* A pilot study of urinary estrogen metabolites (16 alpha-OH E1 and 2-OH E1) in postmenopausal women with and without breast cancer. *Environ Health Perspect* 1997;105(Suppl 3):601-5

97. Stevenson JC. Do we need different galenic forms of estrogens and progestogens? *Menopause* 1996; 243:25-8

98. Pike MC, Peters RK, Cozen W, *et al.* Estrogen-progestin replacement therapy and endometrial cancer. *J Natl Cancer Inst* 1997;89:1110-16

99. Barrett-Connor E. Hormone replacement therapy. *Br Med J* 1998;317:457-61

100. Gupta C, Musto NA, Bullock LP. *In vivo* metabolism of progestins. In Garattini S, Berendes HW, eds. *Pharmacology of Steroid Contraceptive Drugs.* New York: Raven Press, 1977:131-6

101. Hiroi M, Stanczyk FZ, Goebelsmann U, Brenner PF, Lumkin ME, Mishell DR Jr. Radioimmunoassay of serum medroxyprogesterone acetate (Provera) in women following oral and intravaginal administration. *Steroids* 1975;26:373-86

102. Back DJ, Breckenridge AM, Crawford FE. Kinetics of norethindrone in women. II Single-dose kinetics. *Clin Pharmacol Ther* 1978;24:448-53

103. Back DJ, Bates M, Breckenridge AM, Hall JM. The pharmacokinetics of levonorgestrel and ethinylestradiol in women - studies with Ovran and Ovranette. *Contraception* 1981;23:229-39

104. Back DJ, Grimmer SFM, Shenow N, Orme MLE. Plasma concentrations of 3-ketodesogestrel after oral administration of desogestrel and intravenous administration of 3-ketodesogestrel. *Contraception* 1987;35:619-26

105. Tauber U, Tack JW, Matthes H. Single dose of pharmacokinetics of gestodene in women after intravenous and oral administration. *Contraception* 1989;40:461-79

106. Goldstein JL, Brown MS. The low density lipoprotein pathway and its relation to atherosclerosis. *Annu Rev Biochem* 1977;46:897-930

107. Bush TL, Barrett-Connor E, Cowan LD. Cardiovascular mortality and non contraceptive use of estrogens in women. Results from the lipid research clinics programs follow up study. *Circulation* 1987;75:1102-9

108. Stampfer MJ, Colditz A, Willett WC. Postmenopausal estrogen therapy and cardiovascular disease. *N Engl J Med* 1991;325:756-62

109. Sullivan JM, Fowlkes LP. The clinical aspects of estrogen and cardiovascular system. *Obstet Gynecol* 1996;87:365-425

110. Grodstein F, Stampfer M, Manson JE. Postmenopausal estrogen and progestin use and risk of cardiovascular disease. *N Engl J Med* 1996;335:453-61

111. Steinberg D, Parthasarthy S, Carew TE, Khoo JC, Witzum J. Beyond cholesterol. Modifications of low density lipoprotein that increase its atherogenicity. *N Engl J Med* 1989;320:915-24

112. Subbiah MTR, Kessel B, Agrawal M. Antioxidant potential of specific estrogens on lipid peroxidation. *J Clin Endocrinol Metab* 1993;77:1095-7

113. Sack MN, Rader DJ, Cannon RD. Oestrogen and A-O-2 inhibiters of low density lipoproteins in postmenopausal women. *Lancet* 1994;343:269-70

114. Wilcox JG, Sevanian A, Hwang J, Stanczyk FZ, Hodis HN, Lobo RA. Cardioprotective effects of individual conjugated equine estrogens through their possible modulation of insulin resistance and oxidation of low density lipoproteins. *Fertil Steril* 1997;67:57-62

115. Bhavnani BR, Cecutti A, Gerulath A. Are cardio-vascular benefits associated with equine estrogen therapy and red wine consumption a result of the antioxidant properties of their components. *J Soc Gynecol Invest* 1997;4(Suppl 1):106A

116. Bhavnani BR, Cecutti A. Comparison of anti-oxidant effects of Premarin, Premarin plus progestin and generic conjugated estrogen (CES) administration in postmenopausal women. *J Soc Gynecol Invest* 1997;4(Suppl 1):176A

117. Wilcox JG, Hwang J, Gentzschein EK, *et al*. Effect of combined estrogen and progestin therapy in postmenopausal women on endothelium levels and oxidation of LDL. *J Soc Gynecol Invest* 1996; 3(Suppl 2):69A

118. Lacort M, Leal AM, Liza M. Protective effect of estrogens and catechol estrogens against peroxidative membrane damage *in vitro*. *Lipids* 1995;30: 141–6

119. Tang M, Subbiah MTR. Estrogen protects against hydrogen peroxide and arachidonic acid induced DNA damage. *Biochim Biophys Acta* 1996;1299: 155–9

120. Subbiah MTR. Mechanisms of cardioprotection by estrogens. *Proc Soc Exp Biol Med* 1998;217:23–9

121. Paganini-Hill A, Henderson VW. Estrogen deficiency and risk of AD in women. *Am J Epidemiol* 1994;140:256–61

122. Henderson VW, Paganini-Hill A, Emanuel CK, Dunn ME, Buckwalter G. Estrogen replacement therapy in older women. *Arch Neurol* 1994;51: 896–900

123. Tang MX, Jocobs D, Stern Y, *et al*. Effect of oestrogen during menopause on risk and age at onset of Alzheimer's disease. *Lancet* 1996;348:429–32

124. Dehouck B, Fenalt L, Dehouck MP, Pierce A, Torpier G. A new function for LDL receptor. Transcytosis of LDL across the blood-brain barrier. *J Cell Biol* 1997;138:877–89

125. Pitas RE, Boyles JK, Lee SH, Hui D, Weisgraber KH. Lipoproteins and their receptors in the central nervous system. *J Biol Chem* 1987;262: 14352–60

126. Lyras L, Cairus NJ, Jenner A, Jenner P, Halliwell B. An assessment of oxidative damage to proteins, lipids and DNA in brain from patients with Alzheimer's disease. *J Neurochem* 1997;68:2061–9

127. Sayre LM, Zalasko DA, Harris PLR, Perry G, Salomon RG, Smith MA. 4-hydroxynonenal-derived advanced lipid peroxidation end products are increased in Alzheimer's disease. *J Neurochem* 1997;68:2092–7

128. Behl C, Davis JB, Lesley R, Schubert D. Hydrogen peroxide mediates amyloid β-protein toxicity. *Cell* 1994;77:817–27

129. Hulley S, Grady D, Bush T, *et al*. Randomized trial of estrogen plus progestin for secondary prevention of coronary heart disease in postmenopausal women: the Heart and Estrogen/progestin Replacement Study (HERS). *J Am Med Assoc* 1998; 280:605–13

130. Adams MR, Register TC, Golden DL, Wagner JD, Williams JK. Medroxyprogesterone acetate antagonizes inhibitory effects of conjugated equine estrogens on coronary artery athero-sclerosis. *Arterioscler Thromb Vasc Biol* 1997;17: 217–21

131. Chu J, Schweid AI, Weiss NS. Survival among women with endometrial cancer: a comparison of estrogen users and non-users of estrogen. *Am J Obstet Gynecol* 1982;143:569–73

19

Hormone replacement therapy

R. Don Gambrell Jr and Puthgraman K. Natrajan

Introduction

There are about 40 million women in the USA in the menopausal age group, and they will be spending a third of their life deficient in hormones. The age at menopause varies widely, but the average is about 51.4 years. The decline in ovarian function can be rapid in some, slower in others. Some women produce endogenous estrogens sufficient to remain asymptomatic, while others develop a variety of symptoms during the climacteric, a term in current use for the premenopausal, menopausal and postmenopausal period. The symptoms include:

(1) Hot flushes;

(2) Night sweats;

(3) Vaginal dryness;

(4) Insomnia;

(5) Depression.

Hormone replacement therapy (HRT) became popular in the 1960s, but in the 1970s the fear of endometrial cancer decreased its use. The proper use of progestogens has allayed these fears and HRT has regained popularity.

The growing recognition of the dangers of long-term estrogen deficiency leading to the development of osteroporosis and coronary heart disease, and the possible protection against colon cancer and Alzheimer's disease has again brought HRT to the forefront of prevention therapy. There are other hormones that are also becoming popular. Androgens help to alleviate many menopausal symptoms such as fatigue, loss of libido and headaches. Those women who are reluctant to use HRT can take selective estrogen receptor modulators (SERMs) such as raloxifene to help prevent osteoporosis. Women who undergo surgical menopause or premature menopause, and women who have hypogonadism such as gonadal dysgenesis, need to be identified early, and HRT begun, to protect these women from early development of osteoporosis and coronary artery disease.

History

Several centuries ago, Knauer postulated that the ovary has an endocrine function, by demonstrating that in ovariectomized rabbits, atrophy of the uterus was prevented only if the ovaries were transplanted. Many years passed until the isolation of individual hormones such as estrone, estradiol and progesterone in the laboratory.

Estrogen metabolism: biosynthesis and physiology

Estrogens are present in blood plasma partly in free form as estrone and estradiol, and partly conjugated as estrone or estradiol sulfate, and estrone glucuronide. Estrone and estradiol are synthesized in the ovary from acetate and cholesterol. The synthesis from acetate is believed to be cholesterol dependent. Estrogen production varies from minimal values at 5–10 years of age to the maximal values attained during pregnancy. Serum estradiol after the menopause is at one-third to one-half of the level found in adult women during their reproductive life[1]. The highest estrogen secretion in normal non-pregnant women occurs at the time of ovulation and is generally referred to as the 'ovulation peak'. Another peak of a lower level occurs on about the 21st day of the menstrual cycle and is known as the 'luteal peak'. The estrogens secreted by the ovary undergo extensive metabolism in the body. Estrone and estrogen are freely inter-convertible, the conversion of estrogen to estrone being more rapid than the reverse.

Pathophysiology of the menopause

'It is likely that after the menopause all estrogens are derived from peripheral conversion of androgens without secretion by the ovaries.'

Source of estrogens

Apart from the ovary, the adrenals, testes and placenta are implicated in the production of estrogen. After bilateral oophorectomy, significant estrogen levels are found in the blood and urine, the source presumed to be the adrenals. It has been suggested that the adrenals compensate for the loss of estrogens after the menopause by acting as auxiliary glands.

Following the permanent cessation of menses, the concentration of serum estradiol is usually less than 30 pg/ml and does not exhibit the cyclic changes characteristic of menstruating women. Estrone is the major estrogen in postmenopausal women, and has been shown to rise primarily through conversion from adrenal andro-stenedione[2,3]. Present-day studies indicate that the postmenopausal ovary does not produce estrogens *de novo*. This may also be true for the normal adrenal, although adrenal tumors may possess this capacity. Androgens, whether produced by the menopausal ovary or the adrenals or exogenously administered, are converted peripherally to estrogens in varying degrees. The aromatization of androgens by the kidney, liver, brain, muscle and adipose tissue is an important source of estrogens in postmenopausal women[4,5].

Gonadotropin fluctuation from reproductive years to menopause

It is well known that follicle stimulating hormone (FSH) and luteinizing hormone (LH) act together to control follicular development. The ovary in the perimenopausal years is a functional organ. Graafian follicles, mostly in a quiescent state, may still be present for many years after menses have ceased[6]. In the premenopausal years, serum FSH and LH levels often begin to rise, despite normal estrogen levels, because the sensitivity of the feed-back mechanism is altered[7-10]. Later, the ovarian follicles that remain become resistant to the rising gonadotropin levels and amenorrhea sets in. In menopausal women the gonadotropins remain elevated until approximately the seventh decade, after which the levels begin to decline[11].

It is likely that after the menopause all estrogens are derived from peripheral conversion of androgens without secretion by the ovaries[11-16]. That estradiol was mostly converted to estrone was shown by Yen and colleagues when they studied the effect of orally administered micronized estradiol on serum levels[17]. However, Greenblatt and his associates demonstrated that estradiol levels remained high when a bolus of 50 mg of conjugated estrogens was administered intravenously, or pellets of crystalline estradiol were implanted subcutaneously[18]. When a large bolus of estrone or estradiol was administered orally, estrone levels rose considerably while estradiol levels were relatively low[19]. More recently, the distribution of and changes in specific binding sites for FSH and LH in the human ovary have been studied[20]. Rajaniemi and co-workers showed the presence of specific gonadotropin receptors in the ovaries[21,22]. It may be possible that, at the premenopausal stage, this receptor becomes insensitive to the different changes of gonadotropins. However, it is un-known whether follicles that remain in the ovary lose hormone receptors because of atresia or whether atresia results from an insufficient number of hormone receptors.

There is a steady depletion of primary ovarian follicles that begins during fetal life and continues until the menopause[23]. Years before the menopause starts, there is a marked increase in the variability of intermenstrual intervals[24].

The perimenopausal stage varies greatly among women, and this is due to failure of the ovarian follicles to respond to increasing levels of endogenous gonadotropins. Characteristically, unusually long and short cycles are often interspersed. Urinary gonadotropins showed higher levels of LH and a lesser increase in FSH as women approached the menopause[25,26]. Interestingly, a normal urinary estrogen level was found, suggesting an altered feedback mechanism in older women. Nonetheless, follicular maturation occurs, and the corpus luteum functions in the presence of high and sustained gonadotropin concentrations. In perimenopausal women, histological examination of the ovary shows a reduced number of primary follicles, with rare secondary or Graafian follicles or well-developed corpora lutea. When developing ovarian follicles are seen in women in this age group, the follicle and ovary usually appear normal[8]. The hormonal changes observed in older women can be interpreted in the context of the depletion of ovarian follicles. In regularly menstruating perimenopausal women, the hormonal features of follicular maturation are fairly typical of those seen in younger women with the exception of lower levels of estradiol, high levels of FSH and a decrease in the interval from menses to the mid-cycle gonadotropin peak. It has been reported that an elevation of serum FSH could predict the absence of ovarian follicles in patients with primary or secondary amenorrhea prior to surgery[27]. The elevated concentration of serum FSH observed in perimenopausal women may be indicative of a reduced number of functional, residual ovarian follicles. Analysis of serum LH and FSH immediately following oophorectomy has also demonstrated a more rapid increase in FSH and LH[28,29]. The elevated concentrations of FSH may be responsible for the initiation of follicular maturation at more frequent intervals and, hence, for the general decrease in cycle length that is observed in older women. The above studies demonstrated that the potential for hormone secretion by residual follicles in older women diminished, and, early in the menopausal transition, a dissociation in the capacity of estradiol and progesterone secretion was observed with reduced concentrations of progesterone. In later cycles, there was diminished secretion of both hormones. The episodes of vaginal bleeding that occurred after a rise and fall in estradiol but in the absence of measurable increases in progesterone are compatible with what has classically been described as anovulatory vaginal bleeding. Therefore, it is possible to see cycling women with no apparent menopausal symptoms, whose hormonal profile may show 'low normal' estradiol, and 'higher' FSH and LH. It should be taken into consideration that these women can ovulate, and

measures should be taken if they do not want pregnancy.

The premenopausal, menopausal and postmenopausal phases are part of the female climacteric. The symptoms usually seen are secondary to a combination of various factors: hormonal, metabolic, psychogenic and social. Their interaction may affect the severity of symptoms and may create a crisis, either temporary or prolonged. Therefore, symptoms may appear before the onset of the menopause and can endure to the end of life. The reaction most typically seen secondary to the hypoestrogenic state is that of hot flushes. The vasomotor symptoms in menopausal women are temporally associated with the initiation of pulsatile LH release by the pituitary[30,31]. The LH pulses *per se* are not causally related to flush episodes. This has been deduced from the presence of menopausal flushes in hypophysectomized women[32]. It is assumed that neuroendocrine events which govern the pulsatile release of luteinizing hormone-releasing hormone (LHRH) may be linked functionally with the hypothalamic thermoregulatory center. Factors involved in this link may be mechanically involved in the origination of the flush episodes[30].

Urogenital atrophy

The so-called senile vaginitis is simply when the genital epithelium becomes atrophic under the influence of estrogen deprivation, and usually irritation, burning, pruritus and dyspareunia are present. When vaginal secretions decrease, the vagina may shorten and become less distensible[33]. The epithelium may become thin, and trauma is very easily produced. Vulvar changes are also seen to a lesser extent. The lower urinary tract also experiences some changes as it is estrogen-dependent tissue. Dysuria with irritation and burning is a common complaint, and episodic cystitis is also frequently seen in menopausal women.

Psychological factors: mood changes and depression are seen with estrogen deprivation

Psychosomatic changes that are often seen may result indirectly from ·the alteration in the hormonal milieu. Nervousness, depression and anxiety are frequently overlooked or seen as normal in women during the menopause. Headaches are frequently regarded as psychosomatic and not hormone related. Libido usually decreases because of dyspareunia, and is usually treated with lubricants, as not much importance is given to this factor. Sexual dysfunction in the menopausal woman, long regarded by psychologists and sex therapists as entirely psychogenic in origin, has been repeatedly shown to be responsive to hormonal therapy. Relief may be afforded by estrogens for such complaints as vaginal dryness and dyspareunia, and by androgens when loss of sex interest is the basic problem.

Research into biogenic amine neurotransmitters has indicated the existence of a particular amine that may modify human behavior. Studies have shown that its pharmacological manipulation produced behavioral changes, and the anatomical pathway concerned with that behavior appeared to be identified. The concept of the blood–brain barrier explained the mechanisms of transport between the blood and all brain membranes; some substances are able to cross while others cannot[34]. Those that cross have been identified as dopamine and 5-hydroxytryptophan precursors of catecholamine and serotonin[35]. In a study carried out in our clinic in 160 menopausal women with depression, it was found that an improvement in the level of the amino acid tryptophan with estrogen therapy was significant ($p \leq 0.05$). When two pellets of estradiol were given, an improvement in mood changes and depression was seen, as indicated in Table 1. Thus, it may be just as important to treat not

only flushes and night sweats, or atrophic vaginitis, but also psychic changes seen as the mood swings and depression affecting women during this period[36].

Osteoporosis

In recent years, interest in osteoporosis has developed as epidemiological data support the correlation between loss of bone and increased risk of fracture. The final aim of this interest has been prevention of osteoporosis and, hence, prevention of fractures. It must be differentiated from osteopenia which is a normal bone loss process associated with aging. Osteoporosis instead is the pathological state of osteopenia: the bone mass is reduced to the point where the skeleton is unable to perform its function of support, and collapses. Osteoporosis, therefore, is a skeletal disorder characterized by thinner diaphyses and narrower trabeculae, and reduction in the quantity of bone mass predisposes to fracture. Although both sexes have loss of bone mass with aging, it is rare for men to develop symptomatic osteoporosis before age 70. Up to half of all women between the ages of 45 and 75 show signs of osteoporosis. One in three women within this age group has the disease, but by the 75th birthday the number rises to nine in ten. Hip fracture incidence doubles every 5 years after age 60. Therefore, the average woman at menopause has a 40% probability of suffering a hip fracture in her lifetime. Studies have shown that Asian and white women are at a higher risk than women of Hispanic origin or black women[37]. In American women, more than 1 million

Table 1 Tryptophan in depressed menopausal women with loss of libido: free tryptophan values rose following implantation of two pellets of estradiol (25 mg each); improvement of depression and headaches was seen when a pellet of testosterone (75 mg) was added to the regimen of therapy and there was no further lessening of depression; the intensity of libido increased

Therapy	Free tryptophan		Total tryptophan		Level (%)	
	Before therapy	After therapy	Before therapy	After therapy	Libido	Depression[†]
E₂	3.76	4.41*	34.66	35.51	50	70
E₂ + T	0.09	0.19	0.89	1.28	90	70

*$p \leq 0.05$, represents number of patients who estimated an improvement ranging from 25 to 100%; [†]according to Beck scale for depression; E₂, estradiol pellets; T, testosterone pellet

fractures occur annually in this age group, with an estimated care cost of about 12 billion dollars.

Pathophysiology of osteoporosis

Throughout life there is constant remodelling of bone; osteoclasts promote bone resorption that is subsequently followed by repair under the influence of osteoblasts. This remodelling is influenced by several factors: dietetic, mechanical and hormonal. Bone loss is associated with alterations in calcium metabolism, causing a negative calcium balance. By comparing fasting calcium levels in women who had a hysterectomy without oophorectomy with those in women who had bilateral oophorectomy, the increase in resorption of calcium from bone was related to reduced ovarian estrogens. Both fasting plasma and urinary hydroxyproline levels confirmed that the increased calcium excretion was due to increased resorption of calcium from bone. Women undergoing a natural menopause have similar changes in calcium metabolism. The increase in fasting serum or urinary calcium that follows either natural menopause or bilateral oophorectomy is reversible with estrogen therapy. Estrogen therapy inhibits the resorption of calcium from bone, probably mediated through calcitonin. Several clinical studies have shown estrogen effectiveness in preventing osteoporosis[38-40]. In an ongoing study, our preliminary data show that estrogen therapy can decrease the progression of osteoporosis and, therefore, the occurrence of new fractures. Lindsay and colleagues showed that estrogen therapy maintained bone density over 16 years, whereas placebo recipients lost bone[41]. In another study it was found that transdermal estradiol should increase bone density in the spine and hip, and reduce the number of new spine fractures[42]. Weak estrogens such as tamoxifen, which is an estrogen receptor antagonist, have mild estrogenic effects on bone[43]. In 1997 raloxifene, a selective estrogen receptor modulator (SERM), was approved for prevention of osteoporosis, but it is not as effective as conjugated estrogens[44]. It has also been shown that raloxifene can increase bone density[45]. In 'multiple outcome for raloxifene evaluation' (MORE) studies of 7000 patients with osteoporosis, the relative risk of vertebral fracture with raloxifene was 0.48, compared to placebo. Raloxifene also increased bone mineral density by 2-3% in the spine and hip[45]. Estrogen and androgen combinations may also increase bone density, compared to estrogen alone, in some patients[46].

At least eight studies have shown that the addition of a progestogen to estrogen therapy may actually increase bone mass by promoting new bone formation[47-49]. In fact, the addition of a progestogen to estrogen therapy may not only be important for the prevention of osteoporosis, but be even more essential in the treatment of patients with osteoporosis[50]. Christiansen and colleagues, in a cross-over study comparing the effects of estrogen–progestogen therapy with those of placebo, found that bone mineral content measured by densitometry increased during the 3 years of combination therapy, but continued to decrease in the placebo-treated group[48] (Figure 1). When some of the estrogen–progestogen group were changed to a placebo, bone density decreased. The placebo-treated women had an increase in bone mineral content after being changed to estrogen–progestogen therapy. Crilley and associates compared the effects of estrogens only and an estrogen–progestogen combination on the metabolic parameters of bone loss: plasma calcium, urinary calcium/creatinine ratio and hydroxyproline[49]. More recent studies have addressed the presence of estrogen receptors in bone[51]. It may be possible

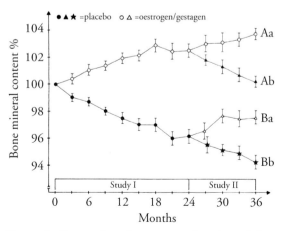

Figure 1 Bone mineral content as function of time and treatment in postmenopausal women. Reproduced with permission from reference 48

that, by this mechanism, estrogen given as replacement therapy will promote new bone formation.

Special care must be taken when LHRH agonists are used, as they produce a menopause-like syndrome with amenorrhea, hot flushes, etc. Use of LHRH agonists was found to result in a decrease in bone mineral density, compared to baseline. This bone loss reverted back to baseline values within 1 year after therapy was stopped[52]. Most physicians use add-back estrogen therapy with these agents.

The National Institutes of Health in a consensus conference sponsored by the Office of Medical Applications of Research, in Bethesda, Maryland, USA recommended the use of estrogens to women whose ovaries are removed before age 50[53]. Estrogens should be given with or without cyclic progesterone for conditions that confer a high risk of osteoporosis, such as the occurrence of premature menopause (natural or induced), and in women where there are not specific contraindications. In addition to estrogen therapy, other recommendations are given by the National Research Council regarding calcium. They suggest 800 mg of elemental calcium per day, but metabolic studies have indicated that this level should be raised to 1000 mg for premenopausal and estrogen-treated women, and for postmenopausal women the recommended dose is 1500 mg. Vitamin D between 500 and 2000 IU per day has been suggested, and an exercise program must be carefully supervised. Walking remains one of the best forms of exercise, and distances may be augmented progressively. All of these factors are the key of prevention in the treatment of osteoporosis. More recent studies have suggested therapy with vitamin D precursors, calcitonin, biphosphonates and fluoride for the treatment of osteoporosis. In 1990 it was reported that, although a marked increase in vertebral mineral density was observed with fluoride, there was no significant reduction in fracture rate, and it may decrease cortical bone mineral density leading to increased skeletal fragility[54]. Therefore, fluoride treatment, irrespective of the side-effects, may not be as effective in the treatment of postmenopausal osteoporosis. However etidronate, a biphosphonate, showed a decrease in the rate of vertebral fracture without the production of serious side-effects[55]. More studies remain to be carried out, to find the perfect element to treat osteoporosis.

Lipids and lipoprotein changes during the menopause and hormone replacement therapy

Coronary artery disease results from abnormalities in vascular endothelium and atherothrombosis, resulting in coronary spasm. Atheromatous plaques may develop in early childhood. The dyslipidemia and platelet aggregation from different causes in adulthood result in microthrombosis in the endothelium and development of atheromatous plaque[56]. Oral estrogen therapy (Premarin®, Estrace®) seems to reverse these processes. There is a 15% rise in high-density lipoprotein (HDI) and a decrease in low-density lipoprotein (LDL), but triglycerides may increase by 20%[57]. If the patient already has hypertriglyceridemia, pancreatitis may occur. Transdermal and parenteral estrogens do not seem to increase triglycerides.

A relationship between sex hormones and an increase in the risk of coronary heart disease was suggested by Kuller[58]. Hypertriglyceridemia as well as hypercholesterolemia have been implicated in the development of atherogenesis[59-61], with emphasis on elevations in cholesterol[61,62]. Carlson and Bottinger[60] in 1972 and Brunzell and colleagues[63] in 1976 thought that triglycerides may be associated with increased risk of atherosclerosis, and more recent studies seem to suggest that triglycerides are an independent risk factor. An increase in cholesterol and triglyceride levels has been noted with increased age. When considering estrogen therapy to counteract this increase, it should be kept in mind that not only do natural estrogens (conjugated estrogens, estradiol pellets, micronized estradiol) and synthetic estrogens (ethinylestradiol, mestranol) have different effects on serum lipid patterns, but in higher dosages they may also produce different lipid responses. Reports have shown that some estrogens more than others increase levels of HDL, suggesting a beneficial effect[61,62]. An increase in very-low-density lipoprotein (VLDL), LDL or both is associated with coronary artery disease, whereas HDL seems to have some protective effect[64-68].

Effect of progestogens on lipids and lipoproteins

Concern has been expressed that added progestogens to estrogen replacement therapy may adversely affect the estrogen-induced benefits on lipids, thus negating the benefit of hormone replacement therapy on heart disease. Most of this concern is based on short-term studies of estrogen–progestogen use. When adequate dosages of estrogen are given, there is no decrease in HDL cholesterol over the long term with added progestogens. Studies utilizing implanted estradiol pellets and oral medroxyprogesterone acetate indicate that the progestogen did not significantly influence beneficial changes in lipoproteins (Figure 2)[69]. In a cross-sectional study of the really long-term effects of hormone replacement on lipids and lipoproteins in 556 postmenopausal women treated for up to 44 years, there were no differences between the unopposed estrogen users and the estrogen–progestogen users[70]. There were no significant differences in mean HDL cholesterol levels between the unopposed estrogen users (67.0 ± 3.94 mg/dl) and the estrogen plus C-21 progestogen users (64.5 ± 4.16 mg/dl) or the estrogen plus C-19 progestogen users (61.0 ± 3.84 mg/dl).

In the 3-year Postmenopausal Estrogen/Progestin Interventions (PEPI) trial, estrogen alone or in combination with a progestogen improved lipoproteins and lowered fibrinogen levels without detectable effects on post-challenge insulin or blood pressure[71]. It may be the dosage of estrogen that is most important in improving the lipid pattern to decrease the risk for cardiovascular disease. In a study comparing different dosages of micronized estradiol, 1, 2 and 4 mg, combined with a standard dosage of norethindrone acetate 1 mg for 11 days, HDL increased in a dose-related fashion but only significantly with the 2 and 4 mg of estradiol[72]. However, there were significant decreases in LDL cholesterol with all three dosages of estradiol plus the progestogen. In another long-term study of up to 20 years of hormone replacement, HDL cholesterol levels were significantly increased in both the conjugated estrogens-only users (1.89 mmol/l) and the users of conjugated estrogens plus medroxyprogesterone acetate (1.88 mmol/l), compared to non-users (1.74 mmol/l)[73]. LDL cholesterol was significantly decreased in both the unopposed estrogen users (3.23 mmol/l) and estrogen–progestogen users (3.38 mmol/l), compared to non-users (3.67 mmol/l). Triglycerides were significantly increased in the unopposed estrogen users (1.31 mmol/l), compared to non-users (1.10 mmol/l), and the added progestogen diminished this response (1.14 mmol/l). This beneficial effect on lipids has also been observed in other studies with added progestogen[70].

In the Heart and Estrogen–progestin Replacement Study (HERS) published recently, there were 2763 women (median age 66.7 years) with proven coronary artery disease and an intact uterus[74]. Half

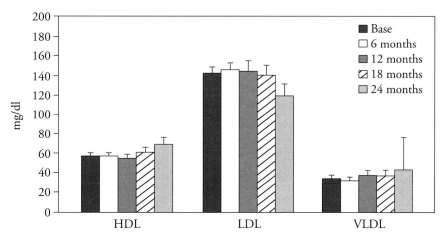

Figure 2 Serum lipoproteins of female patients did not show significant changes after 6–24 months of receiving subcutaneous estradiol pellets when medroxyprogesterone acetate was added

of them received estrogen–progestogen continuously and half received placebo, and there were no significant differences between the two groups in the cardiovascular outcomes. There were more coronary heart disease (CHD) events in the estrogen-treated group in the first year, but fewer in years 4 and 5. In the hormone-treated group, HDL increased by 8% and LDL decreased by 14%, compared to placebo, and more patients in the placebo group also received cholesterol-lowering drugs[74]. Unfortunately, patients received only continuous combined therapy and none of them received estrogen alone or cyclic progestogens or progesterone alone. It is important to remember that the HERS trial does not apply to primary prevention.

In a study of 390 patients using raloxifene (60 mg and 120 mg), conjugated estrogens with medroxyprogesterone acetate and placebo, both raloxifene and HRT decreased LDL (12% and 14%, respectively)[75]. Both dosages of raloxifene significantly lowered lipoprotein(a) by 7–8%, less than the 19% decrease with HRT. Raloxifene did not increase total HDL cholesterol or triglycerides whereas HRT increased HDL by 11% and triglycerides by 20%. However, raloxifene did increase HDL_2 cholesterol by 15–17%. Raloxifene significantly lowered fibrinogen by 12–14%, unlike HRT, which had no effect.

Alzheimer's disease and estrogen

Women are living longer and, hence, they are at a greater risk for Alzheimer's disease. About 3% of women aged 65–74 years are at risk, compared to 47% aged 85 years or older[76]. The pathogenesis is not clear, but estrogen is probably a good antioxidant in the central nervous system (CNS) and may improve cognition. It also may increase cerebral blood flow, enhance synthesis of acetylcholine, decrease levels of apolipoprotein E[77], and enhance cholesterol inhibition as does tacrine[78]. Some authors report a 50% reduction in Alzheimer's disease with estrogen, compared to non-users[77]. Kampen and Sherwin reported increased verbal memory following surgical menopause with estrogen therapy when average plasma estradiol levels were 40 pg/ml[79].

Menopause: comprehensive management

Symptoms that occur during the climacteric phase of a woman's life may begin premenopausally or long before her last menstrual period. The onset of these symptoms fluctuates between the early forties and the late fifties, and used to be considered purely psychoneurotic. The hormonal treatment of menopausal women has been controversial: what to give, when to start and for how long are questions that physicians must answer every day. Should women with symptoms attributed to estrogen deprivation receive hormone replacement therapy? Among many physicians, the idea of the menopause being a physiological phase may result in no treatment for their patients. Others believe that only vasomotor manifestations (hot flushes, sweats) and atrophic vaginitis are caused by estrogen deficiency, and should be treated with oral estrogens in the smallest dosage for the shortest period of time. For women with a uterus, estrogens should be given cyclically with progesterone to induce withdrawal bleeding. But why do women with gonadal dysgenesis who have not been exposed to significant amounts of endogenous estrogens not experience hot flushes even at an advanced age, while women who have been taking hormone replacement therapy for several months and then discontinue it will experience the classical hot flushes[80]? Considering these two observations, it is impossible to say whether the withdrawal syndrome secondary to estrogen deficiency is the cause of the hot flushes, mediated through functional changes of estrogen-sensitive neurons that are linked to the control of pulsatile LHRH secretion and thermoregulation.

Endocrinology views the menopause as a hormone-deficiency state, which therefore should be managed as long as is needed, without a predetermined period of treatment. The human body is programmed to utilize naturally occurring hormones better than synthetic hormones. It is therefore preferable in the long-term management of menopausal women to use natural or biological estrogens, such as estrone and estradiol, rather than synthetic estrogen-like hormones (ethinylestradiol, mestranol and stilbestrol), to avoid ingestion of foreign substances that strain the hepatic and renal enzyme systems in their effort to detoxify, conjugate and secrete their metabolites.

Management of estrogen therapy: pros and cons

It has been the belief that only vasomotor manifestations, hot flashes, sweats, as well as atrophic vaginitis are directly due to estrogen deficiency and should be treated with estrogens; but the consensus has been with the smallest dosage and for the shortest period of time; this is due to alarming past publications in reference to endometrial cancer, breast cancer and venous thromboembolism.

Depending on the severity of symptoms, it may be as well to commence with 0.625–1.25 mg of conjugated estrogens (USP) or 1–2 mg of 17β-estradiol, or their equivalents, for 25 days per month (Table 2). The dosage may be reduced or raised after a 2- or 3-month trial, according to the patient's response. For those who have a return of symptoms during the treatment-free interval, it may be advantageous to use the estrogen continuously. In either case, to induce a withdrawal bleeding and shedding of the endometrium a 12–14-day course of an oral progestogen should be prescribed from days 13 to 25 for the intermittent regimen (Table 3). For those who are adamantly opposed to menses an alternative is available: continuous conjugated estrogens 0.625 mg along with continuous medroxyprogesterone acetate 2.5 mg every day for 365 days each year has been recommended. However, the continuous combined regimen is not fully endometrial-protective, as discussed below. A better regimen to produce amenorrhea is cyclic combined therapy, where the low-dose estrogen and lower dosage of progestogen are both given from the 1st to the 25th of the month. Although there is some troublesome breakthrough bleeding during the first 4–6 months, about 60% of patients will become amenorrheic by 6 months. However, most women will accept the light withdrawal bleeding from the sequential estrogen-progestogen regimen.

Parenteral therapy by intramuscular injection

When oral therapy does not provide the expected relief or, for one reason or another, the patient cannot tolerate the drug, intramuscular injections of a long-acting estrogen with or without an androgen may be administered at 3–6-weekly intervals (Tables 2 and 4). Cyclic oral progestogens should also be prescribed. A therapeutic trial with 1 ml of Depo-Estradiol® is given, and if improvement has not been achieved in 3 weeks, 1 ml of Depo-Testadiol® or 1 ml of Depo-Testosterone® may be given.[81] The addition of an androgen is particularly beneficial for those with persistent fatigue, depression, headaches or poor libido, after initiation of estrogen injections.

Pellet implants

When oral therapy is ineffective and injections are inconvenient or unsatisfactory, pellets may prove quite effective[82–84]. Pellets are implanted subcutaneously with the aid of a trochar under the skin, either in the abdomen 2.5 cm above and parallel to Poupart's ligament, or in the gluteal region. One to four pellets of estradiol (25 mg each) may be implanted at 6-monthly intervals. Estrogen levels are maintained for about 5 months or longer[85] (Figure 3). One or two estradiol pellets and one or two pellets of testosterone (75 mg each) have proved an excellent and much desired combination[83,84]. Cyclic oral progestogen administration is mandatory for all women with uterus intact.

Vaginal creams

Cream or ointments containing estrogens have been employed for many years, especially in cases of atrophic or senile vaginitis. In the management of kraurosis vulvae, an ointment containing either hydrocortisone or one of its analogs should be applied to the vulvar areas once or twice daily along with oral estrogens or vaginal estrogen cream. Vaginal cream may also be used where vaginal dryness causes discomfort during sexual intercourse. When estrogens are contraindicated,

Table 2 Commonly used estrogens

Name	Estrogen	Dosage	Manufacturer
Oral estrogens			
Premarin®	conjugated estrogens	0.3 mg	Wyeth–Ayerst
		0.625 mg	
		0.9 mg	
		1.25 mg	
		2.5 mg	
Estrace®	micronized estradiol	0.5 mg	Bristol-Myers-Squibb
		1.0 mg	
		2.0 mg	
Estratab®	esterified estrogens	0.3 mg	Solvay
		0.625 mg	
		1.25 mg	
		2.5 mg	
Ogen®	estropipate	0.625 mg	Pharmacia & Upjohn
		1.25 mg	
		2.5 mg	
		5.0 mg	
Estinyl®	ethinylestradiol	0.02 mg	Schering
		0.05 mg	
		0.5 mg	
Estrogen vaginal cream and ring			
Premarin® vaginal cream	conjugated estrogens	0.625 mg/g	Wyeth–Ayerst
Estrace® vaginal cream	17β-estradiol	0.1 mg/g	Bristol-Myers-Squibb
Ogen® vaginal cream	estropipate	1.5 mg/g	Pharmacia & Upjohn
Ortho Dienestrol® cream	dienestrol	0.01%	Ortho
Estragard® cream	dienestrol	0.01%	Solvay
Diethylstibestrol suppositories	diethylstilbestrol	0.1 mg/g	Lilly
		0.5 mg/g	
Estring®	estradiol	2 mg total	Pharmacia & Upjohn
Parenteral estrogens			
Depo-Estradiol®	estradiol cypionate	1 mg/ml	Upjohn
		5 mg/ml	
Delestrogen®	estradiol valerate	10 mg/ml	Squibb
		20 mg/ml	
		40 mg/ml	
Estraval®	estradiol valerate	10 mg/ml	Solvay
		20 mg/ml	
Estrape®*	estradiol pellets	25-mg pellet	Bartor
Alora®	transdermal estradiol	0.035 mg/day	Procter & Gamble
		0.075 mg/day	
Estraderm®	transdermal estradiol	0.05 mg/day	Novartis
		0.1 mg/day	
Climara®	transdermal estradiol	0.035 mg/day	Berlex
		0.05 mg/day	
		0.1 mg/day	
Vivelle®	transdermal estradiol	0.0375 mg/day	Ciba–Geneva
		0.05 mg/day	
		0.075 mg/day	
		0.1 mg/day	

*Available from several pharmacies

Table 3 Progestogens

Name	Progestogen	Dosage	Manufacturer
Provera®	medroxyprogesterone acetate	2.5, 5, 10 mg	Pharmacia & Upjohn
Curretab®	medroxyprogesterone acetate	10 mg	Solvay
Cyrin®	medroxyprogesterone acetate	10 mg	Lederle
Amen®	medroxyprogesterone acetate	10 mg	Carnrick
Aygestin®	norethindrone acetate	5 mg	Lederle
Megace®	megestrol acetate	20, 40 mg	Bristol-Myers-Squibb
Ovrette®	norgestrel	0.075 mg	Wyeth-Ayerst
Micronor®	norethindrone	0.35 mg	Ortho
Nor-QD®	norethindrone	0.35 mg	Syntex
Prometrium®	oral micronized progesterone	100 mg	Solvay
–	progesterone vaginal suppositories	25, 50 mg	–

Table 4 Androgens

Name	Androgen	Dosage	Manufacturer
Oral androgens			
Oreton®	methyltestosterone	5 mg	Schering
Metandren®	methyltestosterone	5 mg	Novartis
Halotestin®	fluoxymesterone	2 mg	Upjohn
		5 mg	
Fluoxymesterone	fluoxymesterone	5 mg	Solvay
Injectables			
Depo-Testosterone®	testosterone cypionate	100 mg/ml	Upjohn
		200 mg/ml	
Delatestryl®	testosterone enanthate	100 mg/ml	Squibb
Testopel®	testosterone pellets	75 mg	Bartor
Estrogen-androgen combinations			
Estratest® tablets	esterified estrogens	1.25 mg	Solvay
	methyltestosterone	2.5 mg	
Estratest HS® tablets	esterified estrogens	0.625 mg	Solvay
	methyltestosterone	1.25 mg	
Premarin® with methyltestosterone	conjugated estrogens	1.25 mg	Wyeth-Ayerst
	methyltestosterone	10 mg	
Premarin® with methyltestosterone	conjugated estrogens	0.625 mg	Wyeth-Ayerst
	methyltestosterone	5 mg	
Depo-Testadiol®	estradiol cypionate	2 mg	Upjohn
	testosterone cypionate	50 mg	
Estrapel®	estradiol pellet (given with testosterone pellets)	25 mg	(various pharmacies)

androgens can frequently produce relief, improving energy and sensation of well-being, but in some cases they are not as effective. When estrogens alone are less than effective to restore lost sexual desire or depression, then the addition of an androgen will frequently prove satisfactory (Table 4).

Endometrial cancer

During the menopause, women may present irregular bleeding, caused by proliferation of the endometrium due to non-ovarian estrogen stimulation, as explained above. Because these women do not ovulate, and therefore do not produce progestogens, unopposed estrogen may induce various degrees of hyperplasia of the endometrium and in those with genetical predisposition to adenocarcinoma[86-88] (Figure 4). Progesterone therapy ensures more complete sloughing of the

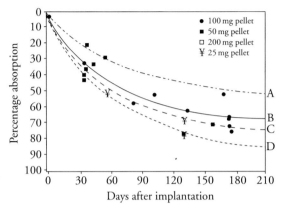

Figure 3 Percentage and mean absorption curve of four pellets of estradiol. Reproduced with permission from reference 85

endometrium, leaving behind fewer cells and glands to continue proliferation that could result in hyperplasia. Therefore, progestogen therapy may introduce a protective factor in the development of cancer[86-89]. The use of medroxyprogesterone acetate 10 mg from day 13 to day 25 is the recommended dosage. Women who complain of heavy bleeding may benefit from norethindrone acetate 5 mg for 13 days, which usually reduces the amount of withdrawal bleeding (Table 3).

It has been known for many years that unopposed estrogen will increase the risk of endometrial hyperplasia and cancer. Estrogen stimulates estradiol and progesterone receptors, and progesterone decreases numbers of both receptors[90]. It has been shown that by using cyclic progestogens 12–14 days per month, the incidence of endometrial hyperplasia and cancer is lower than in patients who do not take any hormones. Among other therapies, continuous combined therapy (Prempro®) has been used to produce

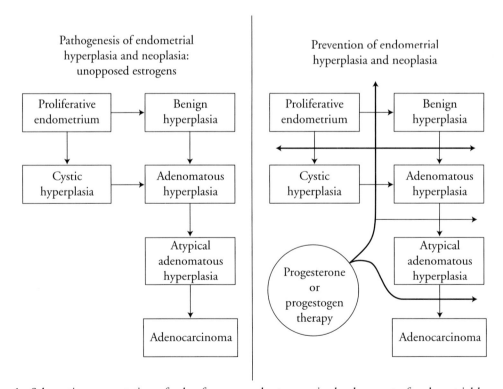

Figure 4 Schematic representation of role of unopposed estrogens in development of endometrial hyperplasia and cancer, and effect of progesterone or progestogens on these pathological changes. Reproduced with permission from reference 86

amenorrhea for the past 15 years, but unfortunately there have been several cases of endometrial cancer with this regimen, even at low values of endometrial thickness measured by ultrasound[89]. Using cyclic combined therapy for 25 days each month may give the receptors a chance to recover and prevent hyperplasia.

Raloxifene has recently been approved for prevention of osteoporosis, and this agent does not seem to stimulate the endometrium. In women who are reluctant to continue menses after the menopause this may be an alternative to estrogen. Tamoxifen is another SERM which has been used as an antiestrogen for breast cancer, but several patients developed endometrial cancer while using this agent for the treatment of breast cancer[91,92].

Breast cancer

Breast cancer is a great cause of concern in relation to hormone therapy with estrogens for physicians and their patients. Carcinoma of the breast is the most frequent malignancy in American women, constituting 29% of all female cancers and 16% of all female cancer deaths[93]. In 1999, it is expected that 176 300 new cases of breast cancer will be diagnosed and 43 300 women will die from this disease. The good news is that the number of new cases is decreasing, down from 184 300 new cases in 1996. The even better news is that the number of deaths has declined from 46 000 during 1995. In contrast to the incidence of cervical, endometrial and ovarian cancers, which peak from the fifth to the seventh decade of life and either remain the same or decline thereafter[86] (Figure 5), the incidence of breast cancer continues to increase as long as women live. There is mounting evidence that estrogen replacement does not increase the risk of breast cancer, even with long-term use[94,95]. Several studies have shown that added progestogen to estrogen replacement may even decrease the risk of this malignancy[96-98]. Studies are now showing that estrogen replacement therapy can be given to breast cancer survivors without any increased risk of recurrences and mortality[99]. When moderate dosages of progestogen are added, either continuously or for 25 days each month, there are fewer recurrences and less mortality[100,101].

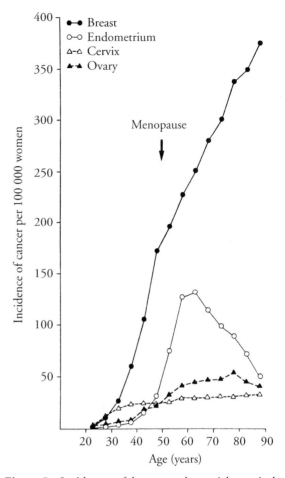

Figure 5 Incidence of breast, endometrial, cervical and ovarian cancer in women according to age. Reproduced with permission from reference 86

Conclusions

The age-old question is do all women need HRT, and when to start therapy and how long to continue? There will be over 40 million women spending an average of 33 years in menopause by the year 2000, and many of these women *will* develop coronary heart disease, osteoporosis, Alzheimer's disease and colon cancer. Should estrogen replacement therapy be used for prevention in all these women?

The most important approach is to educate women about their risks in menopause, and also to discuss the pros and cons of HRT including the development of deep venous thrombosis and cancers. They should be counselled regarding the risks of smoking and its adverse effects on the heart and bone, and attempts should be made to stop them smoking. The benefits of exercise for the heart and bone should be discussed, and minimal weight-bearing exercise, such as walking 2 miles, should be encouraged.

Over the years, typically, physicians have been empirically prescribing HRT based on symptoms, but it is now felt that treatment should be tailored to individual needs. In the USA, fewer than 20% of women take HRT over long periods of time[102].

Tailoring HRT to individuals

There are some women who have moderate to severe symptoms; these patients will approach physicians for therapy, and they are easy to counsel and treat and will continue therapy. There

are many women who continue to produce small amounts of endogenous estrogen, even 5–20 pg/ml, and they seem to have lower incidences of hip fractures and may not need therapy. There are others who are taking high doses of estrogen replacement therapy and continue to lose bone mineral density, and even continue to have symptoms such as vaginal dryness and hot flushes.

Patients should be screened prior to estrogen replacement therapy to establish a baseline FSH level, biochemical markers for bone and a lipid profile, and these should be re-evaluated during the course of therapy before increasing the dosage. If patients do not respond to estrogen therapy alone, androgens should be added. For those who do not wish to take estrogen replacement therapy, alternative therapies such as raloxifene should be offered to protect bone.

References

1. Greenblatt RB, Colle ML, Mahesh VB. Ovarian and adrenal steroid production in postmenopausal women. *Obstet Gynecol* 1986;47:383–7
2. Hammerstein J, Rice BG, Savard K. Steroid hormone formation in the human ovary. Identification of steroids formed *in vitro* from acetate 1014C in the corpus luteum. *J Clin Endocrinol Metab* 1964;24:597–605
3. Mattingly RF, Huang WY. Steroidogenesis of the menopausal and postmenopausal ovary. *Am J Obstet Gynecol* 1969;103:679–93
4. Frieden EH, Patkin JK, Mills M. Effect of follicle stimulating hormone (FSH) upon steroid aromatization *in vitro*. *Proc Soc Exp Biol Med* 1968;129:606–9
5. Longscope C. Steroid production in pre- and postmenopausal women. In Greenblatt RB, Mahesh VB, McDonough PG, eds. *The Menopausal Syndrome*. New York: Medcom Press, 1974:6–11
6. Richards JS, Midgley Ar Jr. Protein hormone action: a key to understanding ovarian follicular and luteal cell development. *Biol Reprod* 1976;14:82–94
7. Adamopoulos DA, Loraine JA, Dove GA. Endocrinological studies in women approaching the menopause. *J Obstet Gynaecol Br Commonw* 1971;78:62–79
8. Costoff A. An ultrastructural study of ovarian changes in the menopause. In Greenblatt RB, Mahesh VB, McDonough PG, eds. *The Menopausal Syndrome*. New York: Medcom Press, 1974:12–28
9. Netter A, Lambert A. Etude hormonal preliminaire de la premenopause. In Bernard I, Kollenc M, Audebert, Imprimerie E, eds. *La Menopause*. Bordeaux: Drouillard, 1975:28
10. Sherman BM, West JH, Korenman SH. The menopausal transition: analysis of LH, FSH, estradiol, and progesterone concentrations during menstrual cycles of older women. *J Clin Endocrinol Metab* 1976;42:629–36
11. Riley GM. Endocrinology of the climacteric. *Clin Obstet Gynecol* 1964;7:432
12. Plotz EJ, Wiener M, Stein AA, *et al.* Enzymatic activities related to steroidogenesis in postmenopausal ovaries of patients with and without endometrial carcinoma. *Am J Obstet Gynecol* 1967;99:182–97
13. Greenblatt RB, Colle ML, Mahesh VB. Ovarian and adrenal steroid production in postmenopausal women. *Obstet Gynecol* 1976;47:383–7
14. Grodin JM, Sitteri PK, McDonald PC. Source of estrogen production in postmenopausal women. *J Clin Endocrinol Metab* 1973;36:207–14

15. Sitteri PK, McDonald PC. Annual Meeting of Society of Physiology. In Greep RO, Astwood E, eds. *Handbook of Physiology and Endocrinology.* Washington, DC: 1973;2:615

16. Poortman J, Thijssen JHH, Schwartz F. Androgen production and conversion to estrogens in normal postmenopausal women and in selected breast cancer patients. *J Clin Endocrinol Metab* 1974;37:101–9

17. Yen SSC, Martin PL, Burnier AM, *et al.* Circulating estradiol, estrone and gonadotropin levels following the administration of orally active 17β-estradiol in postmenopausal women. *J Clin Endocrinol Metab* 1975;40:518–21

18. Greenblatt RB, Colle ML, Mahesh VB. Ovarian and adrenal steroid production in postmenopausal women. *Obstet Gynecol* 1976;47:383–7

19. Greenblatt RB, Natrajan PK, Aksu MF, *et al.* The fate of a large bolus of exogenous estrogen administered to menopausal women. *Maturitas* 1979;2:29

20. Shima K, Kitayama S, Nakano R. Gonadotropin binding in human ovary. *Obstet Gynecol* 1987;69:800–5

21. Rajaniemi HJ, Ronnberg L, Kauppila A, *et al.* Luteinizing hormone receptors in human follicles and corpora lutea during menstrual cycle and pregnancy. *J Clin Endocrinol Metab* 1981;108:307–13

22. Rajaniemi HJ, Midgley AR Jr, Duncan JA, *et al.* Gonadotropin receptors in rat ovarian tissue. III. Binding sites for luteinizing hormone and differentiation of granulosa cells to luteal cells. *Endocrinology* 1977;101:898–910

23. Baker TG. A quantitative and cytological study of germ cells in human ovaries. *Proc R Soc (London)* 1963;158:417

24. Treloar AE, Boynton RE, Benn BG, Brown BW. Variation of the human menstrual cycle through reproduction life. *Int J Fertil* 1967;12:77

25. Papanicolaou AD, Loraine JA, Dove GA, London NB. Hormone excretion patterns in perimenopausal women. *J Obstet Gynaecol Br Commonw* 1969;76:308–16

26. Adamopoulos DA, Loraine JA, Dove GA. Endocrinological studies in women approaching the menopause. *J Obstet Gynaecol Br Commonw* 1971;78:62–79

27. Goldenberg BL, Grudin JM, Rodbard D, Ross GT. Gonadotropins in women with amenorrhea: use of plasma follicle stimulating hormone to differentiate women with and without ovarian follicles. *Am J Obstet Gynecol* 1973;116:1003–12

28. Yen SSC, Tsai CC. The effect of ovariectomy on gonadotropin release. *J Clin Invest* 1971;50:1149–53

29. Monroe SE, Jaffee RB, Midgley AR Jr. Regulation of human gonadotropins. XIII. Changes in serum gonadotropins in menstruating women in response to oophorectomy. *J Clin Endocrinol Metab* 1972;34:420–2

30. Casper RF, Yen SSC, Wilkes MM. Menopausal flushes: a neuroendocrine link with pulsatile luteinizing hormone secretion. *Science* 1979;205:823–5

31. Tatryn IV, Meldrum DR, Lu KH, Frumar AM, Judd HL. LH, FSH and skin temperature during the menopause hot flush. *J Clin Endocrinol Metab* 1979;49:152–4

32. Mulley GM, Tattersall RB. Hot flushes after hypophysectomy. *Br Med J* 1977;1:1062

33. Brown KH, Hammond CB. Urogenital atrophy. *Obstet Gynecol Clin North Am* 1987;15:13–32

34. Thompson RF. Foundations of physiological psychology. New York: Harper and Row, 1967:115

35. Undenfriend S, Weissbach H, Bogdanski DDF. Increase in tissue serotonin following administration of its precursor 5-hydroxytryptophan. *J Biol Chem* 1957;224:803–10

36. Kantor HT, Michael CM, Shore H. Estrogen for older women. *Am J Obstet Gynecol* 1973;116:115–18

37. Cummings ST, Kelsey JL, Nevitt MC, O'Dowd KJ. Epidemiology of osteoporosis and osteoporotic fractures. *Epidemiol Rev* 1985;7:178–208

38. Gallagher JC, Riggs RI, DeLuca HF. Effect of estrogen on calcium absorption and serum vitamin D metabolites in postmenopausal osteoporosis. *J Clin Endocrinol Metab* 1980;51:1359–64

39. Burch JC, Byrd BV, Vaugh WR. Results of estrogen treatment in one thousand hysterectomized women for 14 318 years. In Van Keep PA, Greenblatt RB, Albeaux-Fernet M, eds. *Consensus on Menopause Research.* Lancaster, UK: MTP Press, 1976:164–9

40. Hammond CB, Jelovsek FR, Lee KL, *et al.* Effects of long-term estrogen replacement therapy. I. Metabolic. *Am J Obstet Gynecol* 1979;133:525–36

41. Lindsay R, Hart DM, Baird C, Forrest C. Prevention of spinal osteoporosis in oophorectomized women. *Lancet* 1980;2:1151–3

42. Lufkin EG, Wahner HW, O'Fallon WM, *et al.* Treatment of postmenopausal osteoporosis with transdermal estrogen. *Ann Intern Med* 1992;117:1–9

43. Love R, Mazess RB, Barden HS, *et al.* Effects of tamoxifen on bone mineral density in postmenopausal women with breast cancer. *N Engl J Med* 1992;326:852–6

44. Lufkin EG, Whitaker MD, Argueta R, *et al.* Raloxifene treatment of postmenopausal osteoporosis. *J Bone Miner Res* 1997;12:S150

45. Ettinger B, Black D, Cummings S, *et al.* Raloxifene reduces the risk of incident vertebral fractures: 24-month interim analyses [Abst]. *Osteoporosis Int* 1998;8(Suppl 3):11

46. Watts NB, Notelovitz M, Timmons MC, *et al.* Comparison of oral estrogens and estrogens plus

androgens on bone mineral density, menopausal symptoms, and lipid-lipoprotein profiles in surgical menopause. *Obstet Gynecol* 1995;85:529–37

47. Nachtigall IE, Nachtigall RH, Nachtigall RC, *et al.* Estrogen replacement therapy. I. A 10-year prospective study in the relationship to osteoporosis. *Obstet Gynecol* 1979;53:277–81

48. Christiansen C, Christensen MS, Transbol I. Bone mass in postmenopausal women after withdrawal of oestrogen/progestogen replacement therapy. *Lancet* 1981;1:459–61

49. Crilley RG, Marshall D II, Norlin BEC. The effect of estradiol valerate and cyclic oestradiol valerate/DL-norgestrel on calcium metabolism. *Postgrad Med J* 1978;54:47–9

50. Upton GV. The perimenopause: physiologic correlates and clinical management. *J Reprod Med* 1982;27:1–26

51. Arnett TR, Horton MA, Coston KW, *et al.* Oestrogen receptors and human bone cells; an immunocytochemical study. In Christiansen C, Johanen JS, Riis BJ, eds. *International Symposium on Osteoporosis.* Denmark: 1987;1:519–23

52. Teran AZ, Greenblatt RB. Evaluation of GnRH analog versus Danazol for the treatment of endometrosis.

53. Peck WA, Barrett-Conner E, Buckwalter JA, *et al.* Consensus Conference. Osteoporosis. *J Am Med Assoc* 1984;252:799–802

54. Riggs BL, Hodgson SF, O'Fallon WM, *et al.* Effect of fluoride treatment on the fracture rate in postmenopausal women with osteoporosis. *N Engl J Med* 1990;322:802–9

55. Watts NB, Harris ST, Genant HK, *et al.* Intermittent cyclical etidronate treatment of postmenopausal osteoporosis. *N Engl J Med* 1990;323:73–9

56. Wild RA. Estrogen effects on the cardiovascular tree. *Obstet Gynecol* 1996;87:27S–35S

57. Sullivan JM, Fowlkes LP. The clinical aspects of estrogen and the cardiovascular system. *Obstet Gynecol* 1996;87:36S–43S

58. Kuller LH. Epidemiology of cardiovascular disease: current perspectives. *Am J Epidemiol* 1976;104:425–96

59. Albrink MJ, Man EB. Serum triglycerides in coronary artery disease. *Arch Intern Med* 1959;103:4–8

60. Carlson KA, Bottinger LE. Ischaemic heart disease in relation to fasting values of plasma triglycerides and cholesterol. Stockholm Prospective Study. *Lancet* 1972;1:865–8

61. Kannel WB, Castelli WP, Gordon T, *et al.* Serum cholesterol, lipoproteins and the risk of coronary heart disease: The Framingham Study. *Ann Intern Med* 1971;74:1–12

62. Keys A. Coronary heart disease: the global picture. *Atherosclerosis* 1975;22:149–92

63. Brunzell JD, Schrott MG, Motulsky AG, *et al.* Myocardial infarction in the familiar forms of hypertriglyceridemia. *Metabolism* 1976;25:313

64. Larsson-Cohn U. Lipids and estrogens. In Van Keep PA, Greenblatt RB, Albeaux-Fernet M, eds. *Consensus on Menopause Research.* Lancaster, UK: MTP Press, 1976:51

65. Manninen V, Elo OM, Frick HM, *et al.* Lipid alterations and decline in the incidence of coronary heart disease in the Helsinki Heart Study. *J Am Med Assoc* 1988;260:641–51

66. Gordon T, Castelli WP, Hjortland MC, *et al.* High density lipoprotein as a protective factor against coronary heart disease. The Framingham Study. *Am J Med* 1977;62:707–14

67. Miller GJ, Miller NE. Plasma high-density lipoprotein concentration and development of ischaemic heart-disease: a prospective case–control study. *Lancet* 1975;1:16–19

68. Miller NE, Forde OH, Thelle DS, *et al.* The Thromso heart-study. High density lipoprotein and coronary heart-disease: a prospective case-control study. *Lancet* 1977;1:965–7

69. Teran AZ, Greenblatt RB, Chaddha JS. Changes in lipoproteins with various sex steroids. *Obstet Gynecol Clin North Am* 1987;14:107–19

70. Gambrell RD Jr, Teran A-Z. Changes in lipids and lipoproteins with long-term estrogen deficiency and hormone replacement therapy. *Am J Obstet Gynecol* 1991;165:307–17

71. Writing Group for the PEPI Trial. Effects of estrogen or estrogen/progestin regimens on heart disease risk factors in postmenopausal women. *J Am Med Assoc* 1995;273:199–208

72. Jensen J, Nilas J, Christiansen C. Cyclic changes in serum cholesterol and lipoproteins following different doses of combined postmenopausal hormone replacement therapy. *Br J Obstet Gynaecol* 1986;93:613–18

73. Barrett-Conner E, Wingard DL, Criqui MH. Postmenopausal estrogen use and heart disease risk factors in the 1980s. *J Am Med Assoc* 1989;261:2095–100

74. Hulley SH, Grady D, Bush T, *et al.* Randomized trial of estrogen plus progestin for secondary prevention of coronary heart disease in postmenopausal women. *J Am Med Assoc* 1998;280:605–13

75. Walsh BW, Kuller LH, Wild RA, *et al.* Effects of raloxifene on serum lipids and coagulation factors in healthy postmenopausal women. *J Am Med Assoc* 1998;279:1445–51

76. Ikehara R. Estrogen and Alzheimer's disease: a review and update. *Prim Care Update OB/GYN* 1997;4:228–33

77. Birge SJ. Maintaining mental health with hormone replacement therapy. *Eur Menopause J* 1996;3:164–9

78. Schneider LS, Farlow MR, Henderson VW, *et al.* Effects of estrogen replacement therapy on response to Tacrine in patients with Alzheimer's disease. *Neurology* 1996;46:1580-4

79. Kampen DL, Sherwin BB. Estrogen use and verbal memory in healthy postmenopausal women. *Obstet Gynecol* 1994;83:979-83

80. Yen SSC. The biology of menopause. *Reprod Med* 1977;18:287-96

81. Gambrell RD Jr. *Hormone Replacement Therapy,* 5th edn. Durant, OK: EMIS Medical Publishers, 1997

82. Greenblatt RB, Bryner JR. Estradiol pellet implantation in the management of menopause. *J Reprod Med* 1977;18:307-16

83. Studd JWW. Hormone implants in the climacteric syndrome. In Campbell S, ed. *The Management of the Menopause and Post-Menopausal Years.* Lancaster, UK: MTP Press, 1976:383-5

84. Studd J, Magos A. Hormone pellet implantation for the menopause and premenstrual syndrome. *Obstet Gynecol Clin North Am* 1987;14:229-49

85. Greenblatt RB, Hari LQ. *J Clin Endocrinol* 1942;2: 315

86. Gambrell RD Jr. The menopause: benefits and risks of estrogen–progestogen replacement therapy. *Fertil Steril* 1982;37:457-74

87. Gambrell RD Jr, Massey FM, Castaneda TA, *et al.* Use of the progestogen challenge test to reduce the risk of endometrial cancer. *Obstet Gynecol* 1980;55: 732-8

88. Whitehead MI, Townsend PT, Pryse-Davies J, *et al.* Effects of estrogens and progestins on the biochemistry and morphology of the postmenopausal endometrium. *N Engl J Med* 1981;305: 1599-605

89. Gambrell RD Jr. Strategies to decrease the incidence of endometrial cancer in postmenopausal women. *Am J Obstet Gynecol* 1997;177:1196-207

90. Natrajan PK, Muldoon TG, Greenblatt RB, Mahesh VB. Effect of progestins and estrogen on progesterone receptors of the human endometrium. *J Reprod Med* 1982;27:227-30

91. Lahti E, Blanco G, Kauppila A, *et al.* Endometrial changes in postmenopausal breast cancer patients receiving tamoxifen. *Obstet Gynecol* 1993;81:660-4

92. Fisher B, Constantino J, Redmone C, *et al.* Endometrial cancer in tamoxifen treated breast cancer patients: findings from the National Adjunct Breast and Bowel Project (NSABP) B-14. *J Natl Cancer Inst* 1994;86:527-37

93. Landis SH, Murray T, Bolden S, Wingo PA. Cancer statistics, 1999. *CA Cancer J Clin* 1999;49:8-31

94. Gambrell RD Jr. Hormone replacement therapy and breast cancer risk. *Arch Fam Med* 1996;5:341-8

95. Collaborative Group on Hormonal Factors in Breast Cancer. Breast cancer and hormone replacement therapy: collaborative reanalysis of data from 51 epidemiological studies of 52 706 women with breast cancer and 108 411 women without breast cancer. *Lancet* 1997;350:1047-59

96. Gambrell RD Jr. Use of progestogen therapy. *Am J Obstet Gynecol* 1987;156:1304-13

97. Nachtigall MJ, Smilen SW, Nachtigall RD, *et al.* Incidence of breast cancer in a 22-year study of women receiving estrogen-progestin therapy. *Obstet Gynecol* 1992;80:827-30

98. Stanford JL, Weiss NS, Voigt LF, *et al.* Combined estrogen and progestin hormone replacement therapy in relation to risk of breast cancer in middle-aged women. *J Am Med Assoc* 1995;274: 137-42

99. DiSaia PJ, Grosen EA, Kurosaki T, *et al.* Hormone replacement therapy in breast cancer survivors. A cohort study. *Am J Obstet Gynecol* 1996;174:1494-8

100. Dew J, Eden J, Beller E, *et al.* A cohort study of hormone replacement therapy given to women previously treated for breast cancer. *Climacteric* 1998;1:137-42

101. Natrajan PK, Soumakis K, Gambrell RD Jr. Estrogen replacement therapy in women with previous breast cancer. *Am J Obstet Gynecol* 1999;181:288-95

102. Ettinger B, Li D-K, Klein R. Continuation of postmenopausal hormone replacement therapy: comparison of cyclic versus continuous combined schedules. *Menopause* 1996;3:185-9

20

Routes of hormone replacement therapy

Kelly Parsey

Background

In the United States, the median age of menopause is 51 years with a range of 41–59 years[1]. During the peri- and postmenopause, the natural ovarian production of estradiol decreases, resulting in irregular and, finally, complete cessation of menses. Loss of estrogen also leads to vasomotor instability, loss of bone architecture, genitourinary changes and changes in lipid profiles. Vasomotor instability results in the 'hot flash' experience of flushing and sweating. Although the experience varies in severity between women, approximately 40% of menopausal women seek physician help for this symptom[2]. More insidious, and more devastating in long-term consequences, loss of bone can eventually lead to osteoporosis with fractures of the spine, hip or other bones. It is estimated that over half of all postmenopausal women will develop a spontaneous osteoporotic fracture[1]. Spinal fractures are often painful, and if occurring at several positions cause vertebral collapse with loss of height. Fractures of the hip, however, usually require hip replacement surgery, mean long recovery periods, and often equal a decrease in social function and even survival[1]. The estrogen-depleted vaginal epithelium results in dyspareunia, urinary incontinence and increased risk for urinary tract infections. Repleting the estrogen that is lost can diminish the symptoms, lessen or prevent bone loss and return the vaginal epithelium to a premenopausal state. Additionally, cardiovascular disease increases after the menopause, and 30% of postmenopausal women will die of cardiac disease[1]. Although the data are inconclusive, many epidemiological studies have suggested a reduction in cardiac disease in women who use hormone replacement therapy (HRT). The Nurses' Health Study Cohort found an adjusted relative risk of death from coronary heart disease to be 0.47 for women who were current users of hormones[3].

Current medical opinion on the appropriateness of HRT for the menopausal woman varies, often finding that the medical specialists who deal with the consequences of HRT therapy have the strongest feelings on the issue. The burden of disease from estrogen depletion and the available treatments require that medical opinion leaders attempt to give guidance to the postmenopausal population and their health-care providers on this controversial area. Although the current version of the United States Preventive Services Task Force does not endorse treating every postmenopausal woman with HRT, the task force does recommend counselling every postmenopausal woman on her individual risk of morbidity and her options for treatment[1]. The American College of Obstetricians and Gynecologists, The American Medical Association and the Canadian Medical Association also endorse counselling for all postmenopausal women about the risk and benefit of estrogen therapy[1]. Also, a 1996 European consensus statement indicated that HRT was appropriate for most postmenopausal women[4].

Although the numbers of women entering the menopause are increasing, and there is much evidence to support the use of estrogen repletion, many women are reluctant to use any form of HRT. Those that do start treatment often discontinue quickly, sometimes within the first years[5]. There are numerous reasons for this lack of compliance. As women are taking greater responsibility for their health-care, they want to be fully informed of what medication they use. Often women feel it is not 'natural' to take exogenous estrogens. Many women fear developing breast cancer more than they fear osteoporosis or cardiovascular disease. Still other women may not be informed of the many options in hormone therapies. Health-care providers also may not be aware of different approaches to therapy, so when a woman presents with problems associated with a traditional formulation, she may not be informed of an alternative method. A national telephone survey also found a positive relationship between HRT use and sociodemographic factors, such as geographic location and education[6]. Certainly, incidence of side-effects and ease of use play important roles in compliance with any medication, but when a woman has to plan to use a treatment for potentially 30 years, her satisfaction with the product becomes even more important.

Hormones are available in pill formulations that are familiar to women and are easy to use, with once a day dosing. Estrogen–progesterone combination preparations also exist, increasing the ease of oral dosing and compliance. However, there is still a need for alternative methods of providing HRT. The available routes of estrogen delivery have increased in the past decade to include not only oral estrogen and progestins, either alone or in combination tablets, but also several other options. Transdermal matrix and reservoir delivery systems (patches) now exist and have been extensively studied. Other available but less widely used topical estrogens are topical gels and vaginal creams. With increasing options for HRT, there is sometimes missing information on the benefits and drawbacks of the various therapies. This chapter explores many of the HRT alternatives now available to the menopausal woman and her care provider. The intention is to give an overview of the approach, with literature examples of comparisons between products, measures of efficacy and possible side-effects.

Oral hormone replacement therapy

Oral estrogens have been in use since the 1950s for contraception. They have also been used for over 30 years for replacement of estrogen in women who have undergone premature ovarian failure, particularly in the case of surgical menopause. The majority of women who choose hormone replacement therapy select oral routes of delivery. There

has been much written, and there is much clinical experience with this form of HRT. It is commonly known that estrogen stimulates the endometrial lining, and that proliferation can result in hyperplasia. Atypical hyperplasia is a known precursor for endometrial adenocarcinoma. Prolonged estrogen monotherapy is therefore usually reserved for the postmenopausal woman who has had a hysterectomy. For the woman with an intact uterus, estrogen therapy is combined with a progestin that adds protection against endometrial hyperplasia. The progestin can be added in a cyclical regimen, usually inducing a periodic bleed, or can be given continuously with an attempt to induce amenorrhea. Progestins can be prescribed with estrogen as a separate pill or combined in the same pill. A widely prescribed product in the United States is Prempro® (Wyeth-Ayerst). The components of this combination pill are Premarin® (conjugated equine estrogens) 0.625 mg and Provera® (medroxyprogesterone acetate, MPA) 2.5 mg. For ease of prescribing and improved compliance, the combined pill is a good alternative. The once-a-day dosing is similar to that for oral contraceptives which many women used previously. Absorption is rapid with peak estradiol concentrations being reached in 4–10 h[7]. The half-life is also rapid, and serum levels of estradiol return quickly to pre-dose levels. This means that dosing must be daily, and missing several doses may result in symptoms of estrogen withdrawal.

The types of estrogen vary with the brand of HRT. Other available oral estrogen and progestin compounds are listed in Table 1. One of the concerns about any oral estrogen formulation is that there is significant loss of drug in the gastointestinal tract, necessitating larger initial doses. After the estrogens are absorbed, they are transported to the liver where they undergo first-pass hepatic metabolism resulting in estrone and its conjugates[8]. The use of medications such as phenytoin that induce these hepatic enzymes may result in rapid metabolism of the estrogen and less effective serum levels of estradiol. Estrone is converted to estradiol, but the physiological ratio of estrone to estradiol is 2 : 1, rather than the 1 : 1 ratio of the premenopause. First-pass metabolism has other consequences too. The induction of liver enzymes increases levels of growth hormone, sex steroid

Table 1 Oral formulations of hormone replacement in the United States. Adapted from reference 7

Brand	Estrogen dose (mg)	Progestin dose (mg)	Indication	Dosing
Estrace®	0.5, 1, 2 micronized estradiol		S, O, V	1–2 mg daily*
Estratab®	0.3, 0.625, 2.5 esterified estrogens		S, O, V	1.25 mg daily*
Menest®	0.3, 0.625, 1.25, 2.5 esterified estrogens		S, V	1.25 mg daily*
Ortho-est®	0.75, 1.5 estropipate		S, O, V	0.75–6 mg daily* for symptom control, 0.75 mg daily* for osteoporosis prevention
Premarin®	0.3, 0.625, 0.9, 1.25, 2.5 conjugated estrogens		S, O, V	1.25 mg daily* for symptoms, 0.625 mg daily* for osteoporosis prevention
Amen®		10 MPA	second-degree amenorrhea	10 mg daily for 10 days
Aygestin®		5 norethindrone acetate	second-degree amenorrhea	5–10 mg daily for 10 days
Cycrin®		5, 10 MPA	second-degree amenorrhea	10 mg for 10 days
Prometrium®		100 micronized progesterone	second-degree amenorrhea	400 mg daily for 10 days
Provera®		2.5, 5, 10 MPA	second-degree amenorrhea	10 mg daily for 10 days, 2.5 mg daily continuously
Prempro®	0.625 conjugated estrogens	2.5, 5 MPA	S, O, V	1 tablet daily continuous treatment
Premphase®	0.625 conjugated estrogens	0 or 5 MPA	S, O, V	estrogen only days 1–14, estrogen–MPA days 15–28
Estratest®	1.25 esterified estrogens, 2.5 methyltestosterone		vasomotor symptom relief only	1 tablet daily*

*Cyclic therapy (3 weeks on, 1 week off) is recommended for a woman with an intact uterus unless prescribed with a progestin; S, symptom control; O, osteoporosis prevention; V, vaginal atrophy; MPA, medroxyprogesterone acetate

binding globulin, thyroid binding globulin and cortisol binding globulin[9]. Growth hormone increases insulin secretion, and alterations in clotting factors may predispose to thrombosis.

Transdermal hormone replacement therapy

The permeability of the human skin is designed such that a drug that is expected to cross this to reach the capillary bed should be soluble in both a lipophilic and hydrophilic environment. Estradiol dissolved in alcohol can be delivered across the skin barrier, but is often associated with skin reactions to the alcohol, and is only viable as long as the alcohol does not evaporate. In general, there are two types of patch, with either a reservoir or a matrix design. The reservoir patch contains estradiol dissolved in alcohol in a reservoir inside the patch. The matrix design dissolves the estradiol in the adhesive layer next to the skin. Much of the data that have been collected about patch use have come from European experience with similar products.

A study comparing Climaderm®, a 7-day matrix transdermal patch and Estraderm TTS®, a twice-weekly transdermal reservoir system was conducted in 28 women, measuring serum estradiol levels and symptom relief. The results showed that both systems provided adequate estradiol. The relative bioavailability of the matrix compared to the reservoir system showed them to be bioequivalent, but the matrix patch system resulted in more constant estradiol levels, avoiding the peak and trough effect of changing mid-week[10].

In a comparison of two patches, each delivering 0.05 mg/day estradiol and designed to be dosed twice weekly, the maximum plasma concentrations of estradiol did not differ significantly. However, the Menorest® patch resulted in a significantly higher average serum concentration of estradiol than did Systen®[11]. This difference appeared to be caused by a more rapid decline in estradiol over the dosing period for the Systen system. In previous studies, both systems have been shown to alleviate menopausal symptoms. Given the identical nominal delivery of drug by both systems, but the differences in achieved estradiol levels, it again raises the question of how much estrogen is necessary to be effective. More and more clinical opinions reflect the belief that less drug is better if clinical effectiveness remains. If, however, there is concern for maintaining predictable levels of estradiol in a particular woman, then it may become important to choose a system that can deliver those levels, or at least to follow a woman's estradiol levels if she is not receiving appropriate benefit[8].

Several patches are marketed in the United States and all utilize estradiol, the naturally occurring ovarian estrogen (Table 2). The patch methods of transdermal delivery have been typically designed to provide estrogen to menopausal women to treat climacteric complaints or to prevent bone loss. They are prescribed alone to a woman without a uterus. In a woman with a uterus, an oral progestin is usually prescribed for endometrial protection. This may impact on compliance as it adds to the burden of dosing, requiring that a woman remembers to change a patch either weekly or twice weekly, and to take a pill daily. An estrogen and progestin combined patch is now available. The Combipatch® is indicated for climacteric symptom control and is applied twice weekly (see Combipatch package insert)

Gels and creams

There exists an alternative to estrogen replacement that is neither an oral pill formulation nor a transdermal patch. Although not marketed in the United States, estradiol is available in a gel formulation that can be applied to the skin and, once absorbed, provides the appropriate estrogen replacement without the undesirable side-effects of other routes. In a comparison of permeability of two formulations of hydroalcoholic gel, the delivery of estradiol across the skin was similar, amounting to about 17–18% of the applied dose. The formulations contained different amounts of estradiol, and had different recommended application quantities and areas[12]. Interpretation of clinical benefit or side-effects is therefore difficult. Another 2-year, open-label study compared the efficacy of two transdermal gel doses with that of

Table 2 Available transdermal estradiol patches in the United States. Adapted from reference 7

Brand	Estrogen dose (mg)	Progestin dose (mg)	Indication	Dosing*
Alora® (matrix)	0.05, 0.075, 0.1 estradiol		symptoms	0.05 mg twice weekly
Climara® (matrix)	0.025, 0.05, 0.075, 0.1 estradiol		symptoms, osteoporosis prevention	0.05 mg weekly
Estraderm® (reservoir)	0.05, 0.1 estradiol		symptoms osteoporosis prevention	0.05 mg twice weekly
FemPatch® (matrix)	0.025 estradiol		symptoms	1 patch weekly
Vivelle® (matrix)	0.0375, 0.05, 0.075, 0.1 estradiol		symptoms	0.05 mg twice weekly
Combipatch® (matrix)	0.05 estradiol	0.14, 0.25, norethindrone acetate	symptoms	1 patch twice weekly

*Cyclic therapy (3 weeks on and 1 week off) is recommended for a woman with an intact uterus unless prescribed with a progestin

oral estradiol valerate. Each arm was complemented with oral MPA. The main outcomes were climacteric symptoms, bleeding control, bone metabolism and lipid profiles. In all treatment groups, the climacteric symptoms were reduced over the course of therapy. The percentage of women reporting hot flush symptoms decreased in the 1-mg/day gel group from 89.2 to 6.5% by 24 months. The percentage in the 2-mg/day oral estradiol valerate group decreased from 89.2 to 13.3%. There were no overall differences in any efficacy measures between the groups[13]. A similar study was conducted to compare estradiol gel with an estradiol transdermal patch. In a 12-month, open, randomized study of 120 postmenopausal women, a 1-mg/day gel was compared with a patch delivering 0.05 mg estradiol/day. Main outcomes included clinical symptoms, endometrial effects, total bone mineral density and lipid metabolism. In addition, tolerability was assessed with emphasis on irritation of the skin. The dose of estradiol in either formulation was adjusted for excess estradiol effect or lack of symptom control, and symptom relief was found with both treatments. Hormonal effects on the endometrium were seen in 95.1% of the gel group and in 92.5% of the transdermal group, with no reports of hyperplasia. Serum estrone and estradiol levels were higher in the gel group. Cholesterol was decreased in both groups. Bone mineral density did not change over the year of therapy for either group. Ten subjects in the gel group and eight in the patch group reported adverse events during the study, and, by the study end, 96.4% of the gel group and 90.7% of the patch users reported that the treatments were convenient to use. Two subjects using the gel reported mild itching, and 28 subjects using the patch had skin irritation, usually just erythema and itching, but rarely swelling and peeling[14]. There are few other comparative studies of the irritation of the gel or transdermal formulations, but it is possible that the gel produces less irritation, as it does not require occlusive application like the patches. However, the application requires a large surface area and must be reapplied daily, which may affect compliance and accurate dosing.

Vaginal creams have been available for some time and are used for relief of vaginal itching, dryness, dyspareunia and urethritis. It was once

believed that this route provided benefit without resulting in the systemic absorption that is inherent in oral preparations or in transdermal routes such as patches and gels. This is not accurate. However, the amount absorbed can be altered by the vaginal secretions and vascularization; therefore, the serum levels of estradiol may change daily[9]. Nevertheless, there is a need to provide a progestin to protect the endometrium from estrogen stimulation. Vaginal insertion of the cream is required daily, and some women may find this application inconvenient. Additionally, this route may not be as effective in the relief of hot flushes or prevention of osteoporosis if adequate doses are not applied or are not absorbed. This route of estradiol delivery is usually reserved for reversing atrophic vaginal changes.

Lipids

Estrogen therapy causes changes in serum lipoproteins. Previously it was thought that the decreased risk of cardiovascular disease seen in women, compared to men, was largely the effect of estrogen. This was substantiated by the observation that after the menopause, cardiovascular risk increases and changes occur in lipid profiles such that there is an increase in low-density lipoprotein (LDL) and a decrease in high-density lipoprotein (HDL). This is a plausible biological model, as low-density lipoproteins are atherogenic, and cardiovascular events are thought to be secondary to atheroma formation. Upon further investigation of oral HRT, the evidence suggested that, in women who took oral HRT, total cholesterol and LDL decreased, while HDL increased[15]. This finding supported the estrogen theory of cardiovascular protection. An increase in triglycerides has also been found, but the significance in cardiovascular disease is uncertain. Extreme elevations in triglycerides can cause pancreatitis.

The Randomized Trial of Estrogen Plus Progestin for Secondary Prevention of Coronary Heart Disease in Postmenopausal Women (Heart and Estrogen/progestin Replacement Study, HERS) trial was designed to test the theory that HRT is beneficial in protecting women known to have coronary disease against further cardiovascular events. The concern was that previous epidemiological studies could have been biased in favor of HRT, as women who choose to use HRT may also be in better health or more likely to take care of their health. Women were enrolled who had already demonstrated cardiovascular disease, were treated with oral conjugated estrogens and MPA, and were followed for cardiovascular events for an average of 4.75 years. The underlying assumption was that events occurring in the first 2 years would be due to non-lipid etiologies, and lipid-mediated effects would not be seen for 2 or more years. The primary end-point, occurrence of a cardiovascular event, was not different between the treated and untreated groups. The lipid results were predictable, and, by the first year, LDL decreased in the treated group by 14% and by 3% in the untreated group. HDL increased in the treated group by 8% and decreased in the untreated group by 2%. Mean triglyceride levels increased by 10% in the treated group and by 2% in the untreated group[16]. This finding was somewhat surprising to the medical community, considering the wealth of epidemiological data suggesting a result in favor of HRT. The lipid results were expected, but the overall outcome was not. This is also contrary to current practice guide-lines for lipid management, which advise that anyone who has had a cardiovascular event or has two or more risk factors should receive medication to promote a more protective lipid profile[1]. The results of this large prospective trial make it more difficult to counsel women on whether or not to start HRT.

As the changes in lipids are attributed to the hepatoportal circulation seen with oral HRT, the question has arisen of whether a transdermal route of drug delivery, bypassing the hepatic circulation, would also result in changes in the lipid profile. One transdermal estradiol study did show decreases in total cholesterol, LDL, HDL and triglycerides[15]. Other direct comparisons of oral and transdermal HRT have not found such a clear picture. In a study of 35 women, there were decreases in HDL and the HDL/LDL ratio in both groups, and an increase in LDL in both groups. The total cholesterol level decreased in the transdermal group and increased in the oral group[17]. Finally, a study of 774 women randomized to transdermal estradiol combined with either continuous or sequential, and either high or low doses

of progestin found that total cholesterol decreased in all groups. HDL increased in the sequential progestin group and had a variable outcome in the continuous group. However, HDL$_2$ increased in all groups. LDL decreased, and triglycerides either did not change or decreased in all four groups[18].

This varying information causes confusion, and emphasizes that the effects of HRT, either oral or transdermal, are many. Common practice has now promoted the use of transdermal routes in women who need the benefit of HRT but have tryglyceride elevations that make oral HRT risky. It is becoming more plausible that transdermal therapy could also have beneficial effects on the lipid profile, and that first-pass hepatic circulation may not explain the entire benefit initially thought to be found only with oral therapy. Additionally, the impact of type and delivery of progestin requires further investigation, as most women who use HRT will require combined therapy.

Anticoagulation

A search for the cause of the epidemiological benefit of estrogen replacement on cardiac mortality has led to the investigation of estrogen and progestin effects not only on lipid measures, but also on the possible changes in hemostatic variables. Oral contraceptives have long been associated with an increase in the risk of blood clots, occasionally with fatal complications. The amount of replacement estrogen used in postmenopausal women has been much less, and consequently the clotting complications have been fewer. Assessing the impact of changes in the clotting cascade, including known factors such as fibrinogen, factor VII, tissue plasminogen activator (t-PA), antithrombin III and others, necessitates extended follow-up. Even when women are followed for several months or years, there is not always a consistent answer. Additionally, the impact of different dose routes and hormones is unclear.

One 2-year, prospective cohort study followed 42 women randomly selected from a clinic population while seeking help for menopausal complaints. Transdermal estradiol was prescribed, and hemostatic measurements were assessed at baseline and throughout follow-up. Reference populations were premenopausal women and postmenopausal women not seeking estrogen replacement. In the treated group, plasma fibrinogen concentrations were significantly decreased at 3 months, and were still lower, but not significantly, at the end of treatment. Factor VII antigen concentrations were significantly decreased, and t-PA antigen concentrations were significantly increased at 2 years. There were no significant changes in antithrombin III levels, protein C activity or D-dimer concentrations. The untreated postmenopausal group showed increases in the concentrations of factor VII antigen and plasminogen activator inhibitor-1 (PAI-1) antigen, but no other changes[19]. The overall implication of the outcome was a protective effect of HRT. Another study attempted to elucidate the role of the progestin. Hemostatic measures were compared between 27 women treated with estradiol gel 1 mg/day and MPA 10 mg orally either for 12 days per month or for 12 days every third month. At the end of the 12-month treatment phase, von Willebrand factor antigen, protein C, protein S, PAI-1 and t-PA antigen were not significantly changed by either progestin route. Factor VII was decreased at 3 months by the monthly progestin and by both progestin treatments at 12 months. Fibrinogen was decreased at 3 months by both progestin treatments, but at 12 months in only the monthly progestin group. Antithrombin was decreased at 3 months by both regimens, but at 12 months there was no change in either group. Thrombin–antithrombin III complex and prothrombin fragments 1 and 2 were not significantly changed by either treatment regimen, but at the end of 12 months there were increases in both values in the less-frequent progestin group[20]. Again, the result was in favor of HRT, and no definite effect of progestin route could be seen. A study comparing estradiol gel with oral estradiol valerate, each combined with cyclic micronized progesterone, found increases in prothrombin activation peptide, and decreased antithrombin activity, t-PA and PAI-1 activity with the oral treatment. The gel group did not have these results, and neither group had any other change in a hemostatic variable such as fibrinogen or factor VII[21]. Although this study raises questions about the impact of the oral hormone treatment, the lack of change in fibrinogen or factor VII appears at least to be not prothrombotic. However, in another

study comparing the effects of oral and transdermal estrogen replacement on prostacyclin and thromboxane A_2, oral estradiol 2 mg/day with norethisterone acetate 1 mg/day increased the excretion of thromboxane B_2, but had no effect on prostanoids. The transdermal treatment with estradiol 0.05 mg/day with MPA 10 mg/day had no effect on either the thromboxanes or the prostanoids[22]. This study is difficult to interpret, as the progestins as well as the estrogen treatments were different, but leads to the conclusion that there could be a prothrombotic effect of oral HRT.

Although the outcomes of these trials do not explain the impact of either oral or transdermal estrogen therapy on cardiovascular morbidity, there is some further understanding of the role these treatments play in hemostatic measures. How this translates into actual clinical outcomes remains to be seen. In the HERS trial, women randomized to HRT did not differ in occurrence of a cardiovascular event from women without HRT, but treated women had more cardiovascular events in the first year of therapy. The assumption was that events in the early part of the trial were due to causes other than lipid changes, possibly coagulation disorders. Venous thromboembolic events occurred in 34 women in the treated group and 12 women in the placebo group. The two fatal pulmonary emboli occurred in the treated group. The treated group relative hazard for primary coronary heart disease event in the first year of the study was 1.52 and declined to 0.67 by years 4 and 5[16]. Therefore, the role of HRT in cardiac morbidity remains to be elucidated and, for now, cannot be recommended for secondary prevention in women with coronary heart disease[23]. There is perhaps an early deleterious effect that has not been defined. This study conclusion has been criticized, as the events that were seen were arterial events, and the changes in coagulation would lead to venous thrombotic events[24]. Additionally, it is difficult to know what impact continuous progestins may have on these outcomes. It is unknown whether these results can be extrapolated to all estrogen–progestin combinations or dosing regimens[23].

Given the confusing if not contradicting information regarding HRT and cardiac morbidity and mortality, it is advisable to discuss these issues with women prior to starting therapy, and identify the individual woman's risks and benefits. If there are definite risks and benefits with regard to HRT and cardiac morbidity, the appropriate population for any benefit has yet to be defined.

Insulin sensitivity

As is known with oral estrogen replacement, first-pass hepatic metabolism results in the induction of hepatic enzymes, and estrogen in oral contraceptives also stimulates the secretion growth hormone. The increase in growth hormone results in hyperinsulinemia that has been shown to be a risk factor for atherosclerosis and cardiac morbidity. As already discussed, estrogen replacement therapy epidemiologically appeared to be associated with decreased risk for cardiovascular morbidity, but randomized trials are now starting to find results inconsistent with previous observational data. Neither lipid metabolism nor changes in the co-agulation cascade appear to explain the entire picture. Attention has also been focused on the possible role of hyperinsulinemia in cardiac disease, and the changes induced by estrogen replacement therapy. A 2-month comparative study of 0.1 mg/day transdermal estradiol with or without 10 mg/day of MPA was performed to investigate a possible difference in route of administration on an insulin tolerance test. This was compared with historical data on changes in insulin sensitivity with conjugated equine estrogens. Diet was standardized, and estradiol levels proved that the subjects were compliant with treatment. The previous data on oral estrogens had shown that at 0.625 mg/day the insulin sensitivity improved by 26.3%, but at 1.25 mg/day the sensitivity decreased by 23.9%. The transdermal routes showed differing results. The unopposed transdermal treatment showed improved insulin sensitivity of 13.2%, but the insulin sensitivity decreased by 3.8% when MPA was added[25]. This second study was short in duration, and any change in development of atherosclerosis or other clinical outcome would require much longer follow-up. Another study followed women over 12 months of therapy on either transdermal estradiol 0.1 mg/day or Premarin 1.25 mg/day for 12 weeks. Each treatment was combined with 10 mg MPA

for the last 12 days of each cycle. Oral glucose tolerance tests (GTTs) were performed prior to and after treatment. Growth hormone levels were significantly higher with oral therapy, but the oral GTT did not differ between treatments. Mean insulin levels rose during insulin infusions, but overall did not differ between the groups. Also, although the difference was small, there were significantly lower non-esterified free fatty acids with transdermal treatment compared to oral[26]. Therefore, it is plausible that transdermal estrogens may benefit a woman who is predisposed to glucose intolerance.

Side-effects

Estrogen receptors are found in many tissues including the brain, breast and skin. All estrogens, whether oral or transdermal, produce unwanted effects based on the affinity for the variable estradiol receptors. Known side-effects are bleeding, breast tenderness, nausea, bloating and, for transdermal products, skin irritation. Doses of estrogen required to replace endogenous levels of estradiol are much less than those required to suppress ovulation, so some side-effects may be less concerning for the postmenopausal woman.

There were no significant differences between a reservoir-type system (Estraderm TTS) and a matrix-style transdermal system (Oesclim®) during the sensitization period of a comparative study. During the actual study treatment phase that lasted 4 months, 4.2% of the Oesclim group versus 9.5% of the Estraderm TTS group experienced application-site reactions. Overall numbers of reactions per subject, as well as severity of reaction, and numbers of subjects who experienced reactions were lower with the Oesclim group[10]. A randomized cross-over study comparing the degree of irritation between reservoir and matrix patches found that, of 30 women who discontinued patch wear owing to irritation, 26 were from the reservoir group and four were from the matrix group. Of 41 who reported moderate or severe reaction, 35 were in the reservoir group and six in the matrix group. The likelihood of discontinuation was not affected by the order of patch wear; therefore, if a woman has had a reaction to a reservoir patch, a trial with a matrix patch may be appropriate[27].

Oral versus transdermal

The debate continues regarding the relative benefits and risks of oral versus transdermal therapy. At a consensus conference, prominent gynecologists were asked for their opinions regarding HRT, the risks and benefits, and the possible preferred use of oral or transdermal route of delivery. There was general agreement that, for most women, the benefits outweigh the risks, and that some form of hormone replacement therapy is advisable. Either route is effective in relieving menopausal symptoms, preventing osteoporosis and, when combined with a progestin, protecting the endometrium[8]. From a physiological perspective, oral HRT results in peak and trough levels of estradiol, whereas patch application allows for more continuous delivery of the drug. Estradiol can be dosed as infrequently as once per week by use of the Climara® transdermal matrix patch[28], and estradiol levels can be maintained around 40 pg/ml with a 0.05-mg patch, or around 80 pg/ml with the 0.1-mg dose[7]. It was acknowledged that transdermal estrogens avoid first-pass hepatic metabolism, which could result in benefits for women who develop hypertriglyceridemia or gallstones from oral treatment regimens. Also, a consistent level of serum estradiol may mean that the transdermal route is more appropriate for women who are sensitive to estradiol fluctuations, such as women with migraines or depression[8].

As quality of life is a main reason for compliance, some researchers are looking more closely at the improved quality of life with HRT. Wiklund's group has been studying quality of life for several years, and published the comparative results of five instruments. Two hundred and twenty-three women were randomized to either transdermal estradiol or placebo for 12 weeks of therapy. The Nottingham Health Profile showed improved sleep patterns in both groups, but improvement in social isolation and emotion scores was greater in the estradiol group. The Psychological Well-Being Index also improved for both groups, but to a greater degree for the estradiol group. The Women's Health Questionnaire, a menopause-specific instrument, showed improvement in both groups in total score, anxiety, somatic symptoms and vasomotor symptoms scores, but also improvement in cognitive function, sexual problems, attraction and sleep in the estradiol group, such that the overall benefit was more pronounced with the estradiol treatment. The McCoy Sex Scale showed improvement with estradiol treatment only. Finally, a self-rated symptom scale modelled on the Kupperman index found more improvement in the estradiol group[29].

A comparison study of 0.05 mg/day estradiol transdermal twice weekly and 0.625 mg/day conjugated equine estrogens, each combined with cyclic MPA, evaluated quality of life with the Menopause Specific Quality of Life (MENQOL) questionnaire. Seventy-four subjects were followed for 14 weeks on therapy. The MENQOL found no significant differences between groups, but vasomotor and physical domain scores improved from baseline to 10 weeks. Psychosocial and sexual domain scores also improved, but only achieved statistical significance at 6 weeks. There were no differences between groups. Overall tolerability of treatment regimens was not different. Vaginal bleeding and breast swelling were significant complaints of both groups. The lack of placebo group comparator makes it difficult to know the magnitude of effect of the treatment, and it is impossible to assess the effect of cyclic MPA on the outcomes[30].

Conclusions and directions

The author of the previous edition of this chapter predicted that the future would hold refinement of delivery techniques and increases in treatment options for the menopausal woman[31]. This is now a truth in that there are more routes of delivering estrogen and progestin, and many more products from which to choose. In addition, some of the mechanisms of estrogen effect have been further elucidated. However, as has already been discussed, there are still issues that have been previously over-simplified, and are currently being explored in more depth. There is the probability that the dose of estrogen that is 'effective' and the dose of progestin that is protective will receive further study. The benefit of oral versus transdermal dosing is still being investigated. Also, the impact on cardiovascular disease has to be clarified. One thing is certain: the population continues to age, and these educated peri- and postmenopausal women will not be satisfied with a one-size-fits-all approach to any aspect of their medical care. In response to their needs, it is likely that, for the woman who chooses to use HRT, the choices in dose and route of administration will continue to increase. Support for these women has to exist on a continual basis if they are to remain on HRT. An Estraderm educational study allowed women to telephone an 800 number to speak to a live operator and listen to prerecorded messages about patch use and general menopausal health-care, including topics such as osteoporosis. Women also received informational brochures about topics related to the menopause. The researchers found that increased length of Estraderm use was associated with enrolling in the educational program[5]. Education is probably a large part of HRT compliance, and should be considered a critical part of counselling the postmenopausal woman on her HRT decision. For the health-care provider, this presents the challenge to reassess a woman's needs continually throughout her postmenopausal years, to re-educate her as new products and health-care information become available, and to tailor the HRT therapy over a woman's life span to meet her changing needs.

References

1. US Preventive Services Task Force. *Guide to Clinical Preventive Services*, 2nd edn. Baltimore: Williams & Wilkins, 1996
2. Balfour JA, Heel RC. Transdermal estradiol. A review of its pharmacodynamic and pharmacokinetic properties, and therapeutic efficacy in the treatment of menopausal complaints. *Drugs* 1990;40: 561–82
3. Grodstein F, Stampfer M, Colditz G, *et al.* Postmenopausal hormone therapy and mortality. *N Engl J Med* 1997;336:1769–75
4. Society EM. European consensus development conference on menopause. *Hum Reprod* 1996;11: 975–9
5. Motheral BR, Fairman KA. Patient education programs and continuance with estrogen replacement therapy: evaluation of the women's health exchange. *Menopause* 1998;5:35–42
6. Keating NL, Cleary P, Rossi AS, *et al.* Use of hormone replacement therapy by postmenopausal women in the United States. *Ann Intern Med* 1999; 130:545–53
7. *Physicians' Desk Reference for Prescription Drugs*, 53 edn. New Jersey: Medical Economics, 1999
8. Lobo RA, Ettinger B, Hutchinson KA, *et al.* Estrogen replacement. The evolving role of transdermal delivery. *J Reprod Med* 1996;41:781–96
9. Jewelewicz R. New developments in topical estrogen therapy. *Fertil Steril* 1997;67:1–12
10. Rozenbaum H, Birkhäuser M, De Nooyer C, *et al.* Comparison of two estradiol transdermal systems (Oesclim 50 and Estraderm TTS 50). II. Local skin tolerability. *Maturitas* 1996;25:175–85
11. Reginster JY, Albert A, Deroisy R, *et al.* Plasma estradiol concentrations and pharmacokinetics following transdermal application of Menorest 50 or Systen (Evorel) 50 [Erratum *Maturitas* 1997;28: 193–5]. *Maturitas* 1997;27:179–86
12. Walters KA, Brain KR, Green DM, *et al.* Comparison of the transdermal delivery of estradiol from two gel formulations. *Maturitas* 1998;29:189–95
13. Hirvonen E, Lamberg-Allardt C, Lankinen KS, *et al.* Transdermal oestradiol gel in the treatment of the climacterium: a comparison with oral therapy. *Br J Obstet Gynaecol* 1997;104(Suppl 16):19–25
14. Hirvonen E, Cacciatore B, Wahlström T, *et al.* Effects of transdermal oestrogen therapy in postmenopausal women: a comparative study of an oestradiol gel and an oestradiol delivering patch. *Br J Obstet Gynaecol* 1997;104(Suppl 16):26–31
15. Adami S, Rossini M, Zamberlan N, *et al.* Long-term effects of transdermal and oral estrogens on serum lipids and lipoproteins in postmenopausal women. *Maturitas* 1993;17:191–6
16. Hulley S, Grady D, Bush T, *et al.* Randomized Trial of Estrogen Plus Progestin for Secondary Prevention of Coronary Heart Disease in Postmenopausal Women. *J Am Med Assoc* 1998;280:605–13
17. Erenus M, Kutlay K, Kutlay L, Pekin S. Comparison of the impact of oral versus transdermal estrogen on serum lipoproteins. *Fertil Steril* 1994;61: 300–2

18. Rozenberg S, Ylikorkala O, Arrenbrecht S. Comparison of continuous and sequential transdermal progestogen with sequential oral progestogen in postmenopausal women using continuous transdermal estrogen: vasomotor symptoms, bleeding patterns, and serum lipids. *Int J Fertil Women's Med* 1997;42(Suppl 2):376–87

19. Lindoff C, Peterson F, Lecander I, *et al*. Transdermal estrogen replacement therapy: beneficial effects on hemostatic risk factors for cardiovascular disease. *Maturitas* 1996;24:43–50

20. Kroon UB, Tengborn L, Rita H, Bäckström AC. The effects of transdermal oestradiol and oral progestogens on haemostasis variables. *Br J Obstet Gynaecol* 1997;104(Suppl 16):32–7

21. Scarabin PY, Alhenc-Gelas M, Plu-Bureau G, *et al*. Effects of oral and transdermal estrogen/progesterone regimens on blood coagulation and fibrinolysis in postmenopausal women. A randomized controlled trial. *Arterioscl Thromb Vasc Biol* 1997;17:3071–8

22. Viinikka L, Orpana A, Puolakka J, *et al*. Different effects of oral and transdermal hormonal replacement on prostacyclin and thromboxane A_2. *Obstet Gynecol* 1997;89:104–7

23. Barrett-Connor E, Wenger N, Grady D, *et al*. Coronary heart disease in women, randomized clinical trials, HERS and RUTH. *Maturitas* 1998;31:1–7

24. Speroff L. The Heart and Estrogen/progestin Replacement Study (HERS). *Maturitas* 1998;31:9–14

25. Lindheim SR, Duffy DM, Kojima T, *et al*. The route of administration influences the effect of estrogen on insulin sensitivity in postmenopausal women. *Fertil Steril* 1994;62:1176–80

26. O'Sullivan AJ, Ho KK. A comparison of the effects of oral and transdermal estrogen replacement on insulin sensitivity in postmenopausal women. *J Clin Endocrinol Metab* 1995;80:1783–8

27. Ross D, Rees M, Godfree V, *et al*. Randomised crossover comparison of skin irritation with two transdermal oestradiol patches. *Br Med J (Clin Res Edn)* 1997;315:288

28. Gordon SF, Thompson KA, Ruoff GE, *et al*. Efficacy and safety of a seven-day, transdermal estradiol drug-delivery system: comparison with conjugated estrogens and placebo. The Transdermal Estradiol Patch Study Group. *Int J Fertil Menopausal Stud* 1995;40:126–34

29. Wiklund I, Karlberg J, Mattsson LA. Quality of life of postmenopausal women on a regimen of transdermal estradiol therapy: a double-blind placebo-controlled study. *Am J Obstet Gynecol* 1993;168:824–30

30. Hilditch JR, Lewis J, Ross AH, *et al*. A comparison of the effects of oral conjugated equine estrogen and transdermal estradiol-17β combined with an oral progestin on quality of life in postmenopausal women. *Maturitas* 1996;24:177–84

31. Ellerington MC, Hillard TC, Whitehead MI, Crook D, Stevenson JC. Routes of administration for oestrogen and progestogen replacement therapy. In Eskin BA, ed. *The Menopause: Comprehensive Management*, 3rd edn. New York: McGraw-Hill, 1994:345–64

21

Breast cancer and estrogen replacement therapy

Ian H. Thorneycroft

Introduction

Perhaps the most controversial area of estrogen replacement therapy is whether or not it increases a woman's likelihood of breast cancer, and, if she has had breast cancer, whether or not she is a candidate for estrogen replacement therapy (ERT). In spite of good arguments that ERT should increase breast cancer and its recurrence, the literature does not substantiate these theoretical concerns. Both aspects of the relationship of estrogen to breast cancer are discussed in this chapter. Only the Women's Health Initiative (WHI) in the USA, the Women's International Study of long Duration Oestrogen after Menopause (WISDOM) study in Europe and the Million Women Study will have the power to answer the question to most people's satisfaction[1,2]. The WHI will not be completed until 2007.

Epidemiology of breast cancer

There are many reasons to assume that estrogen and breast cancer are related:

(1) Breast cancer occurs almost exclusively in women;

(2) Early menarche is associated with an increase of breast cancer;

(3) Premature menopause without ERT is associated with a decreased incidence of breast cancer;

(4) Obesity increases breast cancer possibly by peripheral aromatization of androgens to estrogens and decreasing sex hormone binding globulin (SHBG), therefore increasing free estrogens;

(5) Reduced SHBG and, therefore, increased free estrogen levels are also associated with an increased risk of breast cancer (obesity which lowers sex hormone binding levels and increases breast cancer complicates this issue);

(6) Low parity would lower the total estrogen exposure and is associated with increased risk;

(7) The higher the bone density, the higher the rate of breast cancer in menopausal patients;

(8) Antiestrogens such as tamoxifen and raloxifene decrease the incidence of breast cancer.

It is clear, therefore, that there is a logical progression of thought that estrogen has a role in the development of breast cancer. If estrogen has any relationship to breast cancer, it may also be explained by estrogen increasing the number of breast cells (female versus male) and breast cell mitosis, therefore increasing the probability of a malignant cell development. Estrogens would be facilitators, not inducers, in this role. Evidence against estrogens being involved in breast cancer includes:

(1) Two-thirds of breast cancer occurs after the age of 50, at a time in a woman's life when she has exceedingly low estrogen levels;

(2) Patients who have perimenopausal breast cancer are not routinely ovariectomized. The amount of estrogen that they receive from their own ovaries far exceeds that which they will receive with ERT;

(3) Patients who have breast cancer at a young age after treatment can safely proceed with a pregnancy, a very hyperestrogenic stage;

(4) High doses of estrogen have equal efficacy with tamoxifen for suppressing breast cancer recurrence;

(5) Increased alcohol consumption is related to increased breast cancer; alcohol decreases the

metabolism of estrogens and, therefore, decreases estrogen levels.

All of the arguments in favor of estrogen increasing breast cancer incidence assume that estrogens are the only and most important secretion of the

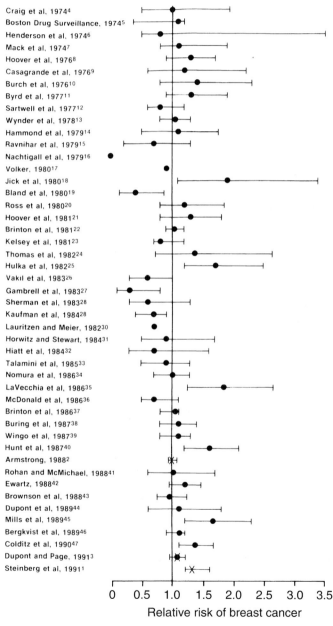

Figure 1 Relative risks and 95% confidence intervals of developing breast cancer during estrogen replacement therapy (ERT) or hormone replacement therapy (HRT). Graph represents most published articles. From reference 3, with permission

ovary. However, the ovary secretes a wide variety of steroids, proteins and growth factors which may be involved in the genesis/promotion of breast cancer in women.

Epidemiological evidence

Ever-use of estrogens

Ever-use refers to those who have ever used estrogen including those who are currently using estrogen. With the above concerns in mind, what are the data? There have been a little over 50 articles in the literature which have addressed this issue. Many articles have totally inadequate numbers to come to any statistically meaningful conclusions. Estrogens have been used widely for over 50 years, and a very clear, consistent and unequivocal relationship has been established with increased endometrial carcinoma and lower cardiac disease; however, no clear relationship to breast cancer has been established. Figure 1 shows the relative risk and 95% confidence intervals of most of the articles on breast cancer and estrogen administration. As can very clearly be seen, there is no consistent increase or decrease in the diagnosis of breast cancer in ever-users of estrogen (current and past users). Table 1 summarizes all of the meta-analyses which have been performed examining ever-use of estrogen and the development of breast cancer[4-11]. Two of these meta-analyses reported small increases with ever-use of estrogen whereas the other six showed absolutely no effect. The study by Steinberg and colleagues did not include the entire literature[8]. The study by Beral and associates[11] was the most complete study and is discussed in more detail throughout this chapter[12]. Nevertheless, it needs to be pointed out that even in these articles which show an increase it is only 14–30%. Any relative risk below 2 is generally considered unreliable and of questionable clinical significance. In Figure 2, the reported relative risks of developing cancer of the endometrium or breast are plotted. Unopposed estrogen clearly and consistently has been reported to increase endometrial cancer; the breast cancer relative risks all oscillate around a value of 1, further pointing out the neutral effect of estrogen on the development of breast cancer when given to menopausal patients.

Table 1 Meta-analyses and risk of developing breast cancer while taking estrogen replacement therapy (ERT)

Study	Number of studies	Relative risk	95% CI
Armstrong, 1988[4]	23	1.01	0.95–1.08
Bates, 1990[5]	11	1.03	0.87–1.17
Sillero-Arenas et al., 1992[6]	28	1.08	0.96–1.20
Dupont and Page, 1991[7]	27	1.06	1.00–1.18
Steinberg et al., 1991[8]	16	1.30	1.20–1.60
Colditz et al., 1993[9]	31	1.02	0.93–1.12
Collins, 1995[10]	37	1.05	1.00–1.11
Beral et al., 1997[11]	47	1.14	1.06–1.20

CI, confidence interval

The meta-analysis conducted by Collins plotted the relative risk of developing breast cancer while taking ERT versus the number of cancer cases in the study[10]. As the number of cases of breast cancer increases to over 300, the relative risk is basically 1. Those studies showing high and low relative risks are the ones with few patients.

Current use

Current use of estrogen is associated with an increased risk of breast cancer in some but not all studies. When former and current users are combined in these studies no increased risk is noted, except in the meta-analysis by Beral[12]. Collins calculated that the relative risk in current users was 1.21 (95% confidence interval 0.96–1.53) and that for past users was 0.97 (95% confidence interval 0.89–1.06) in articles which reported both analyses. Neither estimate is statistically significant. Biologically this makes little sense. Why would only current users rather than past users develop cancer? Could there be a bias favoring the diagnoses of breast cancer during ERT therapy? ERT leads to an increase in surveillance and, therefore, probably detection. Estrogen users have always had more mammography in the Nurses' Health Study, which has consistently shown an increase in breast cancer in current users of ERT[14]. Patients who undergo mammography have a higher rate of breast cancer detection than those that do not[15,16]. It is therefore likely that the increased risk in current users may be explained by the increased use of mammography. This is known as an ascertainment bias. In addition, patients taking

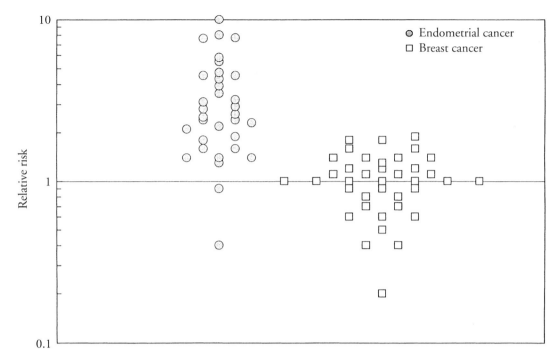

Figure 2 Relative risks of endometrial cancer and breast cancer in patients taking hormone replacement therapy (HRT). Data adapted from reference 13

ERT versus those not taking ERT are more likely to visit a physician and, therefore, more likely to have self-breast examination emphasized and more likely to have a breast examination, both of which will increase the diagnosis of breast cancer.

Length of treatment

Length of ERT treatment has also been associated in some but not all studies with an increased risk and diagnosis of breast cancer. The Nurses' Health and Beral's meta-analyses came to this conclusion[11,14] However, the worst possible scenario is about a 40% increase with prolonged use of 10–15 years. Again, this number is considerably less than a relative risk of 2, and the risk was gone after 5 years in the Beral meta-analysis. It is hard to imagine an effect that takes 10–15 years to develop but is gone in 5 years. The benefits from cardiovascular and Alzheimer's protection far outweigh numerically this length of treatment effect on the breast. Figure 3 from the Collins meta-analysis shows no relationship to duration of use[10]

Appearance of the effect

If estrogen were to induce breast cancer, a relatively slow growing tumor, the appearance is much too rapid for a single mutated malignant cell to grow as a clinically recognizable lesion. It takes probably 10–30 years from induction to detection of a lesion on mammography, which detects lesions earlier than breast examination. The original tumor cell was probably induced long before the menopause, and some estimate time from initial tumor cell development to a 10-mm tumor to be 16 years[17,18].

Disappearance of risk after discontinuation of estrogen

There appears to be a rapid disappearance of this increased relative risk of ERT following the discontinuance of therapy. In the Beral study it was 5 years. If estrogen was an inducer of cancer then the effect should remain for much longer than the 5 years, particularly considering that it takes at least that long for the faster growing tumors to progress from one malignant cell to a detectable breast lesion by mammography.

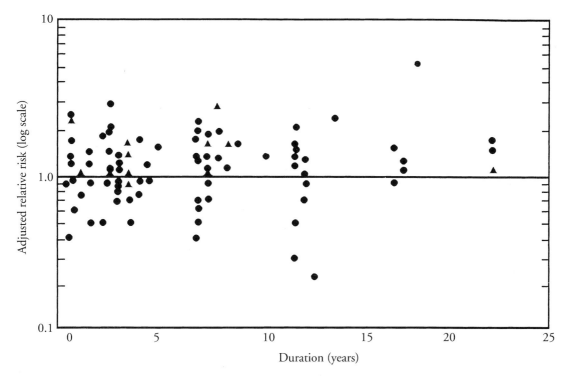

Figure 3 Length of estrogen replacement therapy (ERT) and development of breast cancer. From reference 10, with permission

Tumor characteristic: invasiveness versus in situ disease and grade

The cancer which is detected during ERT in many studies is mainly *in situ* disease, not invasive. Figure 4 shows results of a study in which there clearly was an increase in the diagnosis of *in situ* but not invasive disease[19], and Figure 5 indicates that patients developing breast cancer during estrogen therapy had a 50% reduced chance that it was metastatic[11]. The excess cancer detected in Beral's meta-analysis was explained by an excess of localized disease. Furthermore, the probability of survival, if a woman develops breast cancer, is greater if she is taking estrogen than if she is not taking estrogen (Figure 6). Person and colleagues recently demonstrated a statistically significant reduction in mortality of 50% with ERT use[24]. A recent study demonstrated an increase only in favorable-prognosis breast cancer; overall there was no increase (Figure 7)[25]. Breast cancers detected during ERT are also more differentiated[26].

Dose

There has been no clear dose–response demonstrated, although Persson and colleagues report the highest increase with 'high-dose' estrogen in combination with high-potency progestins[24].

Progestins

It is also unclear at present whether progestins protect against, have no effect on or increase breast cancer. Gambrell[27] has shown a decrease, the Nurses' Health Study[14] and Stanford and co-workers[28] show no effect and Persson and colleagues[24] an increase with a potent progestin in combination with estrogen. More data are clearly needed in this area.

Selective estrogen receptor modulators

Both raloxifene and tamoxifen have been shown to reduce breast cancer[29,30].

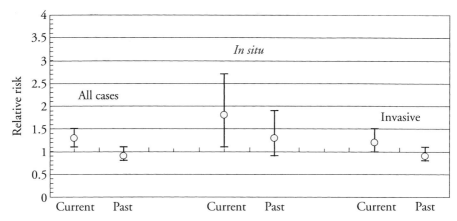

Figure 4   Relative risks and 95% confidence intervals of developing *in situ* versus invasive cancer in patients treated with estrogen replacement therapy (ERT)/hormone replacement therapy (HRT). Current users and past users are shown separately. Adapted from reference 19

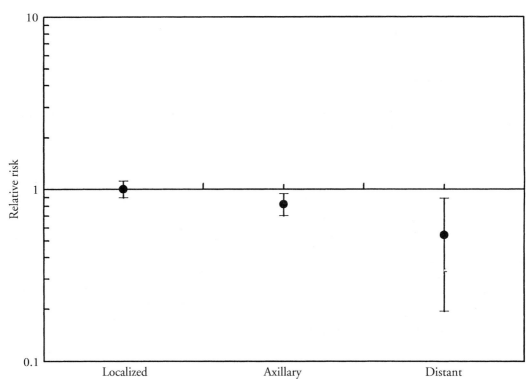

Figure 5   Relative risk of cancer being present in lymph nodes or metastatic at time of diagnosis if patient was taking estrogen replacement therapy (ERT) at time of diagnosis. From reference 11, with permission

Conclusion

Ever-use of estrogens is not associated with any clinically significant increase in breast cancer in spite of theoretical concerns. Current use is associated with an increased rate in some but not all studies and, when present, the risk increases with long-term use. The difference between the findings in current and past users may be due to a detection

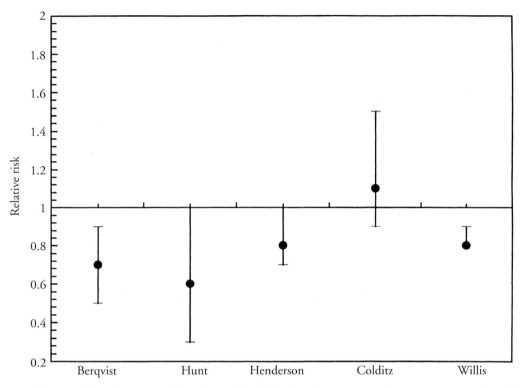

Figure 6 Relative risks and 95% confidence intervals of dying from breast cancer in patients diagnosed with breast cancer while taking estrogen, relative to non-users. Data from references 14, 20–23

bias, particularly since past use is not associated with an increased risk. In the studies which demonstrate an increased rate in current users, the effect disappears too fast after discontinuation to have biological plausibility. For example, it took 15 years for a statistically significant increase to be detected but the increase was gone in 5 years[11]. The detection bias may be from mammography and examination combined with estrogen causing an already existing cancer cell to grow faster, and become clinically apparent earlier. In other words, estrogen may cause an inevitable cancer to be detected earlier. Logical consequences of this would be younger age, less invasive disease and better prognosis and differentiated tumors associated with ERT. The literature substantiates these predictions. The corollary of this would also be better survival, which indeed has been shown in most but not all studies.

Treating patients having a history of breast cancer with estrogens

There are absolutely no data in the literature to suggest that ERT worsens the prognosis or advances the death of patients with a personal history of breast cancer. Metastatic disease will only develop if it was present at the time of diagnosis. All reports in the literature have shown either a decreased recurrence rate or no difference in recurrence rates. The largest study is that from Australia by Eden and associates[31] and is illustrated in Figure 8. There was a reduced recurrence rate in those treated with hormone replacement therapy (HRT). The HRT in the study was the equivalent of 0.625 mg of Premarin® and the equivalent of 50 mg of medroxyprogesterone acetate every day. It would appear, therefore, that in spite of theoretical concerns there is no reason not to give estrogen to patients with a personal history of breast cancer.

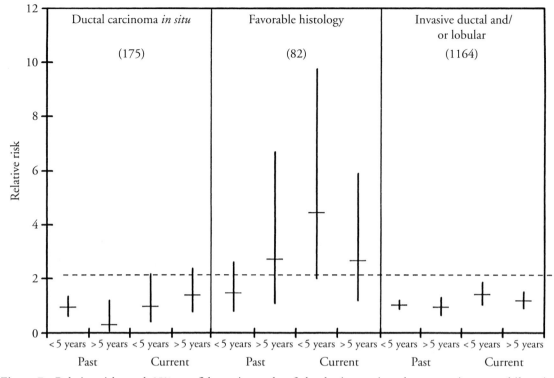

Figure 7 Relative risks and 95% confidence intervals of developing various breast carcinomas while using hormone replacement therapy (HRT) for less than 5 years or more than 5 years. Past use means use more than 1 year ago, current use means currently or within past year. Number in parentheses indicates number of patients with that particular tissue type. Data from reference 25

However, owing to a relative lack of data on either side, one should be very prudent and restrict ERT in patients with a personal history of breast cancer who have severe menopausal symptoms or osteoporosis, or who are at high risk for Alzheimer's or heart disease. Table 2 outlines the author's personal approach with these patients. The first line of therapy is estrogen if they will accept it: if they are concerned then perhaps a lower-dose estrogen such as 0.3 mg of Premarin or Estratab® or a 0.025-mg transdermal estrogen. For vaginal symptoms an Estring® is excellent; the peripheral estrogen levels are unchanged from pretreatment, and it will treat urogenital atrophy[32,33]. If estrogen is unacceptable, treat her bones with Fosamax® first and then Evista®, as Fosamax maintains bone density better and has been shown to decrease hip fracture, whereas raloxifene prevents spine but not hip fractures[34,35]. Cardiac disease has no proven alternative treatment at the present time other than diet and exercise. If raloxifene in the ongoing

Table 2 Management of patient with personal history of breast cancer

No increased recurrence or death reported in literature from ERT. Literature suggests ERT is probably safe

For those still not convinced:
can try low-dose estrogen 0.3 mg orally or 0.025-mg patch
Estring® for vaginal symptoms
Provera® or Megace® for flushes
Fosamax® or Evista® for bone
exercise and diet for cardiovascular prevention
vitamin E and NSAIDs for Alzheimer's prevention
increased fiber for GI cancer protection

None of the above are as good as estrogen

ERT, estrogen replacement therapy; NSAID, nonsteroidal anti-inflammatory drug; GI, gastrointestinal

RUTH (Raloxifene for the Heart) study protects against myocardial infarction then it would be the drug of choice for breast cancer patients after ERT.

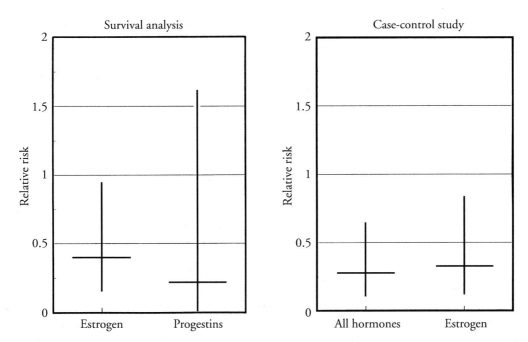

Figure 8 Relative risks and 95% confidence intervals for recurrence of breast cancer in patients treated with hormone replacement therapy (HRT). Estrogen refers to patients who were treated with equivalent of 0.625 mg of Premarin® per day and, on average, equivalent of 50 mg of medroxyprogesterone acetate per day. Progestins refers to patients who were treated with a variety of progestins. Data from reference 31

Raloxifene has not been shown to have beneficial effects on monkey coronary arteries[36]. Tamoxifen, a related compound which does reduce plaque formation in monkeys, leads to about a 15% non-significant reduction in cardiac deaths compared to the 50% cardiac reduction with ERT[30]. It is unlikely that either tamoxifen or raloxifene will have any beneficial effect on Alzheimer's disease. Vitamin E and non-steroidal anti-inflammatory agents should be encouraged in that area.

Conclusion

The literature does not argue that patients with a personal history of breast cancer have any detriment from the utilization of estrogen, but, owing to the lack of extensive data, only those patients with severe menopausal symptoms and those with osteoporosis or high risk for cardiac disease should be given ERT.

References

1. The Women's Health Initiative Study Group. Design of the Women's Health Initiative Clinical Trial and Observational Study. *Controlled Clin Trials* 1998;19:61–109
2. Wren BG. Megatrial of hormonal replacement therapy. *Drugs Aging* 1998; 12:343–8
3. Gambrell RD Jr. Hormone replacement therapy and breast cancer risk. *Arch Fam Med* 1996;5:341–8
4. Armstrong BK. Oestrogen therapy after the menopause – boon or bane? *Med J Aust* 1988;148: 213–14

5. Bates SK. Postmenopausal estrogen replacement therapy and breast cancer. *J Soc Obstet Gynaecol Can* 1990;12:9–12

6. Sillero-Arenas M, Delgado-Rodriguez M, Rodrigues-Canteras R, Bueno-Cavanillas A, Galvez-Vargas R. Menopausal hormone replacement therapy and breast cancer: a meta-analysis. *Obstet Gynecol* 1992;79:286–94.

7. Dupont WD, Page DL. Menopausal estrogen replacement therapy and breast cancer. *Arch Intern Med* 1991;151:67–72

8. Steinberg KK, Thacker SB, Smith SJ, *et al.* A meta-analysis of the effect of estrogen replacement therapy on the risk of breast cancer. *J Am Med. Assoc.* 1991;265:1985–90

9. Colditz GA, Egan KM, Stampfer MJ. Hormone replacement therapy and risk of breast cancer: results from epidemiologic studies. *Am J Obstet Gynecol* 1993;168:1473–80

10. Collins JA. Hormone replacement therapy and breast cancer: what is happening? *J Soc Obstet Gynaecol Can* 1995;17:837–49

11. Beral V, Bull D, Doll R, Key T, Peto R, Reeves G. Breast cancer and hormone replacement therapy: collaborative reanalysis of data from 51 epidemiological studies of 52 705 women with breast cancer and 108 411 women without breast cancer. *Lancet* 1997;350:1047–59

12. Collaborative Group on Hormonal Factors in Breast Cancer. Breast cancer and hormonal contraceptives: collaborative reanalysis of individual data on 53 297 women with breast cancer and 100 239 women without breast cancer from 54 epidemiological studies. *Lancet* 1996;347:1713–27

13. Grady D, Rubin SM, Petitti DB, *et al.* Hormone therapy to prevent disease and prolong life in postmenopausal women. *Ann Intern Med* 1992;117:1016–37

14. Colditz GA, Hankinson SE, Hunter DJ, et al. The use of estrogens and progestins and the risk of breast cancer in postmenopausal women. *N Engl J Med* 1995;332:1589–640

15. White E, Lee CY, Kristal AR. Evaluation of the increase in breast cancer incidence in relation to mammography use. *J Natl Cancer Inst* 1990;82:1546–52

16. McCaul KD, Branstetter AD, Schroeder DM, Glasgow RE. What is the relationship between breast cancer risk and mammography screening? A meta-analytic review. *Health Psychol* 1996;15:423–9

17. Fournier D, Weber E, Hoeffken W, Bauer M, Kubli F, Barth V. Growth rate of 147 mammary carcinomas. *Cancer* 1979;45:2198–207

18. Friberg S, Mattson S. On the growth rates of human malignant tumors: implications for medical decision making. *J Surg Oncol* 1997;65:284–97

19. Schairer C, Byrne C, Keyl PM, *et al.* Menopausal estrogen and estrogen-progestin replacement therapy and risk of breast cancer (United States). *Cancer Causes Control* 1994;5:491–500

20. Bergkvist L, Adami H, Persson I, Hoover R, Schairer C. The risk of breast cancer after estrogen and estrogen-progestin replacement. *N Engl J Med* 1989;321:293–7

21. Hunt K, Vessey M, McPherson K. Mortality in a cohort of long-term users of hormone replacement therapy: an updated analysis. *Br J Obstet Gynaecol* 1990;97:1080–6

22. Henderson BE, Paganini-Hill A, Ross RK. Decreased mortality in users of estrogen replacement therapy. *Arch Intern Med* 1991;151:75–8

23. Willis DB, Calle EE, Miracle-McMahill HL, Heath CW Jr. Estrogen replacement therapy and risk of fatal breast cancer in a prospective cohort of postmenopausal women in the United States. *Cancer Causes & Control* 1996;7:449–57

24. Persson I, Yuliano SG, Bergkvist L, Schairer C. Cancer incidence and mortality in women receiving estrogen and estrogen–progestin replacement therapy – long-term follow-up of a Swedish cohort. *Int J Cancer* 1999;67:327–32

25. Gapstur S, Morrow M, Sellers T. Hormone replacement therapy and risk of breast cancer with a favorable histology: results of the Iowa Women's Health Study. *J Am Med Assoc.* 1999;281:2091–141

26. Bilimoria MM, Winchester DJ, Sener SF, Motykie G, Sehgal UL, Winchester DP. Estrogen replacement therapy and breast cancer: analysis of age of onset and tumor characteristics. *Ann Surg Oncol* 1999;6:200–7

27. Gambrell RD Jr. Estrogen replacement therapy and breast cancer risk: a new look at the data. *Female Patient* 1993;18:50–62

28. Stanford JL, Weiss NS, Voigt LF, Daling JR, Habel LA, Rossing MA. Combined estrogen and progestin hormone replacement therapy in relation to risk of breast cancer in middle-aged women. *J Am Med Assoc* 1995;274:137–42

29. Cummings SR, Eckman MH, Krumholz HM, *et al.* The effect of raloxifene on risk of breast cancer in postmenopausal women: results from the MORE randomized trial. *J Am Med Assoc* 1999;281:2189–97

30. Fisher B, Costantino JP, Wickerman DL, *et al.* Tamoxifen for prevention of breast cancer: report of the National Surgical Adjuvant Breast and Bowel Project P-1 Study. *J Natl Cancer Inst* 1998;90:1371–88

31. Eden JA, Bush T, Nand S, Wren BG. A case-control study of combined continuous estrogen–progestin replacement therapy among women with a personal history of breast cancer. *Menopause* 1995;2:67–72

32. Bachmann G, Notelovitz M, Nachtigall L, Birgerson L. A comparative study of a low-dose estradiol vaginal ring and conjugated estrogen cream for postmenopausal urogenital atrophy. *Prim Care Update Obstet Gynecol* 1997;4:109–15

33. Schmidt G, Andersson SB, Nordle O, Johansson CJ, Gunnarsson PO. Release of 17β-oestradiol from a vaginal ring in postmenopausal women. *Gynecol Obstet Invest* 1994;38:253–60

34. Cummings SR, Eckert S, Krueger KA, *et al*. The effect of raloxifene on risk of breast cancer in postmenopausal women: results from the MORE randomized trial. Multiple Outcomes of Raloxifene Evaluation. *J Am Med Assoc* 1999;281:2243–4

35. Ensrud KE, Black DM, Palermo L, *et al*. Treatment with alendronate prevents fractures in women at highest risk: results from the Fracture Intervention Trial. *Arch Intern Med* 1997;157:2617–24

36. Clarkson TB, Anthony MS, Jerome CP. Lack of effect of raloxifene on coronary artery atherosclerosis of postmenopausal monkeys. *J Clin Endocrinol Metab* 1998;83:721–6

Epilogue

Bernard A. Eskin

This summary provides me with an opportunity to review the progress that has occurred since the last edition of *The Menopause: Comprehensive Management*. While the entire body of work accomplished in this field over the last 20 years is formidable, the greatest improvement may still be the continued growth of interest in improving women's health in an aging society. From this objective has evolved the medical advances that we have described.

Life phases of women

The clinical phases of a woman's life are shown in Figure 1. This graph represents the monthly mean levels of estradiol, which has maximal activity on the estrogen α receptor. All these phases are important; however, the book has given particular attention to those related to the menopause. The transition is recognized by the onset of mild to moderate menopausal symptomatology, usually unexpected and denied. Represented as a wavy irregular line on the graph, the transition and the premenopause show the interaction of the neuroendocrine and ovarian secretions by maintaining functional, but decreasing, estrogen titers. These disruptions are usually symptomatic and lead into irregular menses, increasing infertility and other 'change-of-life' symptomatology.

The classical 'menopause' follows and is defined as the last uterine (endometrial) bleed. The postmenopause immediately begins and continues until, on the basis of the variable endocrine findings, the increased luteinizing hormone (LH) and follicle stimulating hormone (FSH) levels diminish. Thus, the premenopause, menopause and postmenopause together represent the perimenopause in this evolving cycle. Beyond this point and becoming increasingly important is the *geripause*. I have suggested that this label should be substituted for such inconclusive expressions as frail and elderly, climacteric or senescent. It is my opinion that these women have been understudied and definitely undertreated. This population is increasing in the United States and elsewhere. They

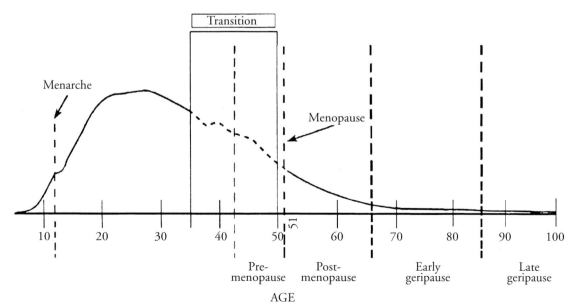

Figure 1 Lifetime estrogen levels

are demanding recognition and should receive it. The chapter introducing the geripause provides information that all physicians treating women should read and consider.

Aging and the menopause

The predetermination of aging still remains a constant. New findings concerning molecular biology from cloned animals and certain human diseases show a mathematical pattern, which, while complex, is still persistently on course (Chapter 1). Reproductive outcomes remain elusive as far as gene predetermination, probably multifaceted. Both neuroendocrine and ovarian tissues are responsible, but the relative influences of each are not defined.

As stated above in the previous section, the geripause presents a new entity for study. The elderly menopausal woman takes on many new problems and health hazards. Little is known of her therapeutic needs. Maintenance of hormonal replacement is only now being utilized and evaluated (Chapter 2). The prevalence of disability is presented and methodology for enhancing quality of life is an extremely important new focus. The geriatric principles are quintessential, but individuality in handling this age group is required.

Prevalence of mature-age pregnancies continues despite warnings from perinatologists and obstetricians over the years (Chapter 3). Choosing to forego early adult pregnancy has led to many difficult and sometimes unhappy gestational experiences. The use of specific cautionary treatments has improved the morbidity of these pregnancies. However, the harsh physiological demands of pregnancy may still be a difficult task in the late reproductive years.

Appreciation of the pathology of the menopause is essential (Chapter 4), since it represents the total changes that include both aging and hormonal loss. Tissue re-evaluation after replacement is often useful since these two depleting entities can be separated by the results and the prognosis can more easily be determined.

Chapter 5 provides a new approach to sexuality, by measuring a woman's sexual capacity as she ages and by going beyond just suggesting the usual cookbook therapies. Wary of the 'use it or lose it' philosophy, the newer types of advice and use of pharmacotherapies (Viagra®, etc.) provide a unique method. Sexuality in its many forms provides an acceptable way of personal enjoyment for older individuals.

Endocrinology of the menopause

The function of the thyroid gland, a most solicitous endocrine, varies throughout a woman's life. It is perhaps the most difficult hormone with which to deal clinically, particularly in the menopause (Chapter 6). Thyroid screening, primarily by thyroid stimulating hormone (TSH), should be performed at premenopause and menopause, since thyroid disease can be elusive, yet the symptomatology pervasive.

The perimenopause described in Chapter 7 shows an evident drop in the level of reproductive hormones. The series of events differs remarkably timewise, although the sequence seems to be easily defined. By using experiences from *in vitro* fertilization and ovulation stimulation, this diminishing ability of the ovary to respond to FSH (see Figure 1) is analyzed.

Chapter 8 describes the endocrinology of the menopause. It provides the endocrine relationships of the hypothalamic–pituitary axis, adrenal androgen production, inhibin production and peripheral hormonal conversion. Correlating these interchanges with the endocrine system provides evidence that the cellular aging process is an important player in the timing of the menopause.

Characteristically, fertility becomes unattainable after the series of perimenopausal events described in this section. However, the availability of new endocrine and reproductive techniques has provided a bridge to gestation for women, even beyond ages we might have anticipated (Chapter 9). This chapter updates the reader on fertility technologies (ART) which can attain pregnancies in older women. Arguments that indicate that the 'older' woman of today is healthier and better able to accept these hazards to her health will require trials and statistical implementation.

Clinical problems in the menopause

Osteoporosis (Chapter 10) remains the most disastrous and incapacitating problem that can be blamed on menopause. Many causative factors expressed would include the relative thinness (compared to males) of the lower vertebral and pelvic bones and the increased need for nutritional maintenance with calcium and other minerals in pregnancy. Sensitive testing systems have become available and, although false-positive results occur, these are able to show a need for therapy. Treatment remains basic (calcium, vitamin D), but is now fortified by hormone replacement. Other therapies, such as alendronate, calcitonin, raloxifene and tibolone are considered viable substitutes.

Cardiovascular disease has had a shaky but relevant history (Chapter 11). Women entering the perimenopause show a marked increase in all forms of cardiovascular disease. Increased serum cholesterol levels, because of the loss of estrogen, were considered to be the major cause. However, after several trials, only about 15% of the etiology could be assigned to cholesterol. There are numerous factors that have been presented in this chapter. Several large multicenter studies are actively pursuing the action of estrogen on cardiovascular disease.

Exercise is an essential component for maintaining good health in the menopause (Chapter 12). Sedentary life commonly occurs with aging and many believe that continuing to work, regardless of the level of activity, suffices as exercise. However, it is also important that each healthy patient should reward herself with the opportunity to continue physical regimens for maintaining the quality of her health. A moderate intensity, graded exercise program is an important prescription for menopausal fitness.

Diagnoses of gynecological (Chapter 13) and urological (Chapter 14) symptoms are more variable and often elusive in the menopause. Gynecological problems include unexpected vaginal bleeding when diagnoses of malignancy are present. Women in this age group are often embarrassed with their problems of urinary incontinence. The availability of medical/surgical devices or urinary/gynecological surgical procedures with minimal anesthetic has permitted health care through reconstructive techniques. Women now seek assistance more often and satisfaction seems to be improving.

The need for early diagnosis and treatment of breast disease ranks high in the care of menopausal women. Despite a decreasing mortality, malignant breast disease has a higher morbidity in women after the menopause than in her reproductive years. Thus, it is essential to make early diagnosis and prevent disaster.

Cognitive changes in the menopause provide a new chapter (Chapter 16) which deals with menopausal women and the effects of both dementia and depression. Evaluating normal intellectual loss due to aging remains difficult because of individual differences. Defining whether menopause is responsible can be associated only with hormonal vicissitudes in treatment or cyclicity. Little evidence has been seen to establish a common pattern with menopause; however, estrogen and progesterone seem to evoke some depression, especially when higher progesterone doses are given. At present, there is no evidence of any deleterious effects of estrogen on cognitive or emotional function, while the effect on Alzheimer's disease seems to augment psychopharmacological interventions.

Nutritional needs change with aging. The value of tasteful diets containing desirable elements is often overlooked when preparing meals for only one or two (Chapter 17). The media are constantly detailing diets which are directed towards impossible goals and some diets may actually be harmful. However, careful dietary instructions are useful and provide a basis for good living. Included in this chapter are alternative therapies for menopausal symptoms which may be useful for some patients.

Therapy of the menopause

The many therapies for menopausal women vary from generalized replacement hormones to specific treatment of both hormone dysfunction and aging problems. Chapter 18 deals with replacement therapies and the chemistry of these pharmaceuticals. Many of the contraindications have been clarified and somewhat accepted. There are no substantial data on long-term risks involved in hormone replacement therapies (Chapter 19). However, in cases of breast cancer, treatment should be carefully restricted, especially where estrogen receptors in the tumor are elevated.

Far from the unrestrained use of estrogen replacement, initiated in the 1960s, a sensitive and sensible approach to replacement therapy for the menopause has evolved. This improved treatment is directed to the functional losses that are clinically evident and those perceived by the patient. While new forms of estrogen are available, so are hormone modulators and specific therapies directed towards related disorders. Most evident is a need to educate women concerning the risks in her particular case if she chooses not to have estrogen replacement (Chapter 21). Then it is important that this same care be used to explain what risks she may take if she chooses to take estrogen replacement. Thus, the option is chosen on the basis of a careful analysis of need and risk, which is tailored to the individual patient. If treatment is given with hormone replacement therapy, a choice of delivery systems is available (Chapter 20). Consideration for the patient and her needs is most important in order to maintain her interest in continuing the therapy. As new products become available, particularly those that may assist in tailoring the medication to the patient's needs, she should be re-assessed.

Conclusions

The purpose of studying the hormonal changes that occur during a woman's lifetime is to help her cope with undesirable conditions and improve her quality of life. As indicated throughout this textbook, increasing remedial opportunities continue to arise. Future research should be directed towards the specificity of medications for reducing each of the medical problems indicated. Substitute therapies must be developed for those women who cannot take hormone replacement therapy, as prophylaxis is unavailable for those with many serious ailments. Separation of hormonal problems from those seen in aging is difficult, but, with increased longevity, we may have an opportunity to evaluate these entities more carefully.

By my next edition, I expect many new advances in our care that will provide an improved quality of life for the menopausal *and* geripausal woman. Appropriately, I conclude this edition with a thoughtful poem by Dr Richard Edgren.

Lines

(Composed at 35,000 feet above the Midwest and returning from a CMA meeting, July 27, 1994)
We are said to be drowning in a sea of estrogen
Let's thank the goddess for this estrogen!
Because of it we are here
    The eggs from which we came were ovulated in response to a surge of estrogen
    The sperm that fertilized that egg was deposited during estrogen-controlled behavior
    The fertilized egg was pushed through the oviduct by estrogen-controlled movements
    The zygote implanted in an endometrium that developed under the impact of estrogen and progesterone
    The pregnancy continued in a uterus that functioned under the influence of estrogen and progesterone
    The fetus was expelled by estrogen-stimulated uterine contractions after the cessation of the progesterone block
    The infant was nurtured by milk from a breast that developed in response to estrogen
    The female children became women under the influence of estrogen
And the whole cycle started over again!
As the woman ages, the endogenous estrogen is supplanted by exogenous estrogen that
    Helps to keep her on an even emotional keel
    Suppresses hot flushes
    Permits normal sleep patterns
    Prevents osteoporotic fractures
    Protects against cardiovascular accidents
In short – VIVE L'ESTROGEN!

Richard A. Edgren, PhD

Index